BF724.8 .R43 2004

0134106384826

Recent advanc
 psychology a
    2004.

ADVANCES IN CELL AGING AND GERONTOLOGY
VOLUME 15

Recent Advances in Psychology and Aging

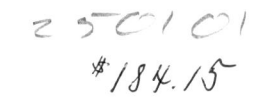

ADVANCES IN CELL AGING AND GERONTOLOGY
VOLUME 15

Recent Advances in Psychology and Aging

Volume Editors:

Paul T. Costa, Jr.
Laboratory of Personality and Cognition
National Institute on Aging
Baltimore, MD 21224
USA

Ilene C. Siegler
Duke University, Department of Psychiatry
and Behavioral Sciences
Durham, NC 27710
USA

ELSEVIER

Amsterdam – Boston – Heidelberg – London – New York – Oxford
Paris – San Diego – San Francisco – Singapore – Sydney – Tokyo

ELSEVIER B.V.
Sara Burgerhartstraat 25
P.O. Box 211, 1000 AE
Amsterdam, The Netherlands

ELSEVIER Inc.
525 B Street, Suite 1900
San Diego, CA 92101-4595
USA

ELSEVIER Ltd
The Boulevard, Langford Lane
Kidlington, Oxford OX5 1GB
UK

ELSEVIER Ltd
84 Theobalds Road
London WC1X 8RR
UK

© 2004 Elsevier B.V. All rights reserved.

This work is protected under copyright by Elsevier B.V., and the following terms and conditions apply to its use:

Photocopying
Single photocopies of single chapters may be made for personal use as allowed by national copyright laws. Permission of the Publisher and payment of a fee is required for all other photocopying, including multiple or systematic copying, copying for advertising or promotional purposes, resale, and all forms of document delivery. Special rates are available for educational institutions that wish to make photocopies for non-profit educational classroom use.

Permissions may be sought directly from Elsevier's Rights Department in Oxford, UK: phone (+44) 1865 843830, fax (+44) 1865 853333, e-mail: permissions@elsevier.com. Requests may also be completed on-line via the Elsevier homepage (http://www.elsevier.com/locate/permissions).

In the USA, users may clear permissions and make payments through the Copyright Clearance Center, Inc., 222 Rosewood Drive, Danvers, MA 01923, USA; phone: (+1) (978) 7508400, fax: (+1) (978) 7504744, and in the UK through the Copyright Licensing Agency Rapid Clearance Service (CLARCS), 90 Tottenham Court Road, London W1P 0LP, UK; phone: (+44) 20 7631 5555; fax: (+44) 20 7631 5500. Other countries may have a local reprographic rights agency for payments.

Derivative Works
Tables of contents may be reproduced for internal circulation, but permission of the Publisher is required for external resale or distribution of such material. Permission of the Publisher is required for all other derivative works, including compilations and translations.

Electronic Storage or Usage
Permission of the Publisher is required to store or use electronically any material contained in this work, including any chapter or part of a chapter.

Except as outlined above, no part of this work may be reproduced, stored in a retrieval system or transmitted in any form or by any means, electronic, mechanical, photocopying, recording or otherwise, without prior written permission of the Publisher.
Address permissions requests to: Elsevier's Rights Department, at the fax and e-mail addresses noted above.

Notice
No responsibility is assumed by the Publisher for any injury and/or damage to persons or property as a matter of products liability, negligence or otherwise, or from any use or operation of any methods, products, instructions or ideas contained in the material herein. Because of rapid advances in the medical sciences, in particular, independent verification of diagnoses and drug dosages should be made.

First edition 2004

Library of Congress Cataloging in Publication Data
A catalog record is available from the Library of Congress.

British Library Cataloguing in Publication Data
A catalogue record is available from the British Library.

ISBN: 0-444-51495-3
ISSN: 1566-3124 (Series)

∞ The paper used in this publication meets the requirements of ANSI/NISO Z39.48-1992 (Permanence of Paper).
Printed in The Netherlands.

TABLE OF CONTENTS

Overview   vii
Paul T. Costa, Jr. and Ilene C. Siegler

Chapter 1
Aging and the Seven Sins of Memory 1
Benton H. Pierce, Jon S. Simons and Daniel L. Schacter

Chapter 2
Age-related Changes in Visual Attention 41
David J. Madden and Wythe L. Whiting

Chapter 3
**Studies of Aging, Hypertension and Cognitive Functioning:
With Contributions from the Maine-Syracuse Study**................. 89
Merrill F. Elias, Michael A. Robbins, Marc M. Budge, Penelope K. Elias,
Barbara A. Hermann and Gregory A. Dore

Chapter 4
A Life Span View of Emotional Functioning in Adulthood and Old Age 133
Susan T. Charles and Laura L. Carstensen

Chapter 5
Personality and Self-esteem Development Across the Life Span 163
Kali H. Trzesniewski, Richard W. Robins, Brent W. Roberts
and Avshalom Caspi

Chapter 6
**The Evolving Concept of Subjective Well-being: The Multifaceted
Nature of Happiness** 187
Ed Diener, Christie Napa Scollon and Richard E. Lucas

Chapter 7
A Cultural Lens on Biopsychosocial Models of Aging 221
James S. Jackson, Toni C. Antonucci and Edna Brown

List of Contributors 243

Overview
Paul T. Costa and Ilene C. Siegler

The title of this book gives an important clue to the advances being celebrated. The psychology of aging developed as an important subspecialty that was recognized with the founding of *Psychology and Aging* by the American Psychological Association in 1985. Of the many advances in the past 18 years, the main one may be that aging content has become a regular part of mainstream psychology. The chapters in the present volume give evidence of the importance of aging content and issues in mainstream psychological research, including cognitive neuroscience represented by the chapters on aging and memory by Pierce, Simons, and Schacter (Chapter 1); and visual attention by Madden and Whiting (Chapter 2); longitudinal studies of hypertension's impact on cognition by Elias and colleagues (Chapter 3); emotional functioning by Charles and Carstensen (Chapter 4); and Trzesniewski, Robins, Roberts, and Caspi on self-esteem and personality across the life span (Chapter 5). The impact of psychological research in gerontology and aging is also dramatically prominent in the areas of emotions, personality, and subjective well-being as seen in the chapters on subjective well-being by Diener, Scollon, and Lucas (Chapter 6). Exciting new attempts at reconsidering and reconceptualizing basic biopsychosocial models to integrate psychological and cultural perspectives on race, ethnicity, and racial minority populations are advanced in the concluding chapter by Jackson, Antonucci, and Brown (Chapter 7). Their efforts to promote a biopsychosocially informed ethnic research matrix to health and aging issues might well succeed in advancing research and public policy of ethnic and racial differences in aging related processes.

These chapters all share a concern with life span views of development and present data from broad cross-sectional age ranges from college students through the 80s (although there is relatively little data on the extreme old – those in their 90s and 100s). Another important addition in these chapters is attention to data from international comparisons where available.

Longitudinal data are featured where possible. The attention to methods, noting which findings are longitudinal and which cross-sectional, is important and useful. Most of the present authors are careful to observe this important distinction and draw appropriate inferences regarding difference or change. Age differences found in cross-sectional studies cannot separate out the impact of birth cohort and time of measurement from maturational age effects. Age changes refer to findings from longitudinal or prospective cohort studies. Maturational changes are seen but may reflect limitations from selections of the particular birth cohorts studied and the secular effects of when measurements were made.

The present chapters concern normal development and non-pathological behavior. There is little concern with psychiatric illness. The chapters cover normal range emotions and subjective well-being but not anxiety and mood disorders nor other psychiatric disorders; self-esteem and personality traits are discussed but not personality disorders. Similarly, in the cognitive domain, individuals with disordered cognition due to dementia or other illness are not the primary focus of interest. Primary foci include fundamental attentional memory and cognitive processes. Let us turn to a more specific overview of each chapter.

Chapter 1 by Benton H. Pierce, Jon S. Simons, and Daniel L. Schacter provides an absorbing and highly accessible framework or categorization of the breakdowns of memory. The importance of memory in everyday life is difficult to overstate. Its successes provide a sense of personal history, knowledge of facts and concepts, and learning of complex skills. But there are also phrases calling attention to memory's fragile side, its "indiscretions," shortcomings, or transgressions. These authors point out that memory is not a unitary function or monolith. There are many different kinds of memory and each kind of memory has its unique failure. Schacter and his colleagues employ a catalog of seven basic "sins" of memory: transience, absent-mindedness, blocking, misattribution, suggestibility, bias, and persistence to systematically examine age-related memory problems. Use of the seven sins framework helps to provide insights into the cognitive and neural basis of aging and memory. The first three sins, termed "Sins of Omission," reflect different types of forgetting. Transience – the gradual forgetting over time, first documented in the late 19th century by Hermann Ebbinghaus, – according to Pierce, Simons, and Schacteris is especially troubling to older adults. Absent-mindedness entails inattentive or shallow processing that contributes to weak memories of ongoing events or forgetting to do things in the future; and blocking refers to the temporary inaccessibility of information that is stored in memory. Retrieval blocking – inability to retrieve the names of familiar people – is a particularly vexing form of blocking to many older persons. Another well-known blocking is the tip-of-the-tongue state (TOT). The next four sins – misattribution, suggestibility, bias, and persistence – termed "Sins of Commission," involve distortions, inaccuracies, or intrusions in remembering. Source memory or misattribution involves attributing a recollection or idea to the wrong source; suggestibility refers to memories that are implanted at the time of retrieval; and bias involves retrospective distortions and unconscious influences that are related to current knowledge and beliefs. Finally, persistence refers to pathological remembrances: information or events that we cannot forget, even though we wish we could.

Pierce, Simons, and Schacter introduce a number of memory paradigms used to interrogate memory processes and performance. Many have intriguing or amusing names associated with them, e.g. the false-fame paradigm, the Tipper paradigm, and the thought suppression paradigm. Interference from "Ugly sisters" or the part-set cueing effect and inhibition-induced blocking is relatively intact in advance aged.

Neuropsychological and neuroimaging studies have provided insights into the neural bases of many of the seven sins. Curiously, there exists little neuroimaging evidence concerning retrieval blocking, and no studies in older adults. Misattribution errors can have serious health and social consequences for elderly persons, such as mistakenly thinking one has taken one's medication or identifying a person actually seen in another context during eyewitness testimony. Frontal lobe integrity is a popular hypothesis as a neural basis for these kinds of memory sins. Neuroimaging studies that might identify or highlight age-related brain activation differences in encoding and retrieval processes are needed.

Finally, concepts of motivation and emotion, discussed in the second half of this volume (see Chapter 4 by Charles and Carstensen) are implicated in some of the sins of memory. Charles and Carstensen emphasize that older individuals are more motivated to regulate their emotion than younger individuals and this tendency may contribute to instances of memory bias, particularly choice-supportive source monitoring bias. This bias may help older persons avoid disappointment and regret. The close interplay of cognitive neuroscience concepts and methods, motivation, and emotion and personality constructs and findings is evident in this and other chapters.

Madden and Whiting provide an impressive scholarly review of age-related changes in the visual attention, guided from their perspective of several decades of programmatic and cutting-edge research in attention. Starting with a review of age-related changes in sensory physiology, they elucidate the ways in which these sensory changes contribute to age deficits in visual attention and highlight the importance of context or condition, especially in what they call data-limited conditions, i.e. display duration is near threshold and accuracy is below ceiling. They next consider general and specific effects of attention concluding that the age-related changes in perceptual and cognitive functioning so often observed are the effects of a general mechanism operating throughout the brain and nervous system. Such a general mechanism would be a chief contender to be the basis of cognitive aging. Speed of processing emerges as their general mechanism for age-related changes and they take the reader through a review of Brinley plots or task complexity analysis slopes concluding that age-related slowing is a general phenomenon rather than specific to individual tasks or cognitive functions. Tim Salthouse's alternative methodological approach, which uses an independent measure of information processing speed known as the statistical control approach to generalized slowing, is also discussed in rigorous and careful detail.

Different forms or varieties of attentional control, especially divided attention is a major concern of Madden and Whiting. Two different conceptual paradigms dominate research approaches. Those approaches employ the dual-task paradigm as a tool to determine whether declining attentional resources are responsible for age differences in task performance (i.e. not enough attentional resources for task) – versus older adults having greater difficulty dividing, sharing, or coordinating what resources they possess. Madden and Whiting illustrate that these issues implicate the notion of executive control, but as an essentially broad notion that "encompasses processes such as updating and maintaining information in working memory, shifting between mental sets, and inhibiting irrelevant information" (Madden and Whiting, this volume p. 68).

Madden and Whiting devote a substantial part of their chapter to reviewing the cognitive neuroscience of aging and attention, especially functional neuroimaging studies, some of which were discussed in the memory chapter by Pierce and colleagues. Especially intriguing results concerning increased rCBF prefrontal activation of older vs. younger individuals in a divided attention condition at first appear to contradict decreased involvement of the frontal lobes in certain memory performances (See Pierce, Simons, and Schacter in this volume). However, Madden and Whiting suggest that the surprising age-related increase in prefrontal activation can be interpreted in a way to be consistent with the hypothesis of an age-related decline in prefrontal functioning, by interpreting the pattern of prefrontal activation as increased effort. Thus, younger adults require lower effort levels or a minimum level of executive control in divided attention tasks whereas older adults need to recruit additional attentional functions that are mediated by prefrontal cortical regions. Several other PET studies of memory tasks have been similarly interpreted as compensatory recruitment of prefrontal processing resources not required by younger adults.

The prominence of the prefrontal regions of the brain in neuroimaging studies of age differences in attentional and cognitive performance is in large part due to the large structural and functional changes occurring there, but other cortical and subcortical regions operating in concert with prefrontal systems deserve attention as well. The authors mention basal ganglia as important subcortical nuclei of interest, especially caudate nucleus, as targets in neuroimaging of cortical–subcortical circuits that might address whether specific attentional functions such as inhibition and selection can be distinguished from the more general resource of processing speed.

The following chapter by Merrill Elias and colleagues summarizing recent studies of aging, hypertension, and cognitive functioning draw upon two of this nation's longest-running studies of heart disease risk factors and mental abilities. The first, known as the Maine-Syracuse Studies of Hypertension and Cognitive Functioning, began in 1975, and has received continuous funding since 1977. The second is the famous Framingham Heart Study. The author and his colleagues have virtually pioneered this important area at the intersection of health, disease, aging, and cognitive functioning. Their contribution to this volume serves as a primer for those new to the area and a roadmap for tackling unresolved issues for other active investigators. Their five goals are, to discuss the importance of studying hypertension and cognitive function to aging research; identifying major methodological issues that must be addressed to move forward; summarizing the contributions of cross-sectional and longitudinal studies for our understanding of the relations between hypertension, aging, and cognitive function; examining these findings in the broader context of patient-treatment and public health or policy perspectives; and placing their findings in the broader context of cardiovascular risk to the preservation of cognitive functioning with advancing age.

A continuing issue for longitudinal studies is: What can be new about a study that has been ongoing for 30 or more years? How can such data still be relevant and useful? The chapter by Elias et al. gives a clear answer. They have been studying the relation of hypertension and its' treatment to cognitive decline over the lifespan. Current concerns with the relations between normal cognitive decline, age associated memory impairment, vascular dementia, Alzheimer's dementia, and vascular cognitive impairment make their data more useful. While their primary cohort is still too young to be experiencing sufficient rates of dementia to test directly, their work holds promise to verify their important hypotheses in the next 5-year data collection period. A second area concerns a pair of surprising and even provocative findings. The first is dubbed the "young adult phenomenon," is that younger hypertensive individuals appear to be more vulnerable to the effects of hypertension on cognitive functioning than older hypertensive individuals. The authors argue that the greater vulnerability of younger individuals might be due to different mechanisms relating hypertension or blood pressure to cognitive functioning in different age segments of the adult population. As noted by the authors, diastolic blood pressure rises until about age 45 and then levels off, while systolic blood pressure continues to rise and systolic hypertension becomes increasingly prevalent in the elderly. They advance the notion that endothelial dysfunction might be the mechanism for the link between hypertension and cognitive functioning at younger age segments, while arterial stiffness is the mechanism at older ages. Interdisciplinary studies need to pursue this interesting hypothesis.

The second provocative topic is the suggestion that hypertensive treatment may not have the expected impact of reducing the cognitive decline associated with hypertension. The authors point out a number of unresolved issues needing further study, including whether this apparent paradoxical effect is due to the age at which treatment started or whether treatments that are efficacious in lowering blood pressure differ in their cognitive benefits. An additional consideration is the need to identify specific cognitive abilities or processes that are strongly associated with blood pressure. Nearly all cognitive abilities, except for crystallized-verbal abilities that reflect general knowledge and tend to increase with age such as information and vocabulary are associated with hypertension or blood pressure. The construct of Vascular Cognitive Impairment is highlighted as a promising way to predict which cognitive abilities might be most affected by hypertension and to benefit from its successful treatment.

Chapter 4 by Charles and Carstensen treats emotional functioning from a life span view concentrating on adulthood and old age. Acknowledging emotion's roots in Darwinian terms of biological reactivity, Charles and Carstensen point out that affects and emotions in gerontology were rarely studied scientifically until recently. Importantly, new theoretical perspectives are not burdened with the pejorative assumptions about pervasive declines and decreases thought to accompany aging. This chapter on emotion melds very nicely with the conclusions from the areas of personality and well-being that emotional and personality systems function well and are stable, indeed resilient, and that increases or better the emotional regulation, coping, and overall happiness and life satisfaction increasingly characterize older cohorts.

We editors are delighted that Charles and Carstensen started with the biological foundations of emotion, as it provides a bridge to the cognitive neuroscience fields mentioned in the earlier chapters on memory and attention.

Charles and Carstensen and their colleagues, including Robert Levenson, John Gottman, and Ritchie Davidson, are making seminal contributions to the field of affective neuroscience, and the current contribution by Charles and Carstensen provides compelling testimony that emotions and aging is a vital part of that endeavor. True to their life span orientation, the authors review important concepts from infant and child temperament that link personality traits to affective style. Personality traits of neuroticism and extraversion from the Five-Factor Model of personality are linked to positive affect (PA) and negative affect (NA), which are considered to be the primary affective dimensions of subjective experience. As will be mentioned at greater length in the Chapters 5 and 6 by Trzesniewski et al. on personality and self-esteem and by Diener et al. on well-being, important and powerful links can be forged between personality traits which not only pre-dispose to certain moods and emotional states but also have long-term predictive implications such that level of happiness over many years can be successfully forecast (Costa and McCrae, 1980). The aging literature also shows clearly that there are negligible age differences in life satisfaction and well-being. In fact, Powell Lawton's groundbreaking research established that older persons have a higher balance of positive to negative affect compared to younger persons. Not only are PA and NA relatively independent of one another, they have different patterns of brain activity and independent neuroanatomical pathways.

The neurobiology of emotions and personality is a phenomenally active and growing field, especially studies involving neuroimaging of various cortical and subcortical and limbic structures. Of special interest is the relation between the substantial age-related loss in prefrontal volume and emotional functioning. As Charles and Carstensen point out, the prefrontal cortex is critical not only for executive functioning and social functioning, but also for emotion regulation, with prefrontal damage leading to emotional dysregulation including depression, hostility, and poor emotional judgment. There is a disproportionate age-related loss in prefrontal volumes compared to other brain regions, leading to the plausible expectation that there would be concomitant age-related deficits in emotional functioning, particularly in emotional regulation. But, as the authors write, empirical analyzes do not support this expectation. This discrepancy between maintained or even improved subjective experience in the emotion domain, on the one hand, and decreases in prefrontal lobe cortex volume on the other, is an intriguing question that awaits satisfactory explanation.

We can only highlight the topics skillfully covered by the authors which include emotional expression, social processes and networks, social perceptions, cognitive processes, emotion regulation, general coping strategies, and memory. Particularly valuable is the highlighting of the several strategies that older adults use to regulate their emotions. Older adults are more proactive: that is, they engage in more proactive strategies to avoid negative emotional experiences, specifically in the area of social interactions. Also, they respond with less hostility and aggression to negative emotional experiences, a finding consistent with the personality, coping and aging literature (McCrae, 1982). Moreover, older adults employ complex and insightful cognitions in analyzing emotional problems, often considering multiple perspectives. A highlight of the review of emotions and aging is the expert discussion of various theoretical models that might account for and offer unifying explanations, including socioemotional selectivity theory of Carstensen, cognitive-emotional integration model of Labouvie-Vief and colleagues, Robert Levenson's biological model of lessened physiological reactivity, and inefficient or declining cognitive inhibition mechanisms.

Mention of these models should not lead the reader to think that the picture is a negative one. Far from it. Emotional experience often improves with age, despite the fact that, for the authors, emotions are largely determined by declining biological substrates. As Charles and Carstensen state, there is evidence of improved affective well-being, declines in negative affect over time, and lower rates of affective disorders, especially depression, with aging, even in advanced old age. Indeed, as proclaimed by the authors, the emotion system works, and by advancing our understanding of how emotions unfold or work across the adult life span, we will advance our understanding of the nature of psychological aging.

Personality and Self-Esteem get the life span treatment in the next chapter by a quartet of investigators expert at tackling controversial and hoary issues that have divided and polarized the field of personality and aging. UC Davis psychologists, Kali Trzesniewski and Richard Robins team up with Brent Roberts (who works with the Mills College study as well as doing meta-analyzes) and Avshalom Caspi of Madison, London, and Dunedin, New Zealand, to provide an interesting and balanced overview. Their contribution presents a review of the many longitudinal studies of personality and the life span. According to these authors the picture to date is one of remarkable continuity in personality and the related construct of self-esteem, especially given the "vast array of experiences that impinge upon a lived life." Continuity is based upon longitudinal evidence of moderate test–retest or rank-order stability across multiple measurement times across the life-span. At the same time that such rank-order stability demonstrates continuity in the way persons think, feel, and behave, it does not demonstrate that personality is fixed or immutable.

In publications, discussed, in their chapter, interesting patterns of normative change serve to illustrate what the authors call the organizational role of personality and self-esteem in helping individuals adapt their thoughts, feelings, and behavior to environmental demands and developmental challenges. Their view contrasts with a radically different approach – one which challenges theories of personality change and development over the life span – holds that personality itself shapes lives and gives order, continuity, and predictability to the life course, as well as creating or accommodating change (McCrae and Costa, 2003, pp. 234–235).

In this alternative view, personality or enduring dispositions form a basis for guiding emerging lives.

Trzesniewski and colleagues articulate another important way of viewing the constructs of personality and self-esteem as developmental constructs, in that they demonstrate changes across the life span. They favor environmental or contextual approaches to viewing developmental changes in personality traits. They emphasize the reciprocity between individuals encountering or undergoing "normative developmental transitions" and resulting normative changes in related areas of personality and the self. Interestingly, non-normative changes, which might be even more powerful influences on personality change, are not given much attention. A recent study from the University of North Carolina Alumni Heart Study, using a large cohort of baby boomers, showed that the mid-life event of divorce had one of the largest impacts on mean personality change from among a wide variety of life events (Costa and McCrae, 2000).

The second half of their chapter reviews cross-sectional and longitudinal research on mean-level personality differences and changes or what the authors call normative development of personality across the life span. They also address the impact of socio-contextual factors on personality and self-esteem which is an important and, until relatively recently, neglected topic. In their last section, the authors examine how various life experiences across generations and across individuals lead to varying patterns of personality and self-esteem change. The tension between the normative developmental transition view of personality traits over the life course and the enduring dispositional view is certainly a controversy in this field. The individual difference construct of self-esteem mirrors the debate, with some arguing that self-esteem is trait-like, remaining predominantly stable over time, while others argue that it is a state-like process continually fluctuating in response to environmental stimuli. The authors rely on another meta-analysis of over 50 studies with a combined sample of over 29,000 subjects which found that the median test–retest correlation was moderate in magnitude (0.47). The authors note interesting differences, however, in the trajectories of self-esteem over the life span in comparison to personality. While personality stability shows a linear trend, peaking at around 50, they present data showing a robust curvilinear trend for self-esteem stability, with relatively low stability in childhood, increasing through adolescence until early adulthood, and declining during mid-life and old-age. They interpret the decreasing stability in adulthood and old age as evidence for the effect of life changes and shifting social circumstances typical of later adulthood and old age. They view self-esteem as showing continuing change across the life span but are puzzled by the "large divergence in late adulthood." Sources or causes of change are brought up in their final section, with a heavy emphasis on environmental or socio-contextual factors, including normative and non-normative changes.

At the same time it is clear that longitudinal studies have demonstrated the "relative imperviousness of personality traits to life experiences," (McCrae, 2002, p. 309). Nearly everyone experiences a number of life transitions and major life changes and events in terms of their social relations, occupation, and health. Yet, in terms of their personality traits, their relative stability as well as average level remain largely unchanged, suggesting that personality traits are biologically based enduring dispositions and not merely learned adaptations to external events. When changes in the underlying biological basis occur as in Alzheimer's disease and other neurodegenerative diseases, there are dramatic and well-documented changes in personality associated with changes in the brain attributable to the disease or to traumatic brain injury (Costa et al., 2000).

Environmental events obviously influence personality. We know that a host of environmental influences and events are associated with personality changes, although the causal direction is often frustratingly ambiguous, because personality changes could be the cause, not the effect, of those events. Other important issues awaiting resolution are the intensity and the magnitude of changes associated with various types of events as well as how long they are sustained. Only continued observation of individuals will be able to detect how transient or not socio-contextual influences such as career changes, social movements, religious conversion, and psychotherapy are. Again, longitudinal and or life-course studies are invaluable in pursuit of answers.

The next topic has fascinated philosophers, scientists, and just about everyone else for over 2000 years. For nearly three decades Ed Diener, one of the world's leading researchers on happiness or Subjective Well-Being (SWB), has chronicled and been responsible, in large measure, for an explosive growth in research on this topic. Eid et al. (2003) state that the World Database on Happiness (Veenhoven, 1999) and its component Catalog of Happiness Correlates list more than 6200 findings from 662 studies in 97 nations. Given this outpouring of research, it is more than fitting for Drs. Diener, Scollon, and Lucas to bring conceptual organization and integration of empirical findings.

Readers of their chapter will learn of important new directions that the SWB field is taking, in large part due to the recognition that there are multiple components and not a single core of SWB. Among questions addressed are: (1) the structural components of SWB and how they relate to one another; (2) whether it is the frequency or intensity of affects and thoughts that determines SWB; (3) temporal sequence and stages, and how the picture of SWB changes as one examines different time perspectives; (4) stability and consistency across situations, including whether SWB is a personality characteristic; (5) whether affect or cognition – pleasant feelings or satisfactory evaluations – is more important; (6) what constitutes an adaptive mood system; (7) tradeoffs: Is happiness always the paramount goal? and (8) how best to measure SWB in the elderly.

The authors review age trends in SWB, but their major goal is to orient readers to the evolving and intriguing multifaceted nature of this concept and help achieve a more sophisticated conception and appreciation of SWB. Historically, there have been many interesting tensions in approaching happiness and the Good Life. One of the earliest, began with the pre-Socratic philosopher Democritus' notion that it is the way one reacts to his/her life circumstances, and not what one possesses, that determines one's happiness. This latter view, the authors point out, is referred to as the eudemonia definition of happiness and was championed by Socrates, Plato, and Aristotle, whereby happiness consisted of possessing the greatest goods available. For psychologists and other social scientists concerned with subjective well-being or happiness the tension has been between hedonistic conceptions and cognitive evaluations that reflect purpose, striving, and meaning. Norman Bradburn, more than a quarter-century ago, defined SWB or happiness as the balance between positive and negative affects, a psychological equivalent of the utilitarian principle of maximization of pleasure and minimization of pain. In a recent *Annual Review of Psychology* (2001), Ryan and Deci nicely summarized research from the two general perspectives: the hedonic approach, defined in very similar terms whereby happiness is the attainment of pleasure and the avoidance of pain; and the eudaimonic approach, which they claimed, focuses on meaning and self-realization and defines well-being in terms of the degree to which a person is fully-functioning. Eudaimonic theories, said Ryan and Deci (2001), make the useful distinction between happiness and well-being that is distinct from happiness per se. Interestingly, Carol Ryff and Burton Singer have also challenged hedonistic models of SWB, insisting that mere attainment of pleasure is not enough but the striving for perfection and self-realization is the optimal basis for happiness.

Personality trait models have made important empirical and conceptual advances in understanding SWB from both perspectives. Schmutte and Ryff (1997) hypothesized that such components as environmental mastery, personal growth, and positive relations with others represent aspects of psychological well-being that are related to personality traits. Indeed, Schmutte and Ryff (1997) found that Extraversion (E), Conscientiousness (C), and low Neuroticism (N) from the FFM were correlated with the eudaimonic dimensions of self-acceptance, mastery, and life purpose. Openness to Experience (O) was linked to personal growth. Agreeableness (A) and C were related to positive relationships and low N was linked to autonomy.

From the hedonistic perspective, personality traits have been shown to be among the best predictors of SWB, predicting whether people would feel happy or unhappy about their lives as a whole many years in advance (Costa and McCrae, 1980). Negative affect is independent from positive affect and both are related to global happiness, but to different dimensions of personality. Negative Affect is associated with Neuroticism, whereas Positive Affect is related to Extraversion. The enduring nature of these personality pre-dispositions allows personality trait scores – including those from the independent dimensions of A and C – to predict well-being up to 24 years in advance. Applying the knowledge about maturational patterns of personality traits discussed in Chapter 5 by Trzesniewski et al. we can make predictions about what happens to happiness with age. Negative Affect should decrease between college and middle-adulthood because of the decline in Neuroticism over that period; but Extraversion, and thus Positive Affect, also declines. A and C both increase, which would lead us to predict that adults should be slightly happier than college-age men and women. Many studies on life satisfaction provide support for this prediction. Declines in N and E over the life span are relevant to and support the discussion in Chapter 4 by

Charles and Carstensen on the general blunting of affect, both positive and negative, associated with aging.

Another tension in the literature centers on subjective vs. objective ways of measuring SWB. Some writers disappointed with the relative absence of the effects of "eudemonic" variables such as income, education, occupation, age, race, and sex with self-report measures of SWB question whether such approaches are useful. Even health and most events and life circumstances do not seem to have a long-lasting impact on SWB levels. This state of affairs is problematic only if one expects SWB to reflect actual conditions in a person's life. So when conditions change, self-reports of SWB should reflect these changes, as the authors discuss in their section on stability and consistency. From this perspective, it is not difficult to question whether people's subjective judgments are reliable or valid, or somehow influenced by irrelevant information. As a result, they propose alternative approaches to self-report. The authors urge us to be cautious in interpreting results based solely on self-report methods. Interestingly, they discuss application of informant or observer-reports of target's SWB. But despite the imperfections of self-report measures, the evidence reviewed by Diener and colleagues vindicates the person's judgments or reports as meaningful and valid.

By contrast, as discussed by Diener, Scollon, and Lucas, dispositional factors (personality traits) have dominant influences on SWB. SWB variables also display a substantial degree of stability, but not as large a degree as do most personality traits. How state-like or trait-like SWB measures should be, is unresolved. Most definitions of happiness or SWB emphasize the subjective nature of the construct referring to the fact that it is the individual's own assessment of his or her life-not the judgment of "experts." But not all contemporary researchers are happy with this approach to happiness. Perhaps influenced by economic thinking and concepts such as "utility maximization," this alternative approach does not define happiness in subjective terms but in more tangible, observable, or objective terms. Regardless of the resolution of this tension, subjectively defined psychological well-being remains an important indicator of quality of life and functioning, and is among the most important of outcome variables in gerontology.

James S. Jackson is the Daniel Katz Distinguished Professor of Psychology at the University of Michigan, Director of the prestigious Research Center on Group Dynamics, and an advisor to many national and international organizations including the National Institute on Aging, serving on both the National Advisory Council and the Board of Scientific Counselors. Toni C. Antonucci, also at the University of Michigan and the Institute of Survey Research, a highly influential researcher on attachment, social support, and social relationships over the life span, along with colleague Edna Brown, a Post-doctoral fellow in developmental psychology whose interests are in social relations, aging, health, the caregiving relationship (including the care-receiver), and intergenerational relations, collaborate with Jackson in the concluding chapter (7) of this volume. They present a reconsideration of Engel's biopsychosocial model that they expand into a cultural lens, and extend it to a number of topics.

As with the other contributors to *Recent Advances in Psychology and Aging* Jackson, Antonnucci, and Brown express an urgent need to include a life span developmental perspective in aging research. In addition, they argue that aging needs to include a cultural perspective in research efforts. They call our attention to three major influences on development: normative age-graded systems; normative, history-graded systems; and non-normative systems. These influences interact with the changing ethnic and racial composition of US society, especially racial minority "new" immigrant goups.

These authors also devote attention to how concepts of culture, race, and ethnic groups are to be conceptualized and integrated into the enlarged biopsychosocial model they envision. The consequences for views of human development on public policy hinge on adequate attention to these issues. For them, these perspectives are especially needed to inform quality empirical approaches to issues of aging for racial and ethnic minority groups. A major concern in their chapter is with knowledge and understanding of social relations and health.

Writings about culture usually make it a very complex and inaccessible construct. Jackson and colleagues employ a definition of culture that is at once clear and compelling. They employ a definition, which sees culture embodied not only in formal practices (beliefs, ritual practices, art forms, and ceremonies) but also in informal practices such as language, gossip, stories, and rituals of life. They say that such a definition "emphasizes the role of culture in providing strategies of action, continuity in the ordering of these actions through time and a template for constructing action." Ethnicity and racial identity can be understood in terms of these formal and informal practices. How they vary by ethnic group, gender, and age would certainly be of interest in this context.

Also interesting is the authors' suggestion that concepts of ethnicity and culture be viewed "as mutable and changeable over the life course for different cohorts, with continuity over time and generations." The interplay of these externally imposed social constructions and self-imposed constructions with such psychological characteristics as efficacy, mastery, and self-esteem are important future research topics. These inter-relationships are of intrinsic interest. Health and culture is an important pathway in understanding the aging of different racial and ethnic groups. Jackson et al. discuss dietary customs and racial discrimination as two compelling examples of health and culture.

Social relations occupies a critical role in the culture and life span expanded biopsychosocial model, as one might expect. But culture causes variations here as well. Importantly, the authors give emphasis to the ways in which the cultural milieu influences social exchanges, health, and well-being, arguing that "a culture that encourages the exchange of goods, services, and favors among individuals can have a positive influence on psychological and physical health as well as the aging experience more generally."

Physical and mental health disparities are increasingly being recognized, and national policy makers are encouraged to understand and help develop more responsive policies. Jackson and colleagues argue that these policies must be responsive to life-course considerations and realities of family life if the health of

Blacks and Latinos is to be improved. Attempting to correct simplistic and misleading characterizations, the authors focus on three major themes from the research literature – heterogeneity, vulnerabilities due to societal mal-treatment, and family strengths. It is important to note that recent studies show African/Americans and other race/ethnic groups to be diverse and heterogeneous, having a wide array of group and personal resources. But one should not ignore these facts: minorities face serious obstacles and challenges as they age, they are at greater risk for debilitating, social, psychological, and physical conditions reducing their individual and family life, and "at every point of their life span African-Americans (and many Latino and Native American groups) have greater morbidity and mortality." It is in response to these grave challenges that the authors conclude their chapter by presenting an Ethnic Research Matrix whose elements include ethnicity, national origin, racial group membership, gender, social and economic statuses, age and acculturation; possible mediators of these elements such as coping reactions; and physical and mental health outcomes. The authors argue that this matrix with qualifications spelled out in their chapter "would provide a powerful framework for analyzing physical and mental health disorders, coping and adjustment responses, utilization patterns and a variety of individual and group outcomes."

As Editors, we take pride in this compilation of chapters and hope readers will share our enthusiasm for the progress the field of psychology and aging has made that is heralded by these chapters.

References

Costa, P.T., McCrae, R.R., 1980. Influence of extraversion and neuroticism on subjective well-being: Happy and unhappy people. J. Pers. Soc. Psychol. 38, 688-678.
Costa, P.T., McCrae, R.R., 1984. Personality as a life-long determinant of psychological well-being. In: Malatesta, C., Izard, C. (Eds.), Affective Processes in Adult Development and Aging. Sage Publications, Beverly Hills, CA, pp. 141–150.
Costa, P.T., McCrae, R.R., 2000. Contemporary personality theory. In: Coffey, C.E., Cummings, J.L. (Eds.), Textbook of Geriatric Neuropsychiatry, 2nd ed. American Psychiatric Press, Washington DC, pp. 453–462.
Costa, P.T., Herbst, J.H., McCrae, R.R., Siegler, I.C., 2000. Personality at midlife: Stability, intrinsic maturation, and response to life events. Assessment 7, 365–378.
Eid, M., Riemann, R., Angleitner, A., Borkenau, P., 2003. Sociability and positive emotionality: genetic and environmental contributions to the covariation between different facets of extraversion. J. Pers. 71(3), 319–346.
McCrae, R.R., 1982. Age differences in the use of coping mechanisms. J. Gerontol. 37, 454–460.
McCrae, R.R., 2002. The maturation of personality psychology: Adult personality development and psychological well-being. J. Res. Personal. 36, 307–317.
McCrae, R.R., Costa, P.T., 2003. Personality in Adulthood: A Five-Factor Theory Perspective, 2nd ed. Guilford Press, New York.
Ryan, R.M., Deci, E.L., 2001. On happiness and human potentials: a review of research on hedonic and eudaimonic well-being. Annu. Rev. Psychol. 52, 141–166.
Schmutte, P.S., Ryff, C.D., 1997. Personality and well-being: Reexamining methods and meanings. J. Pers. Soc. Psychol. 73(3), 549–559.
Veenhoven, R., 1999. World database of happiness. Erasmus University, Rotterdam, Netherlands.

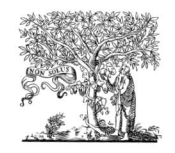

Aging and the seven sins of memory

Benton H. Pierce[1], Jon S. Simons[2] and Daniel L. Schacter[1],*

[1]*Department of Psychology, Harvard University, William James Hall, 33 Kirkland St., Cambridge, MA 02138, USA*
[2]*Institute of Cognitive Neuroscience, University College London, Alexandra House, 17 Queen Square, London WC1N 3AR, UK*

Contents

1. Sins of omission — 2
    1.1. Transience — 2
    1.2. Absent-mindedness — 4
    1.3. Blocking — 8
2. Sins of commission — 12
    2.1. Misattribution — 12
    2.2. Suggestibility — 18
    2.3. Bias — 21
    2.4. Persistence — 24
    2.5. Conclusions — 26
    Acknowledgments — 29
    References — 29

Memory serves many different functions in everyday life, but none is more important than providing a link between the present and the past that allows us to re-visit previously experienced events, people, and places. This link becomes increasingly significant as we age: recollections of past experiences serve as the basis for a process of life review that assumes great importance to many older adults (Coleman, 1986; Schacter, 1996). Not surprising, then, a common worry among older adults is that forgetfulness, which may seem to be increasingly pervasive as years go by, will eventually result in the loss of the precious store of memories that has been built up over a lifetime. While much evidence suggests that various aspects of memory do decline with increasing age, it is clear that performance on some memory tasks remains relatively preserved (Naveh-Benjamin et al., 2001).

*Corresponding author. Tel.: 617-495-3855; fax: 617-496-3122.
E-mail address: dls@wjh.harvard.edu (D.L. Schacter).

It has recently been proposed that the many and various ways in which memory can break down can be divided into seven fundamental categories, or "sins" (Schacter, 1999, 2001). The first three sins – transience, absent-mindedness, and blocking – have been termed "sins of omission," and refer to types of forgetting. Transience involves decreasing accessibility of information over time; absent-mindedness entails inattentive or shallow processing that contributes to weak memories of ongoing events or forgetting to do things in the future; and blocking refers to the temporary inaccessibility of information that is stored in memory. The next four sins – misattribution, suggestibility, bias, and persistence – termed "sins of commission," involve distortions, inaccuracies or intrusions in remembering. Misattribution involves attributing a recollection or idea to the wrong source; suggestibility refers to memories that are implanted at the time of retrieval; and bias involves retrospective distortions and unconscious influences that are related to current knowledge and beliefs. Finally, persistence refers to pathological remembrances: information or events that we cannot forget, even though we wish we could.

While much has been written about memory failures in older adults, age-related memory problems have not been systematically examined from the perspective of the seven sins. Adopting such a perspective could help to sharpen our ideas about age-related memory changes, and could also help to point out areas in which research and ideas are lacking. This chapter provides an overview of the literature on age-related memory changes within the seven sins framework, with the aim of providing insights into the cognitive and neural basis of aging and memory.

1. Sins of omission

1.1. Transience

The gradual forgetting of memories over time is one of the most pervasive of memory's sins. The first experiments to document this fact were carried out by Ebbinghaus in 1885, who taught himself nonsense syllables and then assessed his memory for the items after various delays. He found that, soon after learning, his retention of the syllables diminished rapidly, and as time went on, he retained gradually fewer and fewer of them. The apparent transience of memories is especially troubling to older adults (Craik, 1977), and evidence suggests that the ability to retain information over time is indeed affected by aging. For example, many studies have demonstrated that elderly individuals find it more difficult than younger adults to remember lists of words that they were asked to learn (Huppert and Kopelman, 1989). This may be attributable either to poor acquisition of new information, to degradation of stored memories, or to failure to retrieve information that is still stored in memory.

Evidence suggests that older adults acquire information at a slower rate than younger individuals (Youngjohn and Crook, 1993), and that they are less likely to make use of strategies that promote the formation of rich, elaborate memory traces, even when instructions explicitly encourage this (Simon, 1979; Craik and Byrd, 1982; Rabinowitz and Ackerman, 1982). Investigations of age-related changes in memory retention are complicated by the differences in acquisition between age groups, but researchers have sought to address these difficulties by varying the exposure of young and elderly individuals to the information that is to be remembered so that the groups can be equated on initial remembering, and by comparing within participants the amount of information that can be retrieved initially and after a delay, such that each individual serves as his or her own control. When one or other of these strategies was used to equate initial remembering, several studies found relatively little difference in forgetting rates between young and elderly adults over time (Rybarczyk et al., 1987; Petersen et al., 1992; Giambra and Arenberg, 1993), although others reported evidence of some age-related forgetting that could not be accounted for by acquisition differences (Huppert and Kopelman, 1989; Carlesimo et al., 1997). For example, Huppert and Kopelman (1989) found that elderly adults were significantly worse than young adults at recognizing studied pictures after delays of 24 h and one week, even when performance after a 10-min delay was covaried out.

A great deal of evidence suggests that the success of elderly individuals on memory tests depends, to a large extent, upon the support provided to facilitate retrieval. For example, the age-related deficit of elderly subjects is typically greater on free recall tasks, where they are simply asked to recall studied items in any order that they wish, than on cued recall tasks, where they are provided with a cue about the studied items, such as the fact that they were all animals (Bäckman and Larsson, 1992; Sauzeon et al., 2000). Similarly, performance impairments on tests of recall are very often substantially greater than on recognition tasks, in which participants select items that were studied from amongst non-studied distractors (Craik and McDowd, 1987; Davis et al., 2001). This latter difference may be a reflection of increased retrieval support in recognition tasks, or may be related to the widely held view that while recall tasks depend heavily upon conscious recollection of the study episode, selecting studied items from amongst distractors in a recognition task can be accomplished on the basis of judgments of familiarity (Mandler, 1980; Jacoby and Dallas, 1981). When older adults are given a recognition test in which they are asked whether they "remember" or consciously recollect contextual details about studying an item, or merely "know" the item was studied without conscious recollection (Tulving, 1985), they typically produce far fewer "remember" responses than younger adults, while "know" responses are less affected by age (Parkin and Walter, 1992; Mäntylä, 1993).

While there are often large age-related differences in memory after short delays, evidence suggests that young and elderly adults may perform relatively similar in remembering over longer periods of time. For example, in a study of memory for former one-season TV programs over the previous 15 years, older adults performed significantly worse for programs aired in the most recent five years, but there were far fewer age-related differences for programs from the prior 10-year period (Squire, 1989). Similar results were seen in the recall of personal autobiographical memories over the previous 20 years (Rubin et al., 1986), and over the entire life span (Howes and Katz, 1992). Indeed, some evidence suggests that older adults may remember more episodes from the years of early adulthood (i.e. around ages 10–30) than middle-aged adults (e.g. Rubin and Schulkind, 1997), suggesting that although, over all, there is a tendency for memories to fade over time, episodes from particularly significant periods of life (such as teenage years) may be an exception to the general rule of transience (Conway and Pleydell-Pearce, 2000).

Neuropsychological and neuroimaging studies have provided insights into the neural bases of transience. Studies of patients with brain damage have highlighted the importance of medial temporal lobe regions such as the hippocampus for remembering (Scoville and Milner, 1957; Squire, 1982; Schacter, 1996). Patients with amnesia, such as the well-studied case, HM, who underwent bilateral resection of the hippocampus and surrounding structures to relieve symptoms of severe epilepsy, often exhibit profound transience, able to retain very little information for more than a few minutes (Milner et al., 1968; Corkin, 1984). It is difficult, however, from clinical studies to isolate whether the exhibited transience is attributable to deficits in the encoding, storage, or retrieval of information. Advances in neuroimaging technology using positron emission tomography (PET) and functional magnetic resonance imaging (fMRI) have allowed separate investigation of encoding and retrieval processes.

Recent studies that have examined activations on a trial-by-trial basis have revealed areas in posterior medial temporal lobe, as well as inferior prefrontal cortex, whose level of activation at encoding was higher for information that was subsequently remembered than for information that was subsequently forgotten (Brewer et al., 1998; Wagner et al., 1998; Otten et al., 2001). The involvement of these prefrontal and medial temporal lobe areas at encoding would seem, therefore, to be an important factor in the transience of remembering. It has been theorized that changes in frontal lobe function, and perhaps medial temporal lobe function, contribute to age-related changes in retention (e.g. Moscovitch and Winocur, 1992; Prull et al., 2000). Recent neuroimaging studies have indeed implicated various aspects of frontal lobe function in age-related memory loss (e.g. Schacter et al., 1996c; Cabeza, 2002; Logan et al., 2002), and there is also evidence implicating changes in the medial temporal lobes (Grady et al., 1995; Sperling et al., 2001).

1.2. Absent-mindedness

Although the transience of memories is an abiding concern to older adults, the loss of memories over time is not the only cause of forgetting in everyday life; simple lack of attention during key phases of the remembering process contributes greatly to everyday forgetting. Many people are aware of occasions when, on arriving home, they quickly put their house keys down because the phone was ringing and then, later, had to hunt around for 20 min before finding them again. It is unlikely that this failure to recall the keys' location is attributable to a problem with retention per se, but is instead attributable to insufficient attention being paid to the keys in order to encode their location successfully. It is well established that dividing attention by having subjects perform a concurrent task while they are studying items for a later memory test results in poorer recall and recognition than when the subjects can pay full attention to the items (Craik et al., 1996, 2000).

Evidence suggests that lapses in attention play an important role in the absent-minded errors exhibited by elderly adults. Several studies have shown that when young adults are required to divide attention during encoding, their performance on recall and recognition tests can resemble that of older adults under full attention conditions (Craik and Byrd, 1982; Jennings and Jacoby, 1993). This apparent correspondence between divided attention and aging has been demonstrated in terms of behavioral performance, and also at the neural level. For example, Dywan et al. (1998) recorded event-related potentials (ERPs) in young and elderly adults during encoding, and found that under divided attention conditions, the performance of younger and older adults was similar both behaviorally and electrophysiologically. Likewise, N. D. Anderson et al. (2000), using positron emission tomography (PET), observed left inferior prefrontal activity in young adults associated with encoding under full attention conditions, which was reduced similarly under divided attention conditions and in older adults in the full attention condition.

Although dividing attention during encoding can substantially affect memory performance, it typically has less effect if it occurs during memory retrieval (Naveh-Benjamin et al., 1998). Another factor at encoding that can affect subsequent memory is the "depth of processing" that is carried out on the to-be-remembered information (Craik and Lockhart, 1972). For example, making some kind of semantic decision about a word, such as whether it specifies an abstract or concrete concept, typically results in better memory for that word than simply deciding whether the word is printed in upper or lower case letters (Craik and Tulving, 1975). Evidence suggests that elderly adults are less likely to spontaneously encode items as deeply as younger adults (Simon, 1979; Craik and Byrd, 1982; Rabinowitz and Ackerman, 1982). When they are encouraged to encode information elaboratively, however, subsequent recall can be markedly improved (e.g. Holland and Rabbitt, 1992).

Neuroimaging investigations of depth of processing effects have converged with the divided attention studies described above in identifying left prefrontal regions as being implicated in absent-minded encoding errors (Kapur et al., 1994; Wagner et al., 1998 experiment 1; Baker et al., 2001; Otten et al., 2001). For example, Kapur et al. (1994) observed activation in left inferior prefrontal cortex when comparing semantic (deciding if a word specified a living or nonliving item) and nonsemantic (deciding if a word contained the letter "a") encoding tasks. Similarly, a recent study that compared encoding-related activation associated with living/nonliving and alphabetic decisions about words found greater activation during the semantic task in prefrontal, as well as in medial temporal, regions (Otten et al., 2001). Interestingly, this same study found that a subset of these regions, left inferior prefrontal cortex and left anterior hippocampus, exhibited greater activation for words that were subsequently remembered than for words that were subsequently forgotten. Together, these results suggest that the absent-minded memory errors often seen in elderly adults may be the result of reduced activity in these left prefrontal, and perhaps medial temporal, regions.

In addition to encoding factors that may be responsible for absent-minded memory errors in older adults, retrieval factors may also play an important role. One situation in which the influence of such factors can be observed is that of prospective memory, or the realization of delayed intentions (Ellis, 1996). Different types of prospective memory tasks may be differentially affected by aging. For example, Einstein and colleagues (e.g. Einstein and McDaniel, 1990; Einstein et al., 1992) proposed a distinction between "event-based" and "time-based" prospective memory tasks. Event-based tasks refer to those in which a future action is to be performed when a particular external event occurs (e.g. giving someone a telephone message). These can be contrasted with time-based tasks in which one must perform a specific action at a specific time or after a certain time period has elapsed. Einstein and McDaniel (1990) suggested that minimal age differences would be found in event-based tasks because such tasks contain external cues that guide retrieval. However, in time-based memory tasks, no external cues are available, requiring one to use self-generated cues to prompt retrieval. This type of memory task in which a high level of self-initiated processing is required would be expected to produce the largest age differences.

Although several studies did, indeed, find an absence of age differences in event-based prospective memory tasks (e.g. Einstein et al., 1995; D'Ydewalle et al., 2001), other studies have reported significant age-related declines in these tasks (e.g. Maylor, 1996; Park et al., 1997). Einstein et al. (1997) suggested that this inconsistent age-related pattern of event-based prospective memory might be attributable to the nature of the background tasks that participants engage in until the prospective memory cue occurs. By increasing the demands of background activities (e.g. adding a digit-monitoring task), Einstein et al. showed that age-related declines in prospective memory emerged that were absent with less demanding background activity. In addition, Einstein et al. examined the effects of this increased background activity at encoding and at retrieval and found that age differences in prospective memory increased only when the digit-monitoring task was administered at retrieval. These results suggest that demanding ongoing activities, which tax the cognitive resources of older adults, add a working memory load that becomes more difficult for older adults to handle in conjunction with the to-be-performed action.

One implication of these findings is that prospective memory tasks that must be delayed over a substantial period of time may prove especially taxing for older adults, perhaps leading to prospective memory deficits even without a demanding secondary task at retrieval. As Einstein et al. (2000) have pointed out, many everyday prospective memory tasks must be delayed or postponed until there is an opportunity to perform them. For example, one may remember to make an important telephone call while in the back yard, but have to wait until in the house to actually make the call. Einstein et al. (2000, 2002) have examined the effects of maintaining intentions on prospective memory performance in older adults using a laboratory paradigm they call a "retrieve-delay" task. In this paradigm participants are required to wait for a brief period of time after encountering a target event before executing the appropriate action. Results of these studies showed that delaying execution of an intention, as briefly as 5 s, leads to substantial prospective memory forgetting in the older adults, even when the delay contained no concurrent activities. Furthermore, this age-related decline in prospective memory performance persisted even after some older adults received strong instructions to rehearse the intention during the delay period. These results suggest that older adults' impaired performance in this task stems in part from their difficulty in keeping representations activated (Einstein et al., 2002). As Einstein et al. suggest, older adults would be advised to "do it or lose it."

Previous discussion examined the involvement of the frontal lobes during encoding processes and the potential link between these processes and absent-minded errors in older adults. However, frontal lobe involvement, and in particular, anterior prefrontal cortex, may also be important during retrieval processes required for older adults' successful performance on prospective memory tasks (e.g. Bisiacchi, 1996; Glisky, 1996; West, 1996; Burgess and Shallice, 1997; Burgess et al., 2000, 2001). One hypothesis concerning this form of memory focuses on the requirement to monitor the environment for a cue that signals the intended action to be performed (Bisiacchi, 1996; Burgess and Shallice, 1997). Such processes may be mediated by a supervisory attentional system linked to frontal lobe functioning (Shallice and Burgess, 1991; Burgess and Shallice, 1997). Furthermore, it has been proposed that once the environmental cue has been encountered and noticed, retrospective memory is required to search for the intended action (McDaniel, 1995; Einstein and McDaniel, 1996), a largely voluntary and strategic retrieval process that may require the involvement of prefrontal systems (Shimamura et al., 1991; Moscovitch, 1994). Other hypotheses concerning the role of the frontal lobes in prospective memory have also been proposed (Mäntylä, 1996; Burgess and Shallice, 1997; McDaniel et al., 1998, 1999).

Evidence consistent with the view that the frontal lobes, to a greater extent than other brain regions such as the medial temporal lobe, may be critical for prospective memory emerged from an aging study by McDaniel et al. (1998). These authors divided participants into four groups on the basis of their scores on two composite measures: one that assessed frontal lobe function, and the other that assessed medial temporal lobe function. McDaniel and colleagues found that high-functioning older adults on the frontal measure performed significantly better on a prospective memory task than did the low-functioning group. For the medial temporal groups, there was no significant difference in prospective memory performance between high-functioning and low-functioning older adults. McDaniel et al. suggested that these results support the general consensus that the frontal lobes play a key role in prospective memory (see Cherry and LeCompte, 1999 for other evidence of individual differences in older adults' prospective memory performance).

More direct evidence of frontal lobe involvement in absent-minded memory errors come from both human lesion cases (Burgess et al., 2000) and neuroimaging studies (Okuda et al., 1998; Burgess et al., 2001). Wes and Covell (2001), for example, recorded event-related potentials (ERPs) in younger and older adults while participants performed a prospective memory task. The researchers observed age-related reductions in the amplitude of ERP modulations related to prospective memory, suggesting that reduced efficiency of a frontally mediated neural system in older adults contributes to their prospective memory failures. Okuda et al. (1998) provided additional evidence of frontal involvement in prospective remembering in a PET study with younger adults. Participants were required to perform a routine task (repeating spoken words) during scanning. In the prospective memory condition, participants were also required to also retain a planned action (to tap when prespecified words appeared) while performing other activities. Okuda et al. observed activation in a number of brain regions during prospective remembering, most notably the surface of the right frontal lobe (dorsolateral and ventrolateral regions), the front of the left frontal lobe (frontal pole), and inner parts of the frontal lobe near the midline. The importance of the frontal pole area for prospective memory was confirmed in two more recent PET studies by Burgess and colleagues (Burgess et al., 2001; Burgess et al., in press). Like the study by Okuda et al., these experiments contrasted conditions in which a cognitively-demanding task was undertaken that either did, or did not, require subjects to maintain a delayed intention to be acted upon when a particular cue was provided. Burgess et al. demonstrated that involvement of the region of the frontal pole in prospective memory was material- and stimulus-non-specific, was involved more in the maintenance than in the execution of the delayed intention, and could not be explained by differences in the difficulty of the two cognitively demanding tasks.

1.3. Blocking

When asked to report their most troublesome cognitive difficulty, older adults often cite an inability to retrieve the names of familiar people (Lovelace and Twohig, 1990). This inability to gain access to a target item after being given cues related to the sought-after information has been termed retrieval blocking (Roediger and Neely, 1982). Because one is aware of the block as it occurs, blocking represents an especially compelling sin of memory and a particular source of frustration in seniors.

Perhaps the best example of blocking is the tip-of-the-tongue state (TOT), an experience in which one is certain that information is in memory but is temporarily unable to retrieve it (Brown, 1991). A number of studies have confirmed that TOTs tend to increase with age (e.g. Maylor, 1990; Burke et al., 1991; Brown and Nix, 1996; Heine et al., 1999). These TOT increases in older adults have been observed in naturalistic situations involving diaries or questionnaires (Burke et al., 1991, Study 1; Heine et al., 1999; Brown, 2000; James and Burke, 2000), as well as in laboratory studies using names of famous people (e.g. Maylor, 1990) and rare words (e.g. Brown and Nix, 1996). It is worth noting, however, that despite reporting more TOTs than their younger counterparts, older adults appear to be equally capable of eventually resolving these TOT experiences if given enough time (Brown and Nix, 1996; Heine et al., 1999).

Explanations for higher TOT reports among elderly adults have focused primarily on two alternative hypotheses. The first, termed the inhibition hypothesis (Burke et al., 1991), states that TOT experiences are due in large part to the existence of interfering items or "interlopers" that hinder memory retrieval (e.g. Jones and Langford, 1987; Jones, 1989). These interlopers were originally called "ugly sisters" by Reason and Lucas (1984), referring to Cinderella's undesirable but dominating older sisters. These ugly sisters are incorrect items that are either semantically or phonologically related to the sought-after target and occur recursively through the retrieval attempt. If older adults are less able to inhibit task-irrelevant thoughts (e.g. Hasher and Zacks, 1988; Zacks et al., 2000), they may be especially susceptible to the effects of these interfering items, resulting in an increased likelihood that a TOT state will be induced.

According to the inhibition hypothesis, older adults should experience more interlopers during TOT states than young adults. However, most studies that have examined this issue have found that older adults are less likely to generate such competing items during attempted retrieval (Cohen and Faulkner, 1986; Burke et al., 1988, 1991; but see Brown and Nix, 1996). These findings lend support to an alternative hypothesis of age-related TOT increases known as the *transmission-deficit hypothesis* (Burke et al., 1991), based on the notion that activation of the target word is incomplete (Brown, 1991). A key aspect of Burke et al.'s hypothesis is that words or concepts can be represented as interconnected nodes of information (semantic, lexical, and phonological nodes). According to Burke et al. (1991), aging weakens the connections between these nodes, reducing the transmission of activation from lexical nodes to connected phonological nodes, resulting in a reduced likelihood of phonological activation and an increase in TOT experiences.

A review of studies examining TOT states in older adults supports Burke et al.'s (1991) transmission-deficit hypothesis (Brown, 2000). As predicted by the hypothesis, older adults experience fewer related words (interlopers), as well as lower levels of partial information concerning the target word.

Although inhibition of competing items may not be a significant factor in increased TOT reports among elderly adults, other evidence suggests that inhibitory deficits may play a role in other blocking phenomena commonly found among seniors. For example, Hartman and Hasher (1991) devised a garden-path sentence task to assess whether older adults would be less likely to suppress or inhibit information that was highly familiar but no longer relevant. In this task, participants generated a final word for a series of sentences (e.g. the word "bowl" for the sentence "She ladled the soup into her ____"). For critical sentences, the participant-generated word was replaced by a plausible, but much less likely ending word (e.g. "lap"). Participants were instructed to remember the final word for a later memory test. On a later indirect memory test, participants were asked to provide endings for a series of new sentences that were moderately predictive of their final words (e.g. "Scotty licked the bottom of the ____" and "The kitten slept peacefully on her owner's ____"). Accessibility of the alternative endings was measured by how often participants used them to complete the new sentences above a baseline completion rate (priming).

Using this task, several studies have found that priming patterns differ across younger and older adults. Whereas younger adults show reliable above baseline completion using the target endings but not for disconfirmed endings (Hartman and Hasher, 1991; Hartman and Dusek, 1994; Hasher et al., 1997; May et al., 1999), older adults exhibit priming for both types of items (Hartman and Hasher, 1991; Hartman and Dusek, 1994; May and Hasher, 1998; Hasher et al., 1999; May et al., 1999). These findings suggest that when instructed during the study task to remember only the target items, younger participants are able to inhibit or suppress the disconfirmed endings. Older adults, on the other hand, apparently are less able to inhibit the self-generated endings and show priming for those items as well as for the target items (but see Hartman, 1995 for a noninhibitory interpretation of the sentence completion data).

Less efficient inhibitory processes in older adults result in a sort of "mental clutter" in which extraneous information interferes with task relevant goals, producing a deleterious effect on memory performance (Zacks et al., 2000). For example, age-related increases have been found in the "fan effect" (Cohen, 1990; Gerard et al., 1991), which refers to the finding that the more associations that are linked to a concept, the more difficult is retrieval of any one association (i.e. the greater the "fan") (Zacks et al., 2000). Age deficits in inhibitory control have also been found in "directed forgetting" tasks in which older adults are less able than younger adults to suppress the processing and retrieval of items cued as to be forgotten (Zacks et al., 1996).

Older adults also show greater difficulty in ignoring distracting information in a selective attention task known as the negative priming or Tipper paradigm (Tipper, 1991). In this task, two stimuli are presented and participants are instructed to select one and ignore the other. On the next trial, the previously ignored distractor becomes the target, a task in which younger adults are slowed, thereby demonstrating "negative priming." Older adults, in contrast, fail to show reliable negative priming in this task (Hasher et al., 1991; McDowd and Oseas-Kreger, 1991, Stoltzfus et al., 1993). Logan and Balota (2000) provided another example of inhibitory control deficits that may be related to increased blocking in older adults. In this study, based on a paradigm devised by Smith and Tindell (1997), orthographically overlapping prime words are presented prior to a word fragment completion task (e.g. the prime word "ANALOGY" presented before the target fragment "A _ L _ _ G Y"). Logan and Balota found that the interfering prime word blocked or hindered retrieval of the target word ("ALLERGY"), an effect that was especially pronounced in older adults. This effect, according to the authors, is attributable to competing sources of spreading activation that are particularly difficult for older adults to control.

Another phenomenon in which inhibition may play a key role in memory blocking resembles the interference from the interlopers or "ugly sisters" mentioned earlier and is known as the "part-set cueing" effect. In part-set cueing, participants encode and retrieve lists of words, but are provided with some retrieval cues that are related to a previously studied word. The part-set cueing effect is the finding that provision of these retrieval cues inhibits or blocks retrieval of the target word, rather than enhances it (e.g. Slamecka, 1968; Roediger, 1974; Sloman et al., 1991). If older adults' inhibitory processes are relatively less efficient, resulting in a greater susceptibility to interference, might they show a greater part-set cueing effect than younger adults? Unfortunately, there are few studies that have explored this issue. Dolan et al. (2002) found that older adults recalled fewer remaining list items than did younger adults when given as few as three study items as cues, thereby demonstrating a relatively greater part-set cueing effect. Hultsch and Craig (1976), however, found a part-set cueing effect in younger but not in older adults, suggesting that the older participants were less susceptible to recall inhibition. Clearly, these conflicting results prompt the need for further research into aging aspects of this phenomenon.

Inhibition may also play a prominent role in a phenomenon somewhat similar to part-set cueing. In this situation, the act of retrieving a studied item can inhibit subsequent recall of related items, a phenomenon referred to as *retrieval-induced forgetting* (e.g. M. C. Anderson et al., 1994; M. C. Anderson and Spellman, 1995). Age differences in such retrieval inhibition have been examined in list-learning studies that showed relatively intact blocking or suppression of non-retrieved items among older adults (e.g. Moulin, 2000). The phenomenon has also been examined in a paradigm involving more complex events such as reviewing photographs depicting events that participants themselves had performed (Koutstaal et al., 1999b). Here again, older adults' memory for non-reviewed events was diminished to a degree similar to that shown by younger adults, supporting the notion that this type of inhibition-induced blocking is relatively intact in advanced age.

In addition to part-set cueing and retrieval-induced forgetting, age equivalence in inhibitory control has been found in other tasks as well. For example, older adults appear as capable as younger adults in suppressing distractors in a spatial location task (Connelly and Hasher, 1993). In this study, younger and older adults were equally slowed in identifying a target stimulus (an "O") in a location that had just been occupied by a distractor (a plus sign), indicating equivalent response suppression in the two age groups. In addition, older adults show no deficits compared to the young when suppressing information that was unconsciously processed and not brought to conscious awareness (Holley and McEvoy, 1996), and actually show an increase compared to younger adults in repetition inhibition (i.e. the *Ranschburg effect*) (Maylor and Henson, 2000). Why then, should such tasks produce no age deficits while age impairments in inhibitory processes are found in other situations, such as garden-path sentences, the directed-forgetting paradigm, and various other tasks? In the latter examples, prior information that was recently relevant is maintained in a relatively accessible state, even though subsequent information or events may have rendered this information irrelevant or even incorrect (Koutstaal et al., 1999b). As Radvansky and Curiel (1998) have suggested, such prior information is both "strong," meaning that it is present at or near the focus of attention, and "wrong," meaning that it is contradictory, inappropriate, or both to current processing goals. Such strong and wrong information places a larger demand on suppression processes, thereby increasing the likelihood of observing an age difference in performance. Conversely, inhibitory tasks that involve automatic suppression of information, such as suppression of non-retrieved items in retrieval-induced forgetting, would be expected to show minimal age differences. Using a retrieval-induced forgetting task, for example, Moulin et al. (2002) found similar levels of inhibition in normal older adult controls and Alzheimer's disease (AD) patients, suggesting that inhibition in this task is automatic. Moulin et al. further suggested that inhibition is a multi-faceted, rather than a unitary construct.

There exists little neuroimaging evidence concerning retrieval blocking, and none of it addresses blocking in older adults. Neuroimaging studies of the TOT phenomenon, perhaps the most common form of blocking, have been difficult to conduct because of the relative infrequency of TOT states. Maril et al. (2001) used event-related fMRI to assess neural activity in younger participants who were attempting to answer general knowledge questions. Results showed that attempted retrieval accompanied by a TOT report was associated with selective activation in the anterior cingulate cortex and right prefrontal cortex, two areas that have been posited as components of a cognitive control system that mediates conflict resolution (Cohen et al., 2000; MacDonald et al., 2000). According to Maril et al., these cognitive control mechanisms may be recruited in an attempt to resolve the TOT induced conflict; impairment of such mechanisms may, therefore, underlie age-related differences in the TOT experience. TOT reports in younger adults are often accompanied by activation of partial information about the sought for target (e.g. the first letter or number of syllables). Older adults, as mentioned earlier, tend to report little partial information about the target and often describe their experience as "drawing a blank" (Cohen and Faulkner, 1986; Burke et al., 1991). The TOT state experienced by older adults, therefore, may be attributable to impairment of the processes associated with conflict detection and retrieval monitoring. Based on Maril et al.'s results, it might be predicted that older adults would show less activation in anterior cingulate and right prefrontal areas during a TOT experience. Evaluation of this prediction awaits future neuroimaging studies of older adults.

2. Sins of commission

2.1. Misattribution

Of the seven sins of memory, perhaps none has been examined in older adults as extensively as misattribution, an error of commission in which some form of memory is present, but is misattributed to an incorrect place, time or person (e.g. Jacoby et al., 1989b; Johnson et al., 1993; Schacter et al., 1998a). It is useful to classify misattribution into three types (Schacter, 1999). The first occurs when one correctly remembers an item or fact from a past experience, but misattributes the item to an incorrect source. This type of memory error is especially prevalent in elderly adults, who have been shown to have difficulty processing contextual information (Burke and Light, 1981; Spencer and Raz, 1995; Light, 1996). For example, older adults have more difficulty than the young in remembering whether information was presented auditorily or visually (Kausler and Puckett, 1981a), in lower or upper case letters (Kausler and Puckett, 1980, 1981a), in a particular color (Park and Puglisi, 1985), or by a male or female presenter (Kausler and Puckett, 1981b).

Source misattributions among elderly adults have been demonstrated in a variety of situations. For instance, Schacter et al. (1997b) found that older adults were prone to confuse whether they had seen an everyday action in a videotape or only in a photograph viewed several days later. Older adults are also more likely to have difficulty remembering which of two speakers presented various information (Schacter et al., 1991), particularly when the speakers are perceptually similar (Ferguson et al., 1992; Johnson et al., 1995). Even when they are permitted additional study exposures to information in order to improve their memory, elderly adults still exhibit impairment at remembering the specific person who presented the information as well as contextual details such as the person's gender (Simons et al., submitted).

Not only do older adults tend to confuse external sources of information more than younger adults, they also tend to have difficulty discriminating between certain events they perceive versus those they just imagine; that is, they have difficulty with reality monitoring (cf. Johnson and Raye, 1981). For example, Henkel et al. (1998) found that older adults had more difficulty than their younger counterparts in remembering which of two perceptually similar objects (e.g. a lollipop and magnifying glass) had been actually perceived or just imagined. Age differences in reality monitoring have also been found in everyday activities such as packing a picnic basket (Hashtroudi, Johnson, and Chrosniak, 1990), possibly because of older adults' tendency to focus on thoughts and feelings at the expense of perceptual aspects of information. According to these authors, this tendency in older adults may arise from a breakdown in inhibitory mechanisms that limit the entrance of irrelevant information into working memory (cf. Hasher and Zacks, 1988). This breakdown, coupled with an increasing importance older adults place on personal experiences and values, may allow personal information such as thoughts and feelings to interfere with retrieval of other contextual information.

The type of source misattribution error described above can have serious consequences in older adults. For example, breakdowns in reality monitoring can lead to confusion regarding whether one has taken prescribed medication or just thought about doing so. In addition, source confusions involving face recognition have important implications for eyewitness testimony. To the extent that older adults mistakenly identify a person who was actually seen in another context, together with their increased tendency to base face recognition judgments more on a general sense of familiarity (Bartlett and Fulton, 1991; Bartlett et al., 1991), the veracity of older adults' eyewitness testimony is brought into question.

A second type of misattribution error is characterized by an absence of any subjective experience of remembering. For example, a spontaneous thought or idea is sometimes misattributed to one's own imagination, when in fact, the thought or idea was encountered in a prior experience (e.g. Schacter, 1987). This inadvertent plagiarism or *cryptomnesia* (e.g. Brown and Murphy, 1989; Marsh and Landau, 1995) is characterized by a lack of awareness of the prior encounter. Although cryptomnesia has not been studied extensively in older adults, age differences have been found in a related misattribution error known as the "false fame effect" (Jacoby et al., 1989a). In this phenomenon, participants first read a list of non-famous names that they are told are non-famous. Later, participants are shown a list containing some of these non-famous names (e.g. Sebastian Weisdorf), along with famous names (e.g. Ronald Reagan) and new non-famous names, and are asked to make fame judgments for each name. The tendency to rate the old non-famous names as famous more than new non-famous names is the false fame effect, arising presumably because the increased familiarity of the old non-famous names is not consciously opposed by recollection that these names are, indeed, non-famous (Jacoby et al., 1989a).

Older adults have been shown to be especially susceptible to the false fame effect (e.g. Dywan and Jacoby, 1990; Jennings and Jacoby, 1993), due to deficits in recollective processes along with familiarity processes that are relatively intact (Jacoby et al., 1996). Age-related increases in the false fame effect have been shown with faces as well as names (Bartlett et al., 1991). It should be noted, however, that these age deficits in spontaneous source monitoring (i.e. monitoring source information in the service of another task) have been shown to essentially disappear when stricter decision criteria are used during the source-monitoring test (Multhaup, 1995).

A third type of misattribution error occurs when one falsely recalls or recognizes an event that never happened. Although false memory research can be traced back at least to Bartlett (1932), who first demonstrated the reconstructive nature of memory, recent studies of such phenomena have focused primarily on a method pioneered by Deese (1959) and later modified and popularized by Roediger and McDermott (1995). In the Deese/Roediger-McDermott paradigm, participants are given a series of word lists containing words highly associated to a critical "theme" word that is not presented. For example, participants may hear or see a list composed of *thread, pin, eye, sewing, thimble*, and other words that converge on the non-presented word *needle*. On a later recall test, Roediger and McDermott reported that participants frequently intruded the critical theme word. Even more striking was the finding that on a subsequent recognition test, participants made false alarms to the critical lures at an astonishing rate (65%–80%). Indeed, false alarms rates to the critical lures were indistinguishable from the hit rates to the actual presented words.

This phenomenon has been studied extensively in older adults (Norman and Schacter, 1997; Tun et al., 1998; Balota et al., 1999; Kensinger and Schacter, 1999). These studies have provided some evidence for age-related increases in false alarm rates to the critical lures, along with false recall rates that are similar, if not slightly greater, than those shown by younger adults. This increased false memory effect in older adults has several potential explanations. One possibility is based on the notion of "implicit associative responses" – the idea that the non-presented critical lure is generated, either consciously or covertly, at the time of study in response to associated words (Underwood, 1965). According to this account, false recognition stems from a failure of reality monitoring, (i.e. a source confusion), where people cannot recollect whether they saw or heard the word at study or generated it themselves (Schacter et al., 1998a). Because of the source-monitoring deficits previously discussed, older adults would appear to be especially susceptible to false recognition of the critical theme words.

Another possibility for elevated false recognition levels in older adults is that they are impaired in their recollection of distinctive, item-specific information. Therefore, older adults rely more heavily than younger adults on memory for the general semantic features of the studied items or their "gist." Koutstaal and Schacter (1997a) provided support for this gist-based account by presenting materials for which source confusions would be highly unlikely. These materials consisted of detailed colored pictures from various categories intermixed with unrelated pictures. When given a recognition test three days later, older adults showed considerably higher levels of false recognition to non-presented pictures from studied categories than did younger adults. This age difference in false recognition was greatest for categories in which a large number of exemplars (18) had been presented for study, with older adults showing approximately twice as many false alarms (60–70%) as younger adults (25–35%). Koutstaal and Schacter suggested that presentation of numerous perceptually and conceptually similar pictures likely increased reliance on memory for the general features or gist of target items in the older adults compared with younger adults who were able to rely more on item-specific recollection of the studied items. Other relevant evidence has been offered supporting a gist-based account of age-related false recognition (e.g. Tun et al., 1998; Kensinger and Schacter, 1999; Koutstaal et al., 1999a).

Given this presumed greater reliance on gist-based responding by older adults and its deleterious effects on false recognition, are there manipulations that can reduce such responding and false recognition? One possibility involves the notion of developing non-overlapping representations of the study items (O'Reilly and McClelland, 1994; McClelland et al., 1995; Schacter et al., 1998a); that is, manipulating encoding conditions to enhance the availability of item-specific or distinctive information for reducing false memories. For example, Koutstaal et al. (1999) attempted to reduce the level of false recognition in older adults in the categorized pictures paradigm through the use of distinctive verbal elaborators at encoding – instructions that called attention to several perceptual and differentiating features of the object, which participants were then asked to notice during subsequent presentation of the object. In this item-by-item scrutiny during test, participants were asked to distinguish between objects that were in some way similar to ones encountered earlier and those that were entirely new, thereby discouraging the use of a gist-based strategy. In each case, additional encoding or retrieval support benefited older adults (in comparison with older controls who received no support). However, despite reduced false recognition in the older adults resulting from these instructional manipulations, their false recognition levels remained above those of the younger adults, even when encouragement to attend to differentiating features of objects was given at both encoding and retrieval. Apparently, more careful scrutiny of items can be beneficial to older adults, but does not eliminate their greater willingness to respond on the basis of general similarity information. It should be noted that findings showing age differences in face recognition (e.g. Bartlett and Fulton, 1991; Bartlett et al., 1991) can also be interpreted as supporting the tendency of older adults to rely on general similarity or resemblance in making recognition judgments.

Another example of distinctive encoding manipulations designed to reduce false recognition in older adults has been highlighted by Schacter and his colleagues. These studies follow the findings of Israel and Schacter (1997), who employed a distinctive encoding manipulation in the converging associates paradigm to reduce false recognition in younger adults. In this manipulation, black and white line drawings accompanied the words in one of the conditions, whereas in the other condition, words were presented alone. False recognition was substantially reduced in the distinctive (pictures plus words) condition compared to the "words-only" condition. Schacter et al. (1999) suggested that false recognition suppression in the picture condition reflected participants' use of a *distinctiveness heuristic*: a mode of responding in which participants demand access to distinctive pictorial information before they are willing to call an item "old." Consequently, the absence of memory for such distinctive information induces participants to call an item "new." Using the same methodology with older adults, Schacter et al. (1999) demonstrated a strong reduction in false recognition responses for words accompanied by distinctive pictorial information relative to a condition in which words were presented alone. These results strongly suggest that older adults can suppress false recognition of semantic associates when using a distinctiveness heuristic. When other mechanisms are involved, however, older adults may fail to show normal suppression. For example, Kensinger and Schacter (1999) employed a method in which lists of semantic associates were presented and tested multiple times. Compared to a single study/test trial, Kensinger and Schacter found that false recognition of critical lures in younger participants was greatly reduced after five study/test trials. Older adults, however, failed to show any false recognition suppression after multiple study/test trials. Benjamin (2001) has extended these findings to a paradigm in which study trials are repeated but test trials are not. These results provide further evidence that older adults are more reliant on general similarity information or gist influences than are younger adults and have less item-specific recollection than younger adults (see Schacter et al., 1998b for a somewhat similar result in amnesic patients).

Absence of false recognition suppression in the Kensinger and Schacter (1999) study mirrors results obtained by Jacoby (Jacoby, 1999a; see also Jacoby, 1999b). Jacoby instructed participants to respond "yes" to words they had heard earlier and "no" to words they had seen earlier, with the read words having been presented multiple times. Although, repetition allowed younger adults to decrease false alarms to words read earlier, older adults demonstrated an opposite effect – false alarms increased as a function of repetition. Older adults apparently fail to use item-specific recollection that accrues from repetition of the study items to reject previously studied words, just as they fail to use repetition of target items in the Kensinger and Schacter (1999) paradigm to reject non-studied but related lure words.

Cognitive neuroscience has begun to make inroads into our understanding of misattribution. Several recent studies examined patterns of neural activity in younger adults using the Deese/Roediger and McDermott false recognition paradigm. Schacter et al. (1996b) investigated false recognition with PET, and Schacter et al. (1997a) and Cabeza et al. (2001) did so again with fMRI. In all three studies, participants heard lists of semantic associates prior to scanning, although in the Cabeza et al. study, participants watched a videotape in which the words were spoken by one of two speakers. Participants were later scanned while they made old/new judgments about previously studied words, the strongly associated critical lures, and unrelated lure words. The main finding from the Schacter et al. (1996b) and Schacter et al. (1997a) studies is that patterns of brain activity were similar for both true and false recognition, with some trends for differences. Cabeza et al. (2001), however, found a dissociation between two regions of the medial temporal lobe as a function of the type of information retrieved. Activity in the hippocampus was similar for true and false items, suggesting that this area is involved in the recovery of semantic information. By contrast, activity in the parahippocampal gyrus was greater for true than for false items, suggesting this area's role in the recovery of perceptual or sensory information.

In all three studies, frontal lobe activation was quite prominent during both true and false recognition, suggesting that frontal regions may be involved in strategic monitoring processes that are invoked when participants attempt to determine whether a related lure word was actually presented earlier at study. These findings mesh well with recent neuropsychological evidence that damage to frontal regions is sometimes associated with increased false recognition (Parkin et al., 1996; Schacter et al., 1996a; Rapcsak et al., 1999). The findings are particularly relevant when addressing misattribution errors in older adults. As previously discussed, impaired source monitoring, which underlies many errors of misattribution, appears to be especially pronounced in older adults. One popular hypothesis concerning age-related deficits in source monitoring focuses on the role of the frontal lobes, with these deficits presumably arising from reduced frontal lobe integrity as a function of aging (Craik et al., 1990; Schacter et al. 1991; Glisky et al., 1995). This hypothesis is supported by structural findings indicating that the frontal lobes are differentially affected by aging (for reviews, see West, 1996; Raz, 2000). Despite the popular notion that frontal lobe impairments underlie age-related deficits in the processing of source or contextual information, it should be noted that much of the supporting evidence has been correlational in nature (e.g. Craik et al., 1990; Glisky et al., 1995).

More direct evidence has been provided by age-related source-monitoring studies using event-related potentials (ERPs). For example, Dywan et al. (2002) measured ERPs in younger and older adults in a repetition-lag paradigm (e.g. Jacoby, 1999a) in which successful rejection of new repeated test items required recollection of the item's context. Using an "exclusion" task (Jacoby, 1996), Dywan et al. found that older adults were much more likely than younger adults to misattribute the familiarity of the repeated new words to the study list, thereby replicating previous findings (e.g. Jacoby, 1999a; Dodson and Schacter, 2002). Furthermore, older adults generated ERP waveforms during the exclusion task that were significantly greater in amplitude at frontal sites than those of younger adults, suggesting to the authors that older adults are less able to quickly or automatically suppress the cortical response to items that are not targets, but are familiar due to repetition. Consequently, older adults must rely more heavily on controlled processes to make these types of source-monitoring decisions. Further direct evidence linking source-monitoring deficits in older adults to frontal functioning was provided in a recent PET study by Cabeza et al. (2000) who examined neural activity in younger and older adults when they were asked to identify which words had appeared in a prior list (item retrieval) or when words occurred within the list (temporal-order retrieval). In the younger participants, right prefrontal regions were activated more during temporal-order retrieval than during item retrieval. In contrast, the older participants did not show this asymmetrical pattern, suggesting that age deficits in context memory are due to frontal dysfunction. Future neuroimaging studies should investigate other types of context or source memory in older adults to provide additional insights into their increased susceptibility to misattribution errors. In particular, direct investigation of frontal lobe activity during the encoding of item and contextual information is important in light of recent neuropsychological evidence suggesting that only a subset of older adults demonstrate source-monitoring deficits (Glisky et al., 2001). According to Glisky et al., impaired source monitoring is not a direct result of aging per se, but rather the result of reduced frontal lobe functioning which is found in a subset of elderly adults. Those individuals appear deficient in initiating the processes necessary to integrate item information with its context during encoding. Future neuroimaging studies are needed to confirm this hypothesized link between reduced frontal lobe activity in older adults and impaired item/context integration, particularly with regard to the suggestions of other researchers who have linked reduced item/context binding in older adults to impaired medial temporal lobe functioning (e.g. Chalfonte and Johnson, 1996; Henkel et al., 1998).

2.2. Suggestibility

Misattribution errors occur when an event or item is perceptually or conceptually similar to a previous one; errors that appear to be especially pronounced in older adults. False memories of entire events may also arise from suggestions that are made when one is attempting to recall an experience that may or may not have occurred. Suggestibility in memory refers to an individual's tendency to incorporate misleading information from external sources into one's personal recollection of an event (Schacter, 2001). These external sources may be other people, written materials or pictures, or even the media. Because the transformation of suggestions into false memories requires misattribution, suggestibility and misattribution are closely related. However, misattribution often occurs in the absence of suggestions, making suggestibility a distinct sin of memory. Given that they are increasingly prone to committing misattribution errors, it is natural to ask whether older adults are also more likely to fall victim to suggestibility. This question is of particular importance from a legal standpoint due to concerns that elderly individuals may lack credibility as eyewitnesses (for reviews, see Bornstein, 1995; Yarmey, 1996). In addition, an increased tendency on the part of senior adults to accept misinformation may make them especially susceptible to certain fraudulent schemes practiced by con artists (Jacoby, 1999).

To experimental psychologists, perhaps the most familiar example of suggestibility comes from the work of Loftus and colleagues concerning the effect of misleading post-event information on memory distortions (e.g. Loftus et al., 1978). In the classic studies of Loftus and colleagues (for a review see Loftus et al., 1995), experimental participants first viewed a slide sequence depicting an automobile accident in which a car stopped at a stop sign. Later, some of the participants were asked what happened after the car stopped at a yield sign. Compared to participants who received no misleading questions, the misled group was more likely to mistakenly claim that it had seen a yield sign. Explanations for this "misinformation effect" have been controversial, although most studies acknowledge that source misattributions play an important role (e.g. Lindsay, 1990; Belli et al., 1992; Zaragoza and Lane, 1994).

Older adults' susceptibility to misleading post-event information has been examined in a number of studies (e.g. Cohen and Faulkner, 1989; Loftus et al., 1992; Coxon and Valentine, 1997; Karpel et al., 2001). Cohen and Faulkner (1989), for example, showed a film of a kidnapping to younger and older adults and then had them read a narrative concerning the film. Compared to a misled younger group, older adults who read an account containing misleading information were more likely to claim that this information had been originally witnessed in the film. Loftus et al. (1992) employed a similar method and also found that older adults were more likely to accept misleading suggestions concerning an event witnessed earlier. However, Loftus et al. found that the older adults also showed much less accurate more for non-misleading items than did the younger age group. This finding suggests that poor memory may prevent older adults from detecting a discrepancy between the post-event information and the original event, thereby making them more likely to be influenced by misleading suggestions.

The notion that age differences in suggestibility are attributable to overall differences in levels of memory is termed the trace strength hypothesis (e.g. Brainerd and Reyna, 1988). Brainerd and Reyna suggested that weak memory traces that result from inadequate learning or accelerated forgetting make the acceptance of misleading post-event information more likely. The results of the Loftus et al. (1992) study appear to support the trace strength hypothesis. However, Loftus et al. did not conduct a correlational analysis on individual scores. It is therefore possible that the older adults who were the most suggestible were not also the least accurate on the non-misleading questions (cf. Coxon and Valentine, 1997). To directly test the trace strength hypothesis, Coxon and Valentine (1997) examined the suggestibility of children, young adults, and elderly adults in a misinformation paradigm and found no relationship between recall accuracy and susceptibility to misleading information. These results, therefore, seem to refute the trace strength hypothesis (but see Marche et al., 2000; Karpel et al., 2001).

As previously discussed, source-monitoring impairments may play an important role in the sin of suggestibility, reflecting the reconstructive nature of memory (e.g. Bartlett, 1932; Bransford and Johnson, 1973). Because of older adults' well-established problems with recollecting the source of their memories (e.g. Schacter et al., 1997c), it is reasonable to assume that these source-monitoring deficits make seniors increasingly likely to accept misleading information (Karpel et al., 2001). However, it is also of interest whether older adults can avoid suggestibility effects under certain conditions, as has been demonstrated in younger adults. For example, Lindsay and Johnson (1989) used a misinformation technique with younger adults in which half the participants received a standard yes/no recognition test for items in the original event. The remaining half of the participants were administered a source-monitoring test in which they were asked to classify items as having been seen in the original event (a picture), the subsequent narrative text, both sources, or neither (i.e. a new item). Participants given the standard yes/no recognition test displayed the typical suggestibility effect; those who had read the misleading text attributed more suggested items to the picture than those who had not been given misleading information. Conversely, the misled participants given the source-monitoring test displayed no suggestibility effect, prompting Lindsay and Johnson (1989) to claim that the source-monitoring test encouraged participants to more carefully examine the information used to make a recognition decision, thereby reducing the suggestibility effect. That is, the source-monitoring test encouraged participants to adopt stricter decision criteria when making source attributions (Johnson et al., 1993).

Multhaup et al. (1999) used a similar method to examine whether older adults would exhibit a reduction in the suggestibility effect, given that adoption of stricter decision criteria through careful source monitoring has been shown to reduce older adults' source misattributions in the false fame paradigm (Multhaup, 1995). Multhaup et al.'s results were as predicted; older adults given a source-monitoring test failed to show the suggestibility effect, in contrast to participants given a yes/no test, who did show the effect. Suggestibility, therefore, may be reduced in older adults when they more carefully consider the source of the misleading information.

In addition to the encoding strength, source-monitoring, and discrepancy detection explanations discussed thus far, Karpel et al. (2001) have suggested that older adults may be relatively more susceptible to the suggestibility effect because of impairments in feature memory and binding (Chalfonte and Johnson, 1996). Because of the difficulty in distinguishing these alternative hypotheses on an empirical level, Karpel et al. argued for a parsimonious explanation based on non-specific (i.e. process-general) effects of age-related memory on suggestibility. Clearly, however, further research is needed to test the relative contributions of these different memory processes.

Despite the theoretical and applied importance of suggestibility, no neuroimaging studies have examined it in any age group. However, as Schacter (2000) has suggested, one possible approach, at least in younger adults, would be to investigate individual differences in suggestibility, building on previous PET studies that have correlated across-individual differences in various behavioral performance levels with patterns of blood flow (e.g. Kosslyn et al., 1996; Nyberg et al., 1996; Alkire et al., 1998). For example, Hyman and Billings (1998) showed that young adults who scored highly on various scales presumed to measure suggestibility were more likely to create false memories of a childhood event. Schacter (2000) proposed that through the use of such a procedure, highly suggestible individuals could be identified who might show reliable differences in brain activity associated with cognitive processes engaged during autobiographical retrieval. It might be possible to identify neural activity that distinguishes between acceptance of misleading post-event information and the correct rejection of such information. Such neural patterns of activity may mirror those found on certain source-monitoring tasks, which would provide further support to the source-monitoring account of age-related increases in suggestibility and would conflict somewhat with Karpel et al.'s (2001) hypothesis that such increases are attributable to non-specific effects of aging.

2.3. Bias

Not only is memory affected by suggestion, it can also be influenced and even distorted by present knowledge, beliefs, and expectations (i.e. schemas; for a review, see Alba and Hasher, 1983). Likewise, recollections of past experiences can be colored by one's current mood and emotional state (Bower, 1992; Ochsner and Schacter, 2000). These distorting influences of current knowledge, beliefs, and feelings on memory for a previous event are referred to as bias (Schacter, 1999, 2001). Biases in recollection have been observed in younger adults in several domains (for reviews, see Dawes, 1988; Ross, 1989; Ross and Wilson, 2000). One of the most common examples of this memory error is the operation of a consistency bias in retrospection, referring to the tendency to exaggerate the consistency between one's past and present attitudes, beliefs, and feelings (e.g. Marcus, 1986; McFarland and Ross, 1987; Levine, 1997; Scharfe and Bartholomew, 1998).

Although very little is known about the operation of such biases in older adults, there are reasons to suspect that increased age may be associated with an increased tendency to bias recollections of past experiences. As Mather and Johnson (2000) have pointed out, older adults are more reliant than their younger counterparts on categorical or schematic information when making source attributions. For example, Hess and Slaughter (1990) found that older adults are more likely than younger adults to falsely recognize objects in a visual scene if those objects were considered likely to have been presented in the scene (e.g. a sink in a kitchen scene). Conversely, older adults were less likely than the young to correctly identify a previously presented object if that object was not typically associated with the scene (e.g. a television in a kitchen scene). In a similar vein, Mather et al. (1999) reported that elderly adults were more likely than younger adults to misattribute the statement, "I was the editor of the paper in high school," to someone who had been previously described as a writer, when in fact the statement had come from a different speaker. When statements were speaker consistent, however, older adults were just as accurate as the young. This greater reliance on stereotypes or other general knowledge when attempting to remember an event may be less effortful (i.e. less cognitively demanding) for older adults than reliance on other types of information, making this bias especially likely to occur (Mather and Johnson, 2000).

Another type of bias that has been explored in older adults involves what Mather and Johnson (2000) have termed choice-supportive asymmetries, describing peoples' tendency to remember the choices they make in a fashion that minimizes negative feelings or regret (Mather et al., 2000). In particular, choice-supportive source monitoring involves attributing (and misattributing) more positive features to the options one chooses and, conversely, attributing (and misattributing) more negative features to the options forgone. To investigate whether older adults are more inclined to engage in choice-supportive source monitoring, Mather and Johnson (2000) presented older and younger adults with various scenarios for which they were asked to make choices (e.g. between two houses or two job candidates), with each option containing both positive and negative features. Participants were asked to review how they felt about the options they chose, to simply review the details of their decisions, or to perform an unrelated filler task. When later instructed to attribute features to the options, older adults attributed significantly more positive features to the options they chose than to the ones they had forgone. Younger adults displayed a similar pattern of choice-supportive source monitoring in the affective review condition, but were less inclined to display the bias in the other two conditions. Furthermore, these age differences persisted even when both age groups were equated on recognition accuracy and identification of source. These results suggest that when people focus on emotional aspects of a past event, their recollections of the event may be biased in an emotionally gratifying direction. As Mather and Johnson (2000) point out, older adults may be more motivated to regulate their emotions than younger adults (for reviews see Blanchard-Fields, 1997; Labouvie-Vief, 1997; Carstensen et al., 1999), making them more likely to engage in choice-supportive source monitoring, a bias that may help them avoid disappointment and regret.

Yet another form of bias that has been examined in older adults refers to the subtle influences of past experience on current judgments about other people or groups. For example, the *fundamental attribution error* (Heider, 1958; Ross and Nisbett, 1991) is the tendency to overestimate the extent to which the outcome of an event is attributable to internal, dispositional factors and to underestimate the contribution of external, situational factors (see Gilbert and Malone, 1995 for a similar construct termed the *correspondence bias*). Several studies have examined age differences in such dispositional biases, with conflicting results. Blanchard-Fields (1996) reported that older adults were more likely than younger adults to attribute the causes of certain events to dispositional factors, but only when the events involved negative relationship situations. Furthermore, there was significant variability within the negative scenarios – some situations produced age differences in attributions, while others did not. Follett and Hess (2002) investigated the fundamental attribution error in young, middle-aged, and older adults, and found that the younger and older groups were more prone to the bias than the middle-age group. These authors suggested that age-related differences in this bias may stem from two factors: (1) variations in the complexity of thought processes hypothesized to underlie the process of attribution (e.g. dialectical thought, preference for complex explanations for events), and (2) reduced cognitive resources in older adults that may reduce their tendency to consider situational factors and make attributional adjustments. However, as Blanchard-Fields (1999) points out, it is important to include other factors when discussing age differences in attributional processes. That is, factors such as stereotypes, schematic beliefs and values, and motivational goals need to be considered along with cognitive processing variables if we are to better understand how this aspect of social cognition changes as we age.

Also of interest in the domain of biases are automatic influences that may bias older adults' assessments of other people. Evidence exists that automatic processes used to make social-cognitive judgments are relatively spared in older adults, whereas mechanisms that rely on controlled processes are impaired (Hess and Follett, 1994; Hess et al., 1996). Hess et al. (1998) examined age differences in the effect of previously activated trait information on judgments about people. Participants were first exposed to a series of positive or negative trait terms in a memory task, and then performed an ostensibly unrelated task in which they were asked to form an impression of a target person while reading a description of his behavior. Hess et al. found that older adults were more likely to form impressions of the target person that were biased toward the previously primed traits, whereas younger adults demonstrated greater awareness of the primed traits and were more likely to correct for the impact of the primes, especially when the source of the priming influence was made available through distinctive contextual cues. These results suggest that in certain situations, such as those involving common advertising schemes, older adults may be more susceptible to unintended influences or biases, particularly with regard to their diminished ability to identify the source of the bias and counteract it (Hess et al., 1998; Hess, 1999).

In a similar vein, von Hippel et al. (2000) found that older adults relied on stereotypes more, and were more prejudiced, than younger adults when evaluating a target person that had been previously described in a certain way (i.e. a student athlete named Jamal or an honors student named John). Compared to young adults, older adults rated John as relatively more intelligent and Jamal as relatively less intelligent. Furthermore, this greater reliance on stereotypes in the elderly adults remained even when they were instructed to ignore the background information on the target individual. von Hippel et al. also found that older adults had more difficulty on an inhibition task, suggesting that along with the historical periods in which older adults came of age, inhibitory deficits also contribute to their greater tendency than younger adults to rely on stereotypes and to be racially biased.

Bias in older adults has been shown to extend even to attitudes toward their own age group. Hummert et al. (2002), for example, recently measured non-conscious or implicit social cognition regarding aging in young adults and two sets of older adults (young–old and old–old). Using an instrument designed to measure attitudes and stereotypes indirectly (the Implicit Association Test; Greenwald, McGhee, and Schwartz, 1998), Hummert et al. found that the old–old participants were actually more biased in favor of youth (and against old age) than were the young participants. Similar findings were reported by Nosek et al. (2002) who collected thousands of responses from respondents who completed the Implicit Association Test at an Internet web site. Although older respondents were more positive toward old relative to young when explicit attitudes were measured, their implicit attitudes revealed a strong negative bias toward old age that was equivalent to that shown by younger respondents. The results of these two studies suggest that an implicit bias toward youth and against old age exists in individuals of all ages. This widespread bias is not surprising when considering that younger and older adults share similar stereotypes regarding aging (e.g. Brewer and Lui, 1984; Hummert et al., 1994; Hummert, 1999).

As with suggestibility, neuroimaging has contributed very little evidence to the study of retrospective biases or the subtle biases inherent in social cognition. Indeed, with respect to many of the retrospective biases typically examined in psychological studies, the long temporal intervals between assessing what people know or believe at Time 1 and the later recollection of what people knew or believe at Time 2 make neuroimaging impractical (Schacter, 2000). However, some of the retrospective biases discussed earlier, which involve much shorter time intervals, may be tractable from a neuroimaging perspective, particularly with regard to aging. For example, the previously discussed work of Mather et al. (1999) may present an especially appropriate way to investigate the neural substrates of bias in older adults.

Mather et al. (1999) examined neuropsychological correlates of stereotype reliance in older adults. These authors found that accurate source identification of statements that were inconsistent with the speaker who read them, a task that presumably requires extensive reflective activity, was correlated with scores on a battery of neuropsychological tests purported to reflect frontal lobe functioning. In contrast, correct attribution of statements that were speaker consistent, a task requiring much less reflective activity during retrieval, was not correlated with frontal scores. Instead, this schema-consistent source monitoring was correlated with scores on a medial temporal lobe battery. In this situation, correct attributions require both the general encoding of the schema about each person and the initial binding and subsequent reactivation of qualitative characteristics (e.g. emotional expression) that were associated with each speaker; these processes may be dependent on medial temporal lobe functioning (e.g. Squire, 1992; Cohen and Eichenbaum, 1993; Johnson and Chalfonte, 1994; Squire and Knowlton, 1995).

Mather et al.'s paradigm appears to be well suited for use in an fMRI study. In particular, direct evidence of reduced frontal-lobe activity when older adults make incorrect source attributions in a schema-inconsistent situation would support the notion that their susceptibility to certain biases may be attributable to impaired frontal-lobe functioning. Another potential area in which to explore age-related biases from a neuroimaging perspective involves those inherent in implicit social cognition. As we have seen, older adults may be particularly susceptible to automatic influences when making certain social judgments. A potential model for examining such biases in older adults could be provided by neuroimaging research on the phenomenon of priming, a type of implicit memory that involves changes in the processing of an object as a result of recent exposure to the object (Tulving and Schacter, 1990). Neuroimaging studies involving younger adults have shown consistent changes in activity in various cortical regions during priming (for reviews, see Schacter and Buckner, 1998; Wiggs and Martin, 1998). Such neural patterns of activity during priming have also been found in older adults (Bäckman et al., 1997). Perhaps the logic and design of such studies in younger adults could be applied to the investigation of biases in implicit social cognition, with a further extension into the examination of such biases shown by older adults.

2.4. Persistence

The first three of memory's sins – transience, absent-mindedness, and blocking – involve forgetting a fact or event that one wants to remember. We have seen that older adults are especially susceptible under certain conditions to these memory errors. The final sin of persistence, however, refers to remembering a fact or event that one would prefer to forget (Schacter, 1999). Persistence is characterized by intrusive recollections of traumatic events, ruminations over negative events and symptoms, and even by chronic fears and phobias.

We have previously discussed that older adults have difficulty inhibiting or suppressing irrelevant information (e.g. Hasher and Zacks, 1988). Particularly relevant are the findings from directed forgetting tasks, in which older adults appear to be less able than their younger counterparts to inhibit information that they were instructed to forget (Zacks et al., 1996). Given these inhibitory deficits, does it follow that older adults are especially prone to unwanted and potentially disabling memories? Unfortunately, there is little evidence pertaining to this issue. For example, traumatic events tend to be remembered repetitively and intrusively (e.g. Herman, 1992; Krystal et al., 1995) and attempts by traumatized individuals to avoid or suppress such unwanted memories are often unsuccessful (for a review, see Koutstaal and Schacter, 1997b). Experimental evidence to this effect has been provided by McNally, Metzger, Lasko, Clancy, and Pitman (1998) who examined "directed forgetting" of traumatic and non-traumatic words in middle-aged women with post-traumatic stress disorder resulting from documented sexual abuse and matched controls who had a history of sexual abuse but no PTSD. Control participants remembered fewer of the trauma-related words that they were instructed to forget than those they had been instructed to remember. PTSD participants, however, showed no directed-forgetting effect, indicating a loss of cognitive control over the encoding and retrieval of trauma-related material. Although no such studies have been conducted with older adults with PTSD, it may be informative to consider that older adults appear to be no more susceptible to negative psychosocial outcomes following traumatic events than younger adults, and in some instances, appear to cope better than their younger counterparts (Hyer, 1999; Weintraub and Ruskin, 1999). This observation suggests that to the extent that repetitive, intrusive memories contribute to the etiology of PTSD, older adults appear to be no more susceptible to such unwanted memories. Whether those older adults with PTSD also show reduced cognitive control over unwanted, traumatic stimuli remains unknown.

Ruminative tendencies represent another example of persistence with potential clinical significance. Excessive rumination over depressive symptoms is associated with, and can contribute to, the prolonging of depressive episodes (Nolen-Hoeksema, 1991). Furthermore, these ruminative tendencies can enhance the persistence of negative memories in individuals with dysphoric moods (Lyubormirsky et al., 1998). Although little is known about the effects of aging on ruminative tendencies, it appears that older adults are no more susceptible than are younger adults, and perhaps are less so. Knight et al. (2000), for example, examined depressed mood and rumination in several age groups both before and after the 1994 earthquake in the Northridge community of Los Angeles. The oldest adults (76+ years of age) showed better psychological adjustment following the earthquake than the two younger groups, including a lesser tendency to ruminate about the earthquake. Perhaps this reduced tendency to ruminate over negative experiences contributes to the enhanced ability of older adults to regulate their emotions, particularly with regard to the frequency of negative emotions (cf. Gross et al., 1997; Isaacowitz et al., 2000).

Other examples of persistence are less extreme than its occurrence in PTSD and depressed mood. For example, studies by Wegner and associates have shown that instructing people not to think about a particular object or item (e.g. do not think about white bears) can result in a rebound effect. That is, items that participants are instructed to suppress are subsequently produced at higher rates than are items for which no suppression instructions were given (Wegner and Erber, 1992). Although we know of no data concerning thought suppression in older adults, the age-related deficits in inhibitory control previously discussed might result in reduced thought suppression ability in seniors. If such reductions were found, an interesting prediction follows that older adults would also show a reduced rebound effect.

Our understanding of persistence, at least in younger adults, has been aided by neuroimaging studies showing the importance of the amygdala in persisting emotional memories. For example, Cahill et al. (1996) performed PET scans while participants viewed emotional or non-emotional films. Amygdala activity during viewing of the emotional films was highly correlated ($+0.91$) with later recall of the emotional films, whereas no correlation was observed for recall of the non-emotional films. In a similar vein, a fMRI study conducted by LaBar et al. (1998) found amygdala activation during acquisition and extinction of conditioned fear. There is reason to believe that similar results may be found in older adults. For example, normal aging is associated with only modest reductions in amygdaloid volume (Smith et al., 1999). In addition, memory in older adults benefits from the emotional arousal level of stimuli (Hamann et al., 2000; Kazui et al., 2000). Furthermore, this memory enhancement effect of emotional stimuli is similar in younger and older adults (Kensinger et al., 2002; also see Carstensen and Turk-Charles, 1994).

It could also be informative to use neuroimaging in future aging studies employing the thought suppression paradigms pioneered by Wegner and associates (e.g. Wegner and Erber, 1992). For example, would similar patterns of neural activity, particularly in prefrontal cortex, be observed in younger and older adults during successful suppression of specified thoughts (e.g. thinking about white bears)? Such similar patterns might be expected based on related fMRI research conducted by Nielsen et al. (2002). In their study, which used a task that required younger and older adults to inhibit prepotent responses to repeated letters, successful inhibition in all age groups was associated with activation in right prefrontal and parietal areas. Furthermore, successful inhibition in the older adults was associated with activation in additional areas in the left hemisphere, particularly in left lateral prefrontal cortex. These findings suggest that elders can compensate for declining performance in inhibition tasks by recruiting additional brain regions (Nielsen et al., 2002; also see Cabeza, 2002). Successful performance during thought suppression tasks, likewise, may be associated with a similar pattern of neural activity in older adults, reflecting the need to recruit additional brain regions to reach a performance level equal to that of younger adults (Cabeza, 2002).

2.5. Conclusions

The increasingly large literature on memory changes in older adults has spawned a variety of theoretical frameworks to account for such changes (e.g. Light, 1996).

In this chapter, we have attempted to add to the literature on memory and aging by examining age-related changes from the perspective of a framework in which everyday memory shortcomings are divided into seven basic "sins" (Schacter, 1999, 2001). We discussed each of these from an aging perspective, including recent findings from cognitive neuroscience that have added to our understanding of such errors in older adults. Let us now review some of the main conclusions concerning aging and each of the seven sins.

The sin of transience – the gradual forgetting of facts and events over time – is observed in older adults to varying degrees. Whereas laboratory tasks have demonstrated convincingly that older adults retain new information less well than younger adults, similar memory performance is observed in both age groups for events from more distant periods, including recall of personal autobiographical memories from particularly significant life periods. Likewise, age differences in the sin of absent-mindedness tend to emerge on some tasks but not others. As the work of Einstein and colleagues have shown (e.g. Einstein et al., 2000, 2002), older adults tend to perform well on prospective memory tasks when such tasks can be carried out with minimal delay and with few background activities that are concurrent. Delaying an intention, however, or imposing other resource demanding activities in conjunction with the to-be performed action, increases the probability that older adults will commit absent-minded errors. The sin of blocking, referring to the temporary inaccessibility of information, is a particularly frustrating memory shortcoming in older adults. The tip-of-the-tongue state – the most thoroughly researched example of blocking – occurs more frequently as we age, due perhaps to an age-related reduction in the phonological activation of target words. Other blocking phenomena that occur more frequently in elderly adults may be due to age-related inhibitory deficits, particularly when the information that must be inhibited or suppressed is relatively accessible.

Misattribution represents a class of memory errors that have been well examined in older adults. This error represents a memory distortion in which some form of memory is present, but is misattributed to an incorrect time, place or person. Older adults were shown to be more likely than their younger counterparts to commit such misattributions across a wide range of situations, including recent findings showing that older adults are sometimes susceptible to false recognition errors in the Deese/Roediger-McDermott paradigm. More research is needed to further examine the causes of older adults' propensity for committing such misattributions, including neuroimaging studies that may highlight age-related brain activation differences in encoding and retrieval processes. The sin of suggestibility, which is closely related to misattribution, is also more prevalent in old age. This finding is not surprising, given that the ability to avoid the influence of suggestions requires one to monitor the source of the suggestive inference, a cognitive process that has been shown to be deficient in older adults (cf. Johnson et al., 1993). As was noted, however, older adults can reduce suggestibility through supporting retrieval instructions that help them focus on the source of the suggestion (Multhaup et al., 1999).

The sin of bias has been documented in older adults, including such examples as the consistency bias (e.g. Hess and Slaughter, 1990), choice-supportive asymmetries

(Mather and Johnson, 2000), the fundamental attribution error (e.g. Follett and Hess, 2002), stereotyping (von Hippel et al., 2000), and even implicit biases toward aging itself (e.g. Nosek et al., 2002). Compared with younger adults, older adults are more susceptible to several of these biases in certain situations. In particular, the memories of older adults tend to be biased when they rely on schematic information or other general knowledge when attempting to remember an event – processes that may be less demanding on older adults' cognitive resources. In addition, older adults may be susceptible to certain automatic influences (e.g. stereotypes) when making assessments of others. Because such automatic processing tends to be relatively spared in old age, whereas more effortful, consciously controlled processes are impaired, older adults may prove more vulnerable to certain advertising ploys in which they fail to identify and counteract the source of the biasing influence. Finally, the sin of persistence appears to be a memory shortcoming that is not manifested in older adults to a greater degree than in younger adults. We suggested that the relatively greater ability of older adults to regulate their emotions implies that certain types of persistence (e.g. depressive ruminations) may actually decrease with advancing age. However, more conclusive evidence supporting this conjecture awaits future studies. Furthermore, laboratory research examining more mundane forms of persistence (e.g. thought suppression of innocuous stimuli) in older adults is needed to determine whether suppression of more traumatic memories generalizes to non-emotional events.

Schacter (1999, 2001) suggested that rather than viewing the seven sins of memory as flaws in system design that the course of evolution should have corrected, these memory errors can be viewed as useful by-products of otherwise adaptive features of memory. When discussed from an aging perspective, it may be useful to view the seven sins of memory as adaptations that have been affected by neurological changes in the aging brain. For example, transience may be viewed as a case of adaptive forgetting (cf. Bjork and Bjork, 1988), in that information that is no longer useful should be forgotten. This type of information, such as old phone numbers or where we parked the car yesterday, is no longer needed and will tend not to be retrieved and rehearsed. Such irrelevant information loses out on the strengthening effects of post event retrieval and thereby becomes less accessible over time. With aging, neurological changes, including those affecting encoding processes, may result in accelerated forgetting of recently learned information. By contrast, certain events from more distant periods may be more personally relevant to older adults, and will have been retrieved and rehearsed much more frequently, thereby proving more resistant to transience.

When examining aging aspects of the three sins that involve distortion of prior experiences – misattribution, suggestibility, and bias – similar ideas can be applied. For example, many instances of misattribution, and at least some instances of suggestibility, involve failure to remember the source of an event – the precise details of where we saw a familiar face, who told us a particular fact, or whether we witnessed an event ourselves or only read or hear about it later. When encoding of such details is incomplete, or when they become inaccessible over time, individuals become vulnerable to the kinds of misattributions associated with false recognition or cryptomnesia, and may also be more prone to incorporating post event suggestions regarding details of an event that is only vaguely remembered. As Schacter (1999) has pointed out, an adapted system would find little need to record specific contextual details of every event that we experience; rather, it would likely retain information that is needed in the environment in which it operates (cf. J. R. Anderson and Schooler, 1991). With advanced age, it may be even less useful to retain the myriad of specific details surrounding our everyday experiences. Furthermore, less efficient neural processes in the aging brain that are involved in the encoding and subsequent retrieval of source-specifying information make it even more likely that older adults will tend to rely on general similarity or gist information when remembering past events. Such reliance on gist at the expense of specific or verbatim information may be a functional strategy for older adults given their diminished cognitive resources, but may make them more vulnerable to certain types of misattribution and suggestibility. Likewise, increased reliance on less cognitively demanding categorical information may make older adults more susceptible to certain biases.

We have seen that cognitive neuroscience has begun to provide information that increases our understanding of these seven memory flaws. Evidence suggests that progressive disruption to the functioning of frontal lobe regions occurs during aging (West, 1996; Raz, 2000), such that older adults show reduced engagement of particular frontal lobe regions, or indeed recruit additional regions, compared with younger adults (Cabeza, 2002; Logan et al., 2002). This frontal lobe disruption may be associated with reductions in the cognitive control of memory processes, to which the memory impairments documented here may be attributable. Future research from a cognitive neuroscience perspective should give us additional insights into how the seven sins of memory are manifested in older adults, including potential neural "signatures" that may identify each type of error in older adults and how such signatures may differ from those found in younger adults. Ultimately, such studies may more clearly identify the basic neural processes involved in the seven sins of memory and how such processes change as we age.

Acknowledgments

Preparation of this chapter was supported by grant AG08441 from the National Institute on Aging.

References

Alba, J.W., Hasher, L., 1983. Is memory schematic? Psychol. Bull. 93, 203–231.
Alkire, M.T., Hairer, R., Fallon, J.H., Cahill, L., 1998. Hippocampal, but not amygdala, activity at encoding correlates with long-term, free recall of non-emotional information. Proc. Natl. Acad. Sci. USA 95, 14506–14510.
Anderson, J.R., Schooler, L.J., 1991. Reflections of the environment in memory. Psychol. Sci. 2, 396–408.
Anderson, M.C., Bjork, R.A., Bjork, E.L., 1994. Remembering can cause forgetting: Retrieval dynamics in long-term memory. J. Exp. Psychol. Learn. Mem. Cogn. 20, 1063–1087.

Anderson, M.C., Spellman, B.A., 1995. On the status of inhibitory mechanisms in cognition: Memory retrieval as a model case. Psychol. Rev. 102, 68–100.

Anderson, N.D., Iidaka, T., Cabeza, R., Kapur, S., McIntosh, A.R., Craik, F.I.M., 2000. The effects of divided attention on encoding- and retrieval-related brain activity: A PET study of younger and older adults. J. Cogn. Neurosci. 12, 775–792.

Bäckman, L., Almkvist, O., Andersson, J., Nordberg, A., Winblad, B., Reineck, R., Långström, B., 1997. Brain activation in young and older adults during implicit and explicit retrieval. J. Cog. Neurosci. 9, 378–391.

Bäckman, L., Larsson, M., 1992. Recall of organizable words and objects in adulthood: Influences of instructions, retention interval, and retrieval cues. J. Gerontol. 47, 273–278.

Baker, J.T., Sanders, A.L., Maccotta, L., Buckner, R.L., 2001. Neural correlates of verbal memory encoding during semantic and structural processing tasks. NeuroReport 12, 1251–1256.

Balota, D.A., Cortese, M.J., Duchek, J.M., Adams, D., Roediger, H.L., McDermott, K.B., Yerys, B.E., 1999. Veridical and false memories in healthy older adults and in dementia of the Alzheimer's type. Cogn. Neuropsychol. 16, 361–384.

Bartlett, F.C., 1932. Remembering: A Study in Experimental and Social Psychology. Cambridge University Press.

Bartlett, J.C., Fulton, A., 1991. Familiarity and recognition of faces in old age. Mem. Cognit. 19, 229–238.

Bartlett, J.C., Strater, L., Fulton, A., 1991. False recency and false fame of faces in young adulthood and old age. Mem. Cognit. 19, 177–188.

Belli, R.F., Windschitl, P.D., McCarthy, T.T., Winfrey, S.E., 1992. Detecting memory impairment with a modified test procedure: Manipulating retention interval with centrally presented event items. J. Exp. Psychol. Learn. Mem. Cogn. 18, 356–367.

Benjamin, A.S., 2001. On the dual effects of repetition on false recognition. J. Exp. Psychol. Learn. Mem. Cogn. 27, 941–947.

Bisiacchi, P.S., 1996. The neuropsychological approach in the study of prospective memory. In: Brandimonte, M., Einstein, G.O., McDaniel, M.A. (Eds.), Prospective Memory: Theory and Applications. Erlbaum, Mahwah, NJ, pp. 297–318.

Bjork, R.A., Bjork, E.L., 1988. On the adaptive aspects of retrieval failure in autobiographical memory. In: Gruneberg, M.M., Morris, P.E., Sykes, R.N. (Eds.), Practical Aspects of Memory: Current Research and Issues, Vol. 1. Wiley, Chichester, England, pp. 283–288.

Blanchard-Fields, F., 1996. Causal attributions across the adult life span: The influence of social schemas, life context, and domain specificity. Appl. Cogn. Psychol. 10, S137–S146.

Blanchard-Fields, F., 1997. The role of emotion in social cognition across the adult life span. In: Schaie, K.W., Lawton, M.P. (Eds.), Annual Review of Gerontology and Geriatrics: Focus on Emotion and Adult Development, Vol. 17. Springer, New York, pp. 238–265.

Blanchard-Fields, F., 1999. Social schematicity and causal attributions. In: Hess, T., Blanchard-Fields, F. (Eds.), Social Cognition and Aging. Academic Press, San Diego, CA, pp. 219–236.

Bornstein, B.H., 1995. Memory processes in elderly eyewitnesses: What we know and what we don't know. Behav. Sci. Law 13, 337–348.

Bower, G.H., 1992. How might emotions affect learning? In: Christianson, S.A. (Ed.), The Handbook of Emotion and Memory: Research and Theory. Erlbaum, Hillsdale, NJ, pp. 3–31.

Brainerd, C.J., Reyna, V.F., 1988. Memory loci of suggestibility development: Comment on Ceci, Ross and Toglia (1987). J. Exp. Psychol. Gen. 117, 197–200.

Bransford, J.D., Johnson, M.K., 1973. Considerations of some problems of comprehension. In: Chase, W. (Ed.), Visual Information Processing. Academic Press, New York, pp. 383–438.

Brewer, J.B., Zhao, Z., Desmond, J.E., Glover, G.H., Gabrieli, J.D.E., 1998. Making memories: Brain activity that predicts how well visual experience will be remembered. Science 281, 1185–1187.

Brewer, M.B., Lui, L., 1984. Categorization of the elderly by the elderly. Pers. Soc. Psychol. Bull. 10, 585–595.

Brown, A.S., 1991. A review of the tip-of-the-tongue experience. Psychol. Bull. 109, 204–223.

Brown, A.S., 2000. Aging and the tip-of-the-tongue experience. Paper presented at the meeting of the American Psychological Society, Miami, FL.

Brown, A.S., Murphy, D.R., 1989. Cryptomnesia: Delineating inadvertent plagiarism. J. Exp. Psychol. Learn. Mem. Cogn. 15, 432–442.

Brown, A.S., Nix, L.A., 1996. Age-related changes in the tip-of-the-tongue experience. Am. J. Psychol. 109, 79–91.

Burgess, P.W., Quayle, A., Frith, C.D., 2001. Brain regions involved in prospective memory as determined by positron emission tomography. Neuropsychologia 39, 545–555.

Burgess, P.W., Scott, S.K., Frith, C.D., 2003. The role of the rostral frontal cortex (area 10) in prospective memory: A lateral vs. medial dissociation. Neuropsychologia 41, 906–918.

Burgess, P.W., Shallice, T., 1997. The relationship between prospective and retrospective memory: Neuropsychological evidence. In: Conway, M.A. (Ed.), Cognitive Models of Memory. MIT Press, Cambridge, MA, pp. 247–272.

Burgess, P.W., Veitch, E., de Lacy Costello, A., Shallice, T., 2000. The cognitive and neuroanatomical correlates of multitasking. Neuropsychologia 38, 848–863.

Burke, D.M., Light, L.L., 1981. Memory and aging: The role of retrieval processes. Psychol. Bull. 90, 513–546.

Burke, D.M., MacKay, D.G., Worthley, J.S., Wade, E., 1991. On the tip of the tongue: What causes word finding failures in young and older adults? J. Mem. Lang. 30, 542–579.

Burke, D., Worthley, J., Martin, J., 1988. I'll never forget what's-her-name: Aging and tip of the tongue experiences in everyday life. In: Morris, P.E., Sykes, R.N. (Eds.), Practical Aspects of Memory: Current Research and Issues, Vol. 2, Clinical and Educational Implications. Wiley and Sons, New York, pp. 113–118.

Cabeza, R., 2002. Hemispheric asymmetry reduction in older adults: The HAROLD model. Psychol. Aging 17, 85–100.

Cabeza, R., Anderson, N.D., Houle, S., Mangels, J.A., Nyberg, L., 2000. Age-related differences in neural activity during item and temporal-order memory retrieval: A positron emission tomography study. J. Cogn. Neurosci. 12, 197–206.

Cabeza, R., Rao, S.M., Wagner, A.D., Mayer, A.R., Schacter, D.L., 2001. Can medial temporal lobe regions distinguish true from false? An event-related functional MRI study of veridical and illusory recognition memory. Proc. Natl. Acad. Sci. USA 98, 4805–4810.

Cahill, L., Haier, R., Fallon, J., Alkire, M., Tang, C., Keator, D., Wu, J., McGaugh, J., 1996. Amygdala activity at encoding correlated with long-term free recall of emotional information. Proc. Natl. Acad. Sci. USA 93, 8016–8021.

Carlesimo, G.A., Sabbadini, M., Fadda, L., Caltagirone, C., 1997. Word-list forgetting in young and elderly subjects: Evidence for age-related decline in transferring information from transitory to permanent memory condition. Cortex 33, 155–166.

Carstensen, L.L., Isaacowitz, D.M., Charles, S.T., 1999. Taking time seriously: A theory of socioemotional selectivity. Am. Psychol. 54, 165–181.

Carstensen, L.L., Turk-Charles, S., 1994. The salience of emotion across the adult life course. Psychol. Aging 9, 259–264.

Chalfonte, B.L., Johnson, M.K., 1996. Feature memory and binding in young and older adults. Mem. Cognit. 24, 403–416.

Cherry, K.E., LeCompte, D.C., 1999. Age and individual differences influence prospective memory. Psychol. Aging 14, 60–76.

Cohen, G., 1990. Recognition and retrieval of proper names: Age differences in the fan effect. Eur. J. Cogn. Psychol. 2, 193–204.

Cohen, G., Faulkner, D., 1986. Memory for proper names: Age differences in retrieval. Br. J. Dev. Psychol. 4, 187–197.

Cohen, G., Faulkner, D., 1989. Age differences in source forgetting: Effects on reality monitoring and eyewitness testimony. Psychol. Aging 4, 10–17.

Cohen, J.D., Botvinik, M., Carter, C.S., 2000. Anterior cingulate and prefrontal cortex: Who's in control? Nat. Neurosci. 3, 421–423.

Cohen, N.J., Eichenbaum, H., 1993. Memory, Amnesia, and the Hippocampal System. MIT Press, Cambridge, MA.

Coleman, P.G., 1986. Ageing and Reminiscence Processes: Social and Clinical Implications. Wiley, New York.

Connelly, L.S., Hasher, L., 1993. Aging and the inhibition of spatial location. J. Exp. Psychol. Hum. Percept. Perform. 19, 1238–1250.

Conway, M.A., Pleydell-Pearce, C.W., 2000. The construction of autobiographical memories in the self-memory system. Psychol. Rev. 107, 261–288.

Corkin, S., 1984. Lasting consequences of bilateral medial lobectomy: Clinical course and experimental findings in HM. Semin. Neurol. 4, 249–259.

Coxon, P., Valentine, T., 1997. The effects of the age of eyewitnesses on the accuracy and suggestibility of their testimony. Appl. Cogn. Psychol. 11, 415–430.

Craik, F.I.M., 1977. Age differences in human memory. In: Birren, J.E., Schall, K. (Eds.), Handbook of the Psychology of Aging. Van Nostrand-Reinhold, New York, pp. 384–420.

Craik, F.I.M., Byrd, M., 1982. Aging and cognitive deficits. In: Craik, F.I.M., Trehub, S. (Eds.), Aging and Cognitive Processes. Plenum, New York, pp. 191–211.

Craik, F.I.M., Govoni, R., Naveh-Benjamin, M., Anderson, N.D., 1996. The effects of divided attention on encoding and retrieval processes in human memory. J. Exp. Psychol. Gen. 125, 159–180.

Craik, F.I.M., Lockhart, R.S., 1972. Levels of processing: A framework for memory research. J. Verbal Learn. Verbal Behav. 11, 671–684.

Craik, F.I.M., McDowd, J.M., 1987. Age differences in recall and recognition. J. Exp. Psychol. Learn. Mem. Cogn. 13, 474–479.

Craik, F.I.M., Morris, L.W., Morris, R.G., Loewen, E.R., 1990. Relations between source amnesia and frontal lobe functioning in older adults. Psychol. Aging 5, 148–151.

Craik, F.I.M., Naveh-Benjamin, M., Ishaik, G., Anderson, N.D., 2000. Divided attention during encoding and retrieval: Differential control effects? J. Exp. Psychol. Learn. Mem. Cogn. 26, 1744–1749.

Craik, F.I.M., Tulving, E., 1975. Depth of processing and the retention of words in episodic memory. J. Exp. Psychol. Gen. 104, 268–294.

Davis, H.P., Trussell, L.H., Klebe, K.J., 2001. A ten-year longitudinal examination of repetition priming, incidental recall, free recall, and recognition in young and elderly. Brain Cogn. 46, 99–104.

Dawes, R., 1988. Rational Choice in an Uncertain World. Harcourt, Brace, Javanovich, San Diego, CA.

Deese, J., 1959. On the prediction of occurrence of particular verbal intrusions immediate recall. J. Exp. Psychol. 58, 17–22.

Dodson, C.S., Schacter, D.L., 2002. Aging and strategic retrieval processes: Reducing false memories with a distinctiveness heuristic. Psychol. Aging 17, 405–415.

Dodson, P.O., Marsh, E.J., Balota, D.A., Roediger III, H.L., 2002. Interference from part-set cues in older and younger adults. Poster presented at the Cognitive Aging Conference, Atlanta, GA.

D'Ydewalle, G., Bouckaert, D., Brunfaut, E., 2001. Age-related differences and complexity of ongoing activities in time-and-event-based prospective memory. Am. J. Psychol. 114, 411–423.

Dywan, J., Jacoby, L.L., 1990. Effects of aging on source monitoring. Differences in susceptibility to false fame. Psychol. Aging 3, 379–387.

Dywan, J., Segalowitz, S., Arsenault, A., 2002. Electrophysiological response during source memory decisions in older and younger adults. Brain Cogn. 49, 322–340.

Dywan, J., Segalowitz, S. J., Webster, L., 1998. Source monitoring: ERP evidence for greater reactivity to nontarget information in older adults. Brain Cogn. 35, 390–430.

Einstein, G.O., Holland, L.J., McDaniel, M.A., Guynn, M.J., 1992. Age-related deficits in prospective memory: Examining the influence of task complexity. Psychol. Aging 7, 471–478.

Einstein, G.O., McDaniel, M.A., 1990. Normal aging and prospective memory. J. Exp. Psychol. Learn. Mem. Cogn. 16, 717–726.

Einstein, G.O., McDaniel, M.A., 1996. Retrieval processes in prospective memory: Theoretical approaches and some new empirical findings. In: Brandimonte, M., Einstein, G.O., McDaniel, M.A. (Eds.), Prospective Memory: Theory and Applications. Erlbaum, Hillsdale, NJ, pp. 115–142.

Einstein, G.O., McDaniel, M.A., Manzi, M., Cochran, B., Baker, M., 2000. Prospective memory and aging: Forgetting intentions over short delays. Psychol. Aging 15, 671–683.

Einstein, G.O., McDaniel, M.A., Richardson, S.L., Guynn, M., Cunfer, A.R., 1995. Aging and prospective memory: Examining the influences of self-initiated retrieval processes. J. Exp. Psychol. Learn. Mem. Cogn. 21, 996–1007.

Einstein, G.O., McDaniel, M.A., Stout, A., Morgan, Z., 2002. Aging and maintaining intentions over brief delays. Poster presented at the Cognitive Aging Conference, Atlanta, GA.

Einstein, G.O., Smith, R.E., McDaniel, M.A., Shaw, P., 1997. Aging and prospective memory: The influence of increase task demands at encoding and retrieval. Psychol. Aging 12, 479–488.

Ellis, J., 1996. Prospective memory or the realization of delayed intentions: A conceptual framework for research. In: Brandimonte, M., Einstein, G.O., McDaniel, M.A. (Eds.), Prospective Memory: Theory and Applications. Erlbaum, Hillsdale, NJ, pp. 1–22.

Ferguson, S.A., Hashtroudi, S., Johnson, M.K., 1992. Age differences in using source-relevant cues. Psychol. Aging 7, 443–452.

Follett, K.J., Hess, T.M., 2002. Aging, cognitive complexity, and the fundamental attribution error. J. Gerontol. Psychol. Sci. 57B, P312–P323.

Gerard, L.D., Zacks, R.T., Hasher, L., Radvansky, G.A., 1991. Age deficits in retrieval: The fan effect. J. Gerontol. Psychol. Sci. 46, P131–P146.

Giambra, L.M., Arenberg, D., 1993. Adult age differences in forgetting sentences. Psychol. Aging 8, 451–462.

Gilbert, D.T., Malone, P.S., 1995. The correspondence bias. Psychol. Bull. 117, 21–38.

Glisky, E., 1996. Prospective memory and frontal lobes. In: Brandimonte, M., Einstein, G.O., McDaniel, M.A. (Eds.), Prospective Memory: Theory and Applications. Erlbaum, Mahwah, NJ, pp. 249–266.

Glisky, E.L., Polster, M.R., Routhieaux, B.C., 1995. Double dissociation between item and source memory. Neuropsychology 9, 229–235.

Glisky, E.L., Rubin, S.S.R., Davidson, P.S.R., 2001. Source memory in older adults: An encoding or retrieval problem? J. Exp. Psychol. Learn. Mem. Cogn. 27, 1131–1146.

Grady, C.L., McIntosh, A.R., Horwitz, B., Maisog, J.M., Ungerleider, L.G., Mentis, M.J., 1995. Age-related reductions in human recognition memory due to impaired encoding. Science 269, 218–221.

Gross, J.J., Carstensen, L.L., Pasupathi, M., Tsai, J., Skorpen, C.G., Hsu, A.Y.C., 1997. Emotion and aging: Experience, expression, and control. Psychol. Aging 12, 590–599.

Hamann, S.B., Monarch, E.S., Goldstein, F.C., 2000. Memory enhancement for emotional stimuli is impaired in early Alzheimer's disease. Neuropsychology 14, 82–92.

Hartman, M., 1995. Aging and interference: Evidence from indirect memory tests. Psychol. Aging 10, 659–669.

Hartman, H., Dusek, J., 1994. Direct and indirect memory tests: What they reveal about age differences in interference. Aging Cogn. 1, 292–309.

Hartman, M., Hasher, L., 1991. Aging and suppression: Memory for previously relevant information. Psychol. Aging 6, 587–594.

Hasher, L., Quig, M.B., May, C.P., 1997. Inhibitory control over no longer relevant information: Adult age differences. Mem. Cognit. 25, 286–295.

Hasher, L., Zacks, R.T., 1988. Working memory, comprehension and aging: A review and a new view. Psychol. Learn. Motiv. 22, 193–225.

Hasher, L., Stoltzfus, E.R., Zacks, R.T., Rypma, B., 1991. Age and inhibition. J. Exp. Psychol. Learn. Mem. Cogn. 17, 163–169.

Hasher, L., Zacks, R.T., May, C.P., 1999. Inhibitory control, circadian arousal, and age. In: Gopher, D., Koriat, A. (Eds.), Attention and Performance XVII-cognitive Regulation of Performance: Interaction of Theory and Application. MIT Press, Cambridge, MA, pp. 653–675.

Hashtroudi, S., Johnson, M.K., Chrosniak, L.D., 1990. Aging and qualitative characteristics of memories for perceived and imagined complex events. Psychol. Aging 5, 119–126.

Heider, F., 1958. The Psychology of Interpersonal Relations. Wiley, New York.

Heine, M.K., Ober, B.A., Shenaut, G.K., 1999. Naturally occurring and experimentally induced tip-of-the-tongue experiences in three adult age groups. Psychol. Aging 3, 445–457.

Henkel, L.A., Johnson, M.K., De Leonardis, D.M., 1998. Aging and source monitoring: Cognitive processes and neuropsychological correlates. J. Exp. Psychol. Gen. 127, 1–18.

Herman, J.L., 1992. Trauma and Recovery. Basic Books, New York.
Hess, T.M., 1999. Cognitive and knowledge-based influences on social representations. In: Hess, T., Blanchard-Fields, F. (Eds.), Social Cognition and Aging. Academic Press, San Diego, CA, pp. 237–263.
Hess, T.M., Follett, K.J., 1994. Adult age differences in the use of schematic and episodic information in making social judgments. Aging Cogn. 1, 54–66.
Hess, T.M., McGee, K.A., Woodburn, S.M., Bolstad, C.A., 1998. Age-related priming effects in social judgments. Psychol. Aging 13, 127–137.
Hess, T.M., Slaughter, S.J., 1990. Schematic knowledge influences on memory for scene information in young and older adults. Dev. Psychol. 26, 855–865.
Holland, C.A., Rabbitt, P.M., 1992. Effects of age-related reductions in processing resources on text recall. J. Gerontol. 47, 129–137.
Holley, P.E., McEvoy, C.L., 1996. Aging and inhibition of unconsciously processed information: No apparent deficit. Appl. Cogn. Psychol. 10, 241–256.
Howes, J.L., Katz, A.N., 1992. Remote memory: Recalling autobiographical and public events from across the lifespan. Can. J. Psychol. 46, 92–116.
Hultsch, D.F., Craig, E.R., 1976. Adult age differences in inhibition of recall as a function of retrieval cues. Dev. Psychol. 12, 83–84.
Hummert, M.L., 1999. A social cognitive perspective on age stereotypes. In: Hess, T., Blanchard-Fields, F. (Eds.), Social Cognition and Aging. Academic Press, San Diego, CA, pp. 175–196.
Hummert, M.L., Garstka, T.A., O'Brien, L.T., Greenwald, A.G., Mellott, D.S., 2002. Using the implicit association test to measure age differences in implicit social cognitions. Psychol. Aging 17, 482–495.
Hummert, M.L., Garstka, T.A., Shaner, J.L., Strahm, S., 1994. Stereotypes of the elderly held by young, middle-aged and elderly adults. J. Gerontol. Psychol. Sci. 49, P240–P249.
Huppert, F.A., Kopelman, M.D., 1989. Rates of forgetting in normal ageing: A comparison with dementia. Neuropsychologia 27, 849–860.
Hyer, L., 1999. The effects of trauma: Dynamics and treatment of PTSD in the elderly. In: Duffy, M. (Ed.), Handbook of Counseling and Psychotherapy with Older Adults. Wiley, New York, pp. 539–560.
Hyman, I.E., Billings, F.J., 1998. Individual differences and the creation of false childhood memories. J. Mem. Lang. 35, 101–117.
Isaacowitz, D.M., Charles, S.T., Carstensen, L.L., 2000. Emotion and cognition. In: Craik, F.I.M., Salthouse, T.A. (Eds.), The Handbook of Aging and Cognition. Erlbaum Associates, Mahwah, NJ, pp. 593–631.
Israel, L., Schacter, D.L., 1997. Pictorial encoding reduces false recognition of semantic associates. Psychon. Bull. Rev. 4, 577–581.
Jacoby, L.L., 1996. Dissociating automatic and consciously controlled effects of study/test compatibility. J. Mem. Lang. 35, 32–52.
Jacoby, L.L., 1999a. Ironic effects of repetition: Measuring age-related differences in memory. J. Exp. Psychol. Learn. Mem. Cogn. 25, 3–22.
Jacoby, L.L., 1999b. Deceiving the elderly: Effects of accessibility bias in cued-recall performance. Cogn. Neuropsychol. 16, 417–436.
Jacoby, L.L., Dallas, M., 1981. On the relationship between autobiographical memory and perceptual learning. J. Exp. Psychol. Gen. 110, 306–340.
Jacoby, L.L., Jennings, J.M., Hay, J., 1996. Dissociating automatic and consciously controlled processes: Implications for diagnosis and rehabilitation of memory deficits. In: Herrmann, D.J., McEvoy, C., Hertzog, C., Hertel, P., Johnson, M.K. (Eds.), Basic and Applied Memory Research: Theory in Context, Vol. 1. Erlbaum, Hillsdale, NJ, pp. 161–193.
Jacoby, L.L., Kelley, C.M., Brown, J., Jasechko, J., 1989a. Becoming famous overnight: Limits on the ability to avoid unconscious influences of the past. J. Pers. Soc. Psychol. 56, 326–338.
Jacoby, L.L., Kelley, C.M., Dywan, J., 1989b. Memory attributions. In: Roediger III, H.L., Craik, F.I.M. (Eds.), Varieties of Memory and Consciousness: Essays in Honor of Endel Tulving. Erlbaum, Hillsdale, NJ, pp. 321–422.
James, L.E., Burke, D.M., 2000. Phonological priming effects on word retrieval and tip-of-the-tongue experiences in young and older adults. J. Exp. Psychol. Learn. Mem. Cogn. 26, 1378–1391.

Jennings, J.M., Jacoby, L.L., 1993. Automatic versus intentional uses of memory: Aging, attention and control. Psychol. Aging 8, 283–293.

Johnson, M.K., De Leonardis, D.M., Hashtroudi, S., Ferguson, S.A., 1995. Aging and single versus multiple cues in source monitoring. Psychol. Aging 10, 507–517.

Johnson, M.K., Raye, C.L., 1981. Reality monitoring. Psychol. Rev. 88, 67–85.

Johnson, M.K., Chalfonte, B.L., 1994. Binding complex memories: The role of reactivation and the hippocampus. In: Schacter, D.L., Tulving, E. (Eds.), Memory Systems 1994. MIT Press, Cambridge, MA, pp. 311–350.

Johnson, M.K., Hashtroudi, S., Lindsay, D.S., 1993. Source monitoring. Psychol. Bull. 114, 3–28.

Jones, G.V., 1989. Back to Woodworth: Role of interlopers in the tip-of-the-tongue phenomenon. Mem. Cognit. 17, 69–76.

Jones, G.V., Langford, S., 1987. Phonological blocking and the tip-of-the-tongue state. Cognition 26, 115–122.

Kapur, S., Craik, F.I.M., Tulving, E., Wilson, A.A., Houle, S., Brown, G.M., 1994. Neuroanatomical correlates of encoding in episodic memory: Levels of processing effect. Proc. Natl. Acad. Sci. USA 91, 2008–2011.

Karpel, M.E., Hoyer, W.J., Toglia, M.P., 2001. Accuracy and qualities of real and suggested memories: Nonspecific age differences. J. Gerontol. Psychol. Sci. 56B, P103–P110.

Kausler, D.H., Puckett, J.M., 1980. Adult age differences in recognition memory for a nonsemantic attribute. Exp. Aging Res. 6, 349–355.

Kausler, D.H., Puckett, J.M., 1981a. Adult age differences in memory for modality attributes. Exp. Aging Res. 7, 117–125.

Kausler, D.H., Puckett, J.M., 1981b. Adult age differences in memory for sex of voice. J. Gerontol. 36, 44–50.

Kazui, H., Mori, E., Hashimoto, M., Hirono, N., Inamura, T., Tanimukai, S., Hanihara, T., Cahill, L., 2000. Impact of emotion on memory: Controlled study of the influence of emotionally charged material on declarative memory in Alzheimer's disease. Br. J. Psychiatry 177, 343–347.

Kensinger, E.A., Brierley, B., Medford, N., Growdon, J.H., Corkin, S., 2002. Effects of normal aging and Alzheimer's disease on emotional memory. Emotion 2, 118–134.

Kensinger, E.A., Schacter, D.L., 1999. When true memories suppress false memories: Effects of ageing. Cogn. Neuropsychol. 16, 399–415.

Knight, B.G., Gatz, M., Heller, K., Bengtson, V.L., 2000. Age and emotional response to the Northridge earthquake: A longitudinal analysis. Psychol. Aging 15, 627–634.

Kosslyn, S.M., Thompson, W.L., Kim, I.J., Rauch, S.L., Alpert, N.M., 1996. Individual differences in cerebral blood flow in area 17 predict the time to evaluate visualized letters. J. Cogn. Neurosci. 8, 78–82.

Krystal, J.H., Southwick, S.M., Charney, D.S., 1995. Post traumatic stress disorder: Psychobiological mechanisms of traumatic remembrance. In: Schacter, D.L. (Ed.), Memory Distortion: How Minds, Brains, and Societies Reconstruct the Past. Harvard University Press, Cambridge, MA, pp. 150–172.

Koutstaal, W., Schacter, D.L., 1997a. Gist-based false recognition of pictures in older and younger adults. J. Mem. Lang. 37, 555–583.

Koutstaal, W., Schacter, D.L., 1997b. Intentional forgetting and voluntary thought suppression: Two potential methods for coping with childhood trauma. In: Dickstein, L.J., Riba, M.B., Oldham, J.M. (Eds.), Review of Psychiatry, Vol. 16. American Psychiatric Press, Washington, DC, pp. 79–121.

Koutstaal, W., Schacter, D.L., Galluccio, L., Stofer, K.A., 1999a. Reducing gist-based false recognition in older adults: Encoding and retrieval manipulations. Psychol. Aging 14, 220–237.

Koutstaal, W., Schacter, D.L., Johnson, M.K., Galluccio, L., 1999b. Facilitation and impairment of event memory produced by photograph review. Mem. Cognit. 27, 478–493.

LaBar, K.S., Gatenby, J.C., Gore, J.C., LeDoux, J.E., Phelps, E.A., 1998. Human amygdala activation during conditioned fear acquisition and extinction: A mixed-trial fMRI study. Neuron 20, 937–945.

Labouvie-Vief, G., 1997. Cognitive-emotional integration in adulthood. In: Schaie, K.W., Lawton, M.P. (Eds.), Annual Review of Gerontology and Geriatrics: Focus on Emotion and Adult Development, Vol. 17. Springer, New York, pp. 206–237.

Levine, L.J., 1997. Reconstructing memory for emotions. J. Exp. Psychol. Gen. 126, 165–177.

Light, L.L., 1996. Memory and aging. In: Bjork, E.L., Bjork, R.A. (Eds.), Memory. Academic Press, San Diego, CA, pp. 443–490.

Lindsay, D.S., 1990. Misleading suggestions can impair eyewitnesses' ability to remember event details. J. Exp. Psychol. Learn. Mem. Cogn. 16, 1077–1083.

Lindsay, D.S., Johnson, M.K., 1989. The eyewitness suggestibility effect and memory for source. Mem. Cognit. 17, 349–358.

Loftus, E.F., Feldman, J., Dashiell, R., 1995. The reality of illusory memories. In: Schacter, D.L. (Ed.), Memory Distortion: How Minds, Brains, and Societies Reconstruct the Past. Harvard University Press, Cambridge, MA, pp. 47–68.

Loftus, E.F., Levidow, B., Duensing, S., 1992. Who remembers best: Individual differences in memory for events that occurred at a science museum. Appl. Cogn. Psychol. 6, 93–107.

Loftus, E.F., Miller, D.G., Burns, H.J., 1978. Semantic integration of verbal information into a visual memory. J. Exp. Psychol. Hum. Learn. Mem. 4, 19–31.

Logan, J.M., Balota, D.A., 2000, April. Blocking word retrieval in younger and older adults. Poster presented at the Cognitive Aging Conference, Atlanta, GA.

Logan, J.M., Sanders, A.L., Snyder, A.Z., Morris, J.C., Buckner, R.L., 2002. Under-recruitment and non-selective recruitment: Dissociable neural mechanisms associated with aging. Neuron 33, 827–840.

Lovelace, E.A., Twohig, P.T., 1990. Healthy older adults' perceptions of their memory functioning and use of mnemonics. Bull. Psychon. Soc. 28, 115–118.

Lyubormirsky, S., Caldwell, N.D., Nolen-Hoeksema, S., 1998. Effects of ruminative and distracting responses to depressed mood on retrieval of autobiographical memories. J. Pers. Soc. Psychol. 75, 166–177.

MacDonald, A.W., Cohen, J.D., Stenger, V.A., Carter, C.S., 2000. Dissociating the role of the dorsolateral prefrontal and anterior cingulate cortex in cognitive control. Science 288, 1835–1838.

Mandler, G., 1980. Recognizing: The judgment of previous occurrence. Psychol. Rev. 87, 252–271.

Mäntylä, T., 1993. Knowing but not remembering: Adult age differences in recollective experience. Mem. Cognit. 21, 379–388.

Mäntylä, T., 1996. Activating actions and interrupting intentions: Mechanisms of retrieval sensitization in prospective memory. In: Brandimonte, M., Einstein, G.O., McDaniel, M.A. (Eds.), Prospective Memory: Theory and Applications. Erlbaum, Hillsdale, NJ, pp. 93–113.

Marche, T.A., Jordan, J.J., Owre, K.P., 2000. Younger adults can be more suggestible than older adults: The influences of learning differences on misinformation reporting. Can. J. Aging 21, 85–93.

Marcus, G.B., 1986. Stability and change in political attitudes: Observe, recall, and "explain". Pol. Behav. 8, 21–44.

Maril, A., Wagner, A.D., Schacter, D.L., 2001. On the tip of the tongue: An event-related fMRI study of semantic retrieval failure and cognitive conflict. Neuron 31, 653–660.

Marsh, R.L., Landau, J.D., 1995. Item availability in cryptomnesia: Assessing its role in two paradigms of unconscious plagiarism. J. Exp. Psychol. Learn. Mem. Cogn. 21, 1568–1582.

Mather, M., Johnson, M.K., 2000. Choice-supportive source monitoring: Do our decisions seem better to us as we age? Psychol. Aging 15, 596–606.

Mather, M., Johnson, M.K., De Leonardis, D.M. 1999. Stereotype reliance in source monitoring: Age differences and neuropsychological test correlates. Cognit. Neuropsychol. 16, 437–458.

Mather, M., Shafir, E., Johnson, M.K., 2000. Misrememberance of options past: Source monitoring and choice. Psychol. Sci. 11, 132–138.

May, C.P., Hasher, L., 1998. Synchrony effects in inhibitory control over thought and action. J. Exp. Psychol. Hum. Percept. Perform. 24, 363–379.

May, C.P., Zacks, R.T., Hasher, L., Multhaup, K.S., 1999. Inhibition in the processing of garden-path sentences. Psychol. Aging 14, 304–313.

Maylor, E.A., 1990. Recognizing and naming faces: Aging, memory retrieval, and the tip of the tongue state. J. Gerontol. Psychol. Sci. 45, P215–226.

Maylor, E.A., 1996. Age-related impairment in an event-based prospective memory task. Psychol. Aging 11, 74–78.

Maylor, E.A., Henson, R.N.A., 2000. Aging and the Ranschburg effect: No evidence of reduced response suppression in old age. Psychol. Aging 15, 657–670.

McClelland, J.L., McNaughton, B.L., O'Reilly, R.C., 1995. Why there are complementary learning systems in the hippocampus and neocortex: Insights from the successes and failures of connectionist models of learning and memory. Psychol. Rev. 102, 419–457.

McDaniel, M.A., 1995. Prospective memory: Progress and processes. In: Medin, D.L. (Ed.), The Psychology of Learning and Motivation, Vol. 33. Academic Press, San Diego, CA, pp. 191–221.

McDaniel, M.A., Robinson-Riegler, B., Einstein, G.O., 1998. Prospective remembering: Perceptually driven or conceptually driven processes? Mem. Cognit. 26, 121–134.

McDowd, J.M., Oseas-Kreger, D.M., 1991. Aging, inhibitory processes, and negative priming. J. Gerontol. Psychol. Sci. 46, P340–345.

McFarland, C., Ross, M., 1987. The relation between current impressions and memories of self and dating partners. Personal. Soc. Psychol. Bull. 13, 228–238.

McNally, R.J., Metzger, L.J., Lasko, N.B., Clancy, S.A., Pitman R.K., 1998. Directed forgetting of trauma cues in adult survivors of childhood sexual abuse with and without posttraumatic stress disorder. J. Abnormal Psychol. 107, 596–601.

Milner, B., Corkin, S., Teuber, H.L., 1968. Further analysis of the hippocampal amnesic syndrome: 14-year follow-up of HM. Neuropsychologia 6, 215–234.

Moscovitch, M., 1994. Memory and working with memory: Evaluation of a component process model and comparisons with other models. In: Schacter, D.L., Tulving, E. (Eds.), Memory Systems 1994. MIT Press, Cambridge, MA, pp. 269–310.

Moscovitch, M., Winocur, G., 1992. The neuropsychology of memory and aging. In: Craik, F.I.M., Salthouse, T.A. (Eds.), The Handbook of Aging and Cognition. Erlbaum, Hillsdale, NJ, pp. 315–372.

Moulin, C.J.A., 2000, April. When it is good to forget: Evidence for intact retrieval inhibition in older adults. Poster presented at the Cognitive Aging Conference, Atlanta, GA.

Moulin, C.J.A., Perfect, T.J., Conway, M.A., North, A.S., Jones, R.W., James, N., 2002. Retrieval-induced forgetting in Alzheimer's disease. Neuropsychologia 40, 862–867.

Multhaup, K.S., 1995. Aging, source, and decision criteria: When false fame errors do and do not occur. Psychol. Aging 10, 492–497.

Multhaup, K.S., De Leonardis, D.M., Johnson, M.K., 1999. Source memory and eyewitness suggestibility in older adults. J. Gen. Psychol. 126, 74–84.

Naveh-Benjamin, M., Craik, F.I.M., Guez, J., Dori, H., 1998. Effects of divided attention on encoding and retrieval processes in human memory: Further support for an asymmetry. J. Exp. Psychol. Learn. Mem. Cogn. 24, 1091–1104.

Naveh-Benjamin, M., Moscovitch, M., Roediger III, H.L., (Eds.), 2001. Perspectives on Human Memory and Aging: Essays in Honor of Fergus Craik. Psychology Press, New York.

Nielsen, K.A., Langenecker, S.A., Garavan, H., 2002. Differences in the functional neuroanatomy of inhibitory control across the adult life span. Psychol. Aging 17, 56–71.

Nolen-Hoeksema, S., 1991. Responses to depression and their effects on the duration of depressive episodes. J. Abnorm. Psychol. 100, 569–582.

Norman, K.A., Schacter, D.L., 1997. False recognition in younger and older adults: Exploring the characteristics of illusory memories. Mem. Cognit. 25, 838–848.

Nosek, B.A., Banaji, M.R., Greewald, A.G., 2002. Harvesting implicit group attitudes and beliefs from a demonstration web site. Group Dynamics: Theory, Research, and Practice 6, 101–115.

Nyberg, L., McIntosh, A.R., Cabeza, R., Nilsson, L.G., Houle, S., Habib, R., Tulving, E., 1996. Network analysis of positron emission tomography regional cerebral blood flow data: Ensemble inhibition during episodic memory retrieval. J. Neurosci. 16, 3753–3759.

Ochsner, K.N., Schacter, D.L., 2000. Constructing the emotional past: A social-cognitive-neuroscience approach to emotion and memory. In: Borod, J. (Ed.), The Neuropsychology of Emotion. Oxford University Press, New York, pp. 163–193.

Okuda, J., Fujii, T., Yamadori, A., Kawashima, R., Tsukiura, T., Fukatsu, R., Suzuki, K., Ito, M., Fukuda, H., 1998. Participation of the prefrontal cortices in prospective memory: Evidence from a PET study in humans. Neurosci. Lett. 253, 127–130.

O'Reilly, R.S.C., McClelland, J.L., 1994. Hippocampal conjunctive encoding, storage, and recall: Avoiding a trade-off. Hippocampus 4, 661–682.

Otten, L.J., Henson, R.N.A., Rugg, M.D., 2001. Depth of processing effects on neural correlates of memory encoding: Relationship between findings from across- and within-task comparisons. Brain 124, 399–412.

Park, D.C., Hertzog, C., Kidder, D., Morrell, R., Mayhorn, C., 1997. The effect of age on event-based and time-based prospective memory. Psychol. Aging 12, 314–327.

Park, D.C., Puglisi, J.T., 1985. Older adults' memory for the color of pictures and words. J. Gerontol. 40, 198–204.

Parkin, A.J., Bindschaedler, C., Harsent, L., Metzler, C., 1996. Pathological false alarm rates following damage to the left frontal cortex. Brain Cogn. 32, 14–27.

Parkin, A.J., Walter, B.M., 1992. Recollective experience, normal aging, and frontal dysfunction. Psychol. Aging 7, 290–298.

Petersen, R.C., Smith, G., Kokmen, E., Ivnik, R.J., Tangalos, E.G., 1992. Memory function in normal aging. Neurology 42, 396–401.

Prull, M.W., Gabrieli, J.E.E., Bunge, S.A., 2000. Age-related changes in memory: A cognitive neuroscience perspective. In: Craik, F.I.M., Salthouse, T.A. (Eds.), The Handbook of Aging and Cognition. Erlbaum, Mahwah, NJ, pp. 91–153.

Rabinowitz, J.C., Ackerman, B.P., 1982. General encoding of episodic events by elderly adults. In: Craik, F.I.M., Trehub, S. (Eds.), Aging and Cognitive Processes. Plenum, New York, pp. 145–154.

Radvansky, G.A., Curiel, J.M., 1998. Narrative comprehension and aging: The fate of completed goal information. Psychol. Aging 13, 69–79.

Rapcsak, S.Z., Reminger, S.L., Glisky, E.L., Kaszniak, A.W., Comer, J.F., 1999. Neuropsychological mechanisms of false facial recognition following frontal lobe damage. Cogn. Neuropsychol. 16, 267–292.

Raz, N., 2000. Aging of the brain and its impact on cognitive performance: Integration of structural findings. In: Craik, F.I.M., Salthouse, T.A. (Eds.), Handbook of Aging and Cognition. Erlbaum, Mahwah, NJ, pp. 1–90.

Reason, J.T., Lucas, D., 1984. Using cognitive diaries to investigate naturally occurring memory blocks. In: Harris, J.E., Morris, P.E. (Eds.), Everyday Memory, Actions, and Absentmindedness. Academic Press, Orlando, FL, pp. 53–69.

Roediger III, H.L., 1974. Inhibiting effects of recall. Mem. Cognit. 2, 261–269.

Roediger III, H.L., McDermott, K.B., 1995. Creating false memories: Remembering words not presented in lists. J. Exp. Psychol. Learn. Mem. Cogn. 21, 803–814.

Roediger, III. H.L., Neely, J.H., 1982. Retrieval blocks in episodic and semantic memory. Can. J. Psychol. 36, 213–242.

Ross, M., 1989. Relation of implicit theories to the construction of personal histories. Psychol. Rev. 96, 341–357.

Ross, L., Nisbett, R.E., 1991. The Person and the Situation: Perspectives of Social Psychology. McGraw-Hill, New York.

Ross, M., Wilson, A.E., 2000. Constructing and appraising past selves. In: Schacter, D., Scarry, E. (Eds.), Memory, Brain, and Belief. Harvard University Press, Cambridge, MA, pp. 231–258.

Rubin, D.C., Schulkind, M.D., 1997. The distribution of autobiographical memories across the lifespan. Mem. Cognit. 25, 859–866.

Rubin, D.C., Wetzler, S.E., Nebes, R.D., 1986. Autobiographical memory across the lifespan. In: Rubin, D.C. (Ed.), Autobiographical Memory. Cambridge University Press, Cambridge, UK, pp. 202–221.

Rybarczyk, B.D., Hart, R.P., Harkins, S.W., 1987. Age and forgetting rate with pictorial stimuli. Psychol. Aging 2, 404–406.

Sauzeon, H., N'kaoua, B., Lespinet, V., Guillem, F., Claverie, B., 2000. Age effect in recall performance according to the levels of processing, elaboration, and retrieval cues. Exp. Aging Res. 26, 57–73.

Schacter, D.L., 1987. Implicit memory: History and current status. J. Exp. Psychol. Learn. Mem. Cogn. 13, 501–518.

Schacter, D.L., 1996. Searching for Memory: The Brain, the Mind, and the Past. Basic Books, New York.

Schacter, D.L., 1999. The seven sins of memory: Insights from psychology and cognitive neuroscience. Am. Psychol. 54, 182–203.

Schacter, D.L., 2000. The seven sins of memory: Perspectives from functional neuroimaging. In: Tulving, E. (Ed.), Memory, Consciousness, and the Brain: The Tallinn Conference. Psychology Press, Philadelphia, PA, pp. 119–137.

Schacter, D.L., 2001. The Seven Sins of Memory: How the Mind Forgets and Remembers. Houghton Mifflin Co., New York.

Schacter, D.L., Buckner, R.L., 1998. Priming and the brian. Neuron 20, 185–195.

Schacter, D.L., Buckner, R.L., Koutstaal, W., Dale, A.M., Rosen, B.R., 1997a. Late onset of anterior prefrontal activity during retrieval of veridical and illusory memories: A single trial fMRI study. NeuroImage 6, 259–269.

Schacter, D.L., Curran, T., Gallucio, L., Milberg, W., Bates, J., 1996a. False recognition and the right frontal lobe: A case study. Neuropsychologia 34, 793–808.

Schacter, D.L., Israel, L., Racine, C.A., 1999. Suppressing false recognition in younger and older adults: The distinctiveness heuristic. J. Mem. Lang. 40, 1–24.

Schacter, D.L., Kaszniak, A.W., Kihlstrom, J.F., Valdiserri, M., 1991. The relation between source memory and aging. Psychol. Aging 6, 559–568.

Schacter, D.L., Koutstaal, W., Johnson, M.K., Gross, M.S., Angell, K.A., 1997b. False recollection induced by photographs: A comparison of older and younger adults. Psychol. Aging 12, 203–215.

Schacter, D.L., Koutstaal, W., Norman, K.A., 1997c. False memories and aging. Trends Cogn. Sci. 1, 229–236.

Schacter, D.L., Norman, K.A., Koutstaal, W., 1998a. The cognitive neuroscience of constructive memory. Annu. Rev. Psychol. 49, 289–318.

Schacter, D.L., Reiman, E., Curran, T., Yun, L.S., Bandy, D., McDermott, K.B., Roediger III, H.L., 1996b. Neuroanatomical correlates of veridical and illusory recognition memory: Evidence from positron emission tomography. Neuron 17, 267–274.

Schacter, D.L., Savage, C.R., Alpert, N.M., Rauch, S.L., Albert, M.S., 1996c. The role of hippocampus and frontal cortex in age-related memory changes: A PET study. NeuroReport 7, 1165–1169.

Schacter, D.L., Verfaille, M., Anes, M.D., Racine, C., 1998b. When true recognition suppresses false recognition: Evidence from amnesic patients. J. Cogn. Neurosci. 10, 668–679.

Scharfe, E., Bartholomew, K., 1998. Do you remember? Recollections of adult attachment patterns. Personal Relationships 5, 219–234.

Scoville, W.B., Milner, B., 1957. Loss of recent memory after bilateral hippocampal lesions. J. Neurol. Neurosurg. Psychiatry 20, 11–21.

Shallice, T., Burgess, P.W., 1991. Deficits in strategy application following frontal lobe damage in man. Brain 114, 727–741.

Shimamura, A.P., Janowsky, J.S., Squire, L.R., 1991. What is the role of frontal lobe damage in memory disorders? In: Levin, H.S., Eisenberg, H.M., Benton, A.L. (Eds.), Frontal Lobe Functioning and Dysfunction. Oxford University Press, Oxford, England, pp. 173–195.

Simon, E., 1979. Depth and elaboration of processing in relation to age. J. Exp. Psychol. Hum. Learn. Mem. 5, 115–124.

Simons, J.S., Dodson, C.S., Bell, D., Schacter, D.L., 2003. Specific and partial source memory in aging: A role for attentional resources? Manuscript submitted for publication.

Slamecka, N.J., 1968. An examination of trace storage in free recall. J. Exp. Psychol. 76, 504–513.

Sloman, S.A., Bower, G.H., Rohrer, D., 1991. Congruency effects in part-list cueing inhibition. J. Exp. Psychol. Learn. Mem. Cogn. 17, 974–982.

Smith, C.D., Malcein, M., Meurer, K., Schmitt, F.A., Markesberv, W.R., Pettigrew, L.C., 1999. MRI temporal lobe volume measures and neuropsychologic function in Alzheimer's disease. J. Neuroimaging 9, 2–9.

Smith, S.M., Tindell, D.R., 1997. Memory blocks in word fragment completion caused by involuntary retrieval of orthographically related primes. J. Exp. Psychol. Learn. Mem. Cogn. 23, 355–370.

Spencer, W.D., Raz, N., 1995. Differential effects of aging on memory for content and context: A meta-analysis. Psychol. Aging 10, 527–539.

Sperling, R.A., Bates, J.C., Cocchiarella, A.J., Schacter, D.L., Rosen, B., Albert, M.S., 2001. Encoding novel face-name associations: A functional MRI study. Hum. Brain Mapp. 14, 129–139.

Squire, L.R., 1982. The neuropsychology of human memory. Annu. Rev. Neurosci. 5, 241–273.

Squire, L.R., 1989. On the course of forgetting in very long-term memory. J. Exp. Psychol. Learn. Mem. Cogn. 15, 241–245.

Squire, L.R., 1992. Memory and the hippocampus: A synthesis from findings with rats, monkeys, and humans. Psychol. Rev. 99, 195–231.

Squire, L.R., Knowlton, B.J., 1995. Memory, hippocampus, and brain systems. In: Gazzaniga, M.S. (Ed.), The Cognitive Neurosciences. MIT Press, Cambridge, MA, pp. 825–837.

Stoltzfus, E.R., Hasher, L., Zacks, R.T., Ulivi, M.S., Goldstein, D., 1993. Investigations of inhibition and interference in younger and older adults. J. Gerontol. Psychol. Sci. 48, P179–P188.

Tipper, S.P., 1991. Less attentional selectivity as a result of declining inhibition in older adults. Bull. Psychon. Soc. 29, 45–47.

Tulving, E., 1985. Memory and consciousness. Can. Psychol. 26, 1–12.

Tulving, E., Schacter, D.L., 1990. Priming and human memory systems. Science 247, 301–306.

Tun, P.A., Wingfield, A., Rosen, M.J., Blanchard, L., 1998. Response latencies for false memories: Gist-based processes in normal aging. Psychol. Aging 13, 230–241.

Underwood, B.J., 1965. False recognition produced by implicit verbal responses. J. Exp. Psychol. 70, 122–129.

von Hippel, W., Silver, L.A., Lynch, M.E., 2000. Stereotyping against your will: The role of inhibitory ability in stereotyping and prejudice among the elderly. Pers. Soc. Psychol. Bull. 26, 523–532.

Wagner, A.D., Schacter, D.L., Rotte, M., Koutstaal, W., Maril, A., Dale, A.M., Rosen, B.R., Buckner, R.L., 1998. Building memories: Remembering and forgetting of verbal experiences as predicted by brain activity. Science 281, 1188–1191.

Wegner, D.M., Erber, R., 1992. The hyperaccessibility of suppressed thoughts. J. Personal. Soc. Psychol. 63, 903–912.

Weintraub, D., Ruskin, P.E., 1999. Posttraumatic stress disorder in the elderly: A review. Harv. Rev. Psychiatry 7, 144–152.

Wes, R., Covell, E., 2001. Effects of aging on event-related neural activity related to prospective memory. Neuroreport 12, 2855–2858.

West, R.L., 1996. An application of prefrontal cortex function theory to cognitive aging. Psychol. Bull. 120, 272–292.

Wiggs, C.L., Martin, A., 1998. Properties and mechanisms of perceptual priming. Cur. Opinion Neurobiol. 8, 227–233.

Yarmey, A.D., 1996. The elderly witness. In: Sporer, S.L., Malpass, R.L., Koehnken, G. (Eds.), Psychological Issues in Eyewitness Identification. Lawrence Erlbaum, Mahwah, NJ, pp. 259–278.

Youngjohn, J.R., Crook, T.H., 1993. Learning, forgetting and retrieval of everyday material across the adult life span. J. Clin. Exp. Neuropsychol. 15, 447–460.

Zacks, R.T., Hasher, L., Li, K.Z.H., 2000. Human memory. In: Craik, F.I.M., Salthouse, T.A. (Eds.), Handbook of Aging and Cognition. Lawrence Erlbaum, Mahwah, NJ, pp. 293–357.

Zacks, R.T., Radvansky, G.A., Hasher, L., 1996. Studies of directed forgetting in older adults. J. Exp. Psychol. Learn. Mem. Cogn. 22, 143–156.

Zaragoza, M.S., Lane, S.M., 1994. Source misattributions and the suggestibility of eyewitness memory. J. Exp. Psychol. Learn. Mem. Cogn. 20, 934–945.

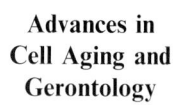

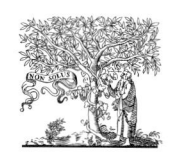

Age-related changes in visual attention

David J. Madden* and Wythe L. Whiting

Duke University Medical Center, Box 2980, Durham, NC 27710, USA

Contents

1. Introduction — *41*
2. Sensory-level processing — *44*
3. General vs. specific effects of attention — *47*
4. Spatial attention, selection, and inhibition — *52*
    - 4.1. Selection by display dimensions — *53*
    - 4.2. Vigilance — *54*
    - 4.3. Movement and distribution of attention — *54*
    - 4.4. Time course effects — *56*
    - 4.5. Attentional inhibition — *57*
5. Practice and the development of automaticity — *60*
6. Varieties of attentional control — *62*
7. Divided attention — *66*
    - 7.1. Different design methodologies — *67*
    - 7.2. Divided attention and memory — *69*
    - 7.3. Time sharing effects — *70*
    - 7.4. Task switching — *71*
8. Cognitive neuroscience of aging and attention — *72*
9. Conclusion — *78*
    - Acknowledgments — *79*
    - References — *80*

1. Introduction

The concept of attention refers to a set of related processes that have important consequences for cognitive functioning. Perhaps the most widely recognized of these processes is selective attention. During many everyday perceptual tasks, such as searching for a familiar face in a crowd, or trying to understand several people

*Corresponding author. Tel.: (919) 660-7537; fax: (919) 684-8569.
E-mail address: djm@geri.duke.edu (D.J. Madden).

talking simultaneously, there is more sensory information available than can be used effectively. In this context, to attend means to select some perceptual events rather than others. Exactly how this selection occurs has been the topic of active research and debate (Duncan, 1993; Pashler, 1998). Proposed mechanisms for selective attention comprise both the enhancement of a sensory signal (Carrasco et al., 2000), the exclusion or inhibition of irrelevant information (Miliken and Tipper, 1998; Dosher and Lu, 2000), and reduction of uncertainty at the decision level (Eckstein et al., 2000). Attention has also been interpreted as involving an intensive dimension, relating to a sense of effort. From this latter perspective, attending to something reflects the allocation of a limited capacity for information processing internal to the observer (Kahneman, 1973; Lavie and Tsal, 1994). A concept related closely to both selection and effort is orienting (Posner, 1980). Attending in this sense refers to the development of a preparation or set for the occurrence of particular events. When preparation is maintained over an extended period of time, attentional effects are interpreted in terms of vigilance (Parasuraman, 1984).

Although researchers design tasks with the purpose of isolating different forms of attentional processing, attention cannot be separated entirely from other cognitive activities such as memory, learning, and problem solving. In working memory tasks, for example, which involve the simultaneous storage and active manipulation of information, attention is an essential component (Baddeley, 1993). In recall and recognition tests of episodic (context-dependent) memory, the success with which an event is remembered depends on the allocation of attention during initial encoding (Craik et al., 2000). Thus, age-related changes in attention will influence older adults' ability to perform a variety of cognitive tasks.

Attention has been a long-standing focus of adult developmental research, leading to a diverse and extensive literature (Hartley, 1992; Madden and Plude, 1993; Groth and Allen, 2000; McDowd and Shaw, 2000). In this chapter, we will be concerned primarily with investigations of attention in the visual modality. Research on age-related changes in auditory attention is reviewed by Kline and Scialfa (1996) and Fozard and Gordon-Salant (2001). We will also be discussing the findings and theories of age-related change in attention in the context of cognitive neuroscience. That is, we will be giving some emphasis to the brain mechanisms responsible for attentional functioning, and to the age-related changes in these neural systems leading to behavioral changes.

Many of the behavioral investigations of age differences in visual attention have used some form of search task, in which participants make a decision regarding the presence of a pre-specified target item in a visual display. Visual search is a category of laboratory tasks that are designed to clarify the component processes involved in identifying objects in real-world environments (Rabbitt, 1984; Eriksen, 1990; Wolfe, 1998). Typically, participants must decide whether some pre-specified target item is present among a display of non-target (distractor) items. A fundamental variable in these tasks is the number of items in the display. Changes in reaction time (RT) and accuracy associated with this variable (i.e. display size effects) represent the rate of search (e.g. increase in RT per individual display item).

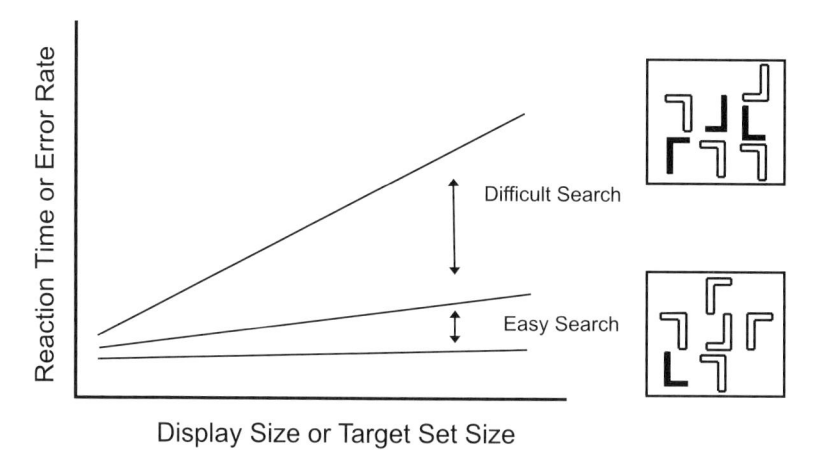

Fig. 1. Different types of visual search tasks (modified from Wolfe, 1998). In a feature search task, the target (e.g. a black upright L) differs from all of the distractors on the same feature dimension (e.g. color). Target identification in this case is performed easily, and the effect of the number of items in the display on RT or error rate (i.e. the display size effect) is minimal. In a conjunction search task, the target is a conjunction of different distractor features, and there is no single feature distinguishing the target. In this case, search for the target is more difficult, and increasing the number of items in the display leads to a corresponding increase in RT or error rate.

Figure 1 illustrates different types of search tasks. Feature search is a particularly easy task in which the target is a singleton, that is, the target differs from all of the distractors on the same feature dimension (e.g. a black upright L among white rotated Ls). The effect of display size is minimal in feature search, and the rate of search, as defined by the slope of the line relating RT to display size is typically very rapid, 10 ms per item or less. Observers performing feature search tasks often report that a singleton target "pops out" of the display. In more difficult search tasks, as when the target is a conjunction of features from different distractors (e.g. an upright black L among black and white rotated Ls), the display size effect is more pronounced, leading to search rates of 30 ms or more per item. The difference in search rate between feature search and conjunction search conditions has been interpreted as reflecting, respectively, the difference between parallel (simultaneous) and serial (item by item) comparison of display items. It currently appears most accurate, however, to view the range of search rates as a continuum representing the efficiency of the search process (Wolfe, 1998). Thus, changes in display size effects can be informative regarding the attentional demands of visual search. Alternatively, the number of target items held in memory can be varied, and search efficiency can be examined through changes in the memory set size effects. Naturally a host of other variables such as the visual quality of the display items, the mapping of the target items to responses, and the participants' degree of experience with the task, also influence performance. Interpretation of the effects of these variables on age differences in visual search and identification tasks has been critical for understanding age-related changes in visual attention.

2. Sensory-level processing

The goal of research on age-related changes in attention is to characterize an internal cognitive process, which is presumably a property of the brain and central nervous system. The recent development of neuroimaging techniques has provided important insights (literally) into the brain mechanisms mediating attentional and other cognitive processes. But in neuroimaging investigations, as well as in behavioral studies, interpretation of the results relies on the measurement of participants' behavioral responses to some observed event, and thus inferences regarding attentional processing depend on the performance of peripheral sensory and perceptual systems. Current theories of visual attention frequently emphasize the continuous flow of information between visual events and observers' decisions (Eriksen and Schultz, 1979). There is a close and, to some extent, unavoidable dependence between sensory and attentional functioning.

Substantial age-related changes occur in the efficiency of a variety of sensory processes, especially in the visual domain. The age-related changes in the physiology of the eye and associated neural pathways combine to yield a general decline in visual image clarity for older adults relative to younger adults (Kline and Scialfa, 1996; Scialfa and Kline, 1996; Fozard and Gordon-Salant, 2001). As Scialfa (1990) noted, these sensory changes do not necessarily imply that all age differences higher-order cognitive functions are reducible to sensory effects. In addition, as we will describe later in this section, low-level sensory processes are themselves influenced by attention. But in the interpretation of attentional and cognitive abilities it is important to recognize the potential role of sensory-level processing as one determinant of age-related changes in performance. Schneider and Pichora-Fuller (2000) have emphasized that perceptual and cognitive systems are highly interrelated rather than highly modular, and that age-related changes in sensory functioning will impact cognitive functioning.

One of the most noticeable age-related visual changes is presbyopia, the loss of the ability to accommodate focus to near objects, which typically occurs between the fourth and fifth decades of life. An age-related increase in the density and hardness of the crystalline lens prevents the change in lens shape necessary for accommodation (Glasser and Campbell, 1999). The changes in the lens also reduce the amount of light transmitted to the retina. Related changes include a decrease in resting pupil diameter, and changes in the vascular and cellular structure of the retina, as well as in the composition of the vitreous body. As a result, there is an increase in scatter of light within the eye and a reduction in retinal illuminance. Under comparable viewing conditions, the retinal illuminance of a 60-year-old eye will be approximately two-thirds lower than that of a 20-year-old eye (Weale, 1961).

These changes in sensory physiology contribute to an age-related decline in several measures of visual function, including best-corrected visual acuity (Pitts, 1982). Whereas 98% of individuals aged 52–64 years possess corrected Snellen acuity of 20/25 or better, only 69% of individuals 75–85 years retain this level of functioning (Kahn, 1977). Acuity, however, primarily represents the ability to spatially resolve high-contrast targets, typically with high luminance. Another way of measuring spatial vision is in terms of the contrast sensitivity threshold, which represents the lowest contrast at which the difference between a homogeneous field and a spatial grating (i.e. an alternating series of light and dark bands) can be detected. The contrast sensitivity threshold, measured in cycles per degree of visual angle, also exhibits age-related decline (particularly at intermediate and higher spatial frequencies) and may be a more sensitive measure of age-related effects than acuity (Greene and Madden, 1987; Haegerstrom-Portnoy et al., 1999). The useful field of view, defined as the spatial extent of the visual field from which an observer can extract information, is also reduced for older adults relative to younger adults (Scialfa et al., 1987; Ball et al., 1988).

In addition to changes in the physiology of the eye, age-related loss of cells occur throughout the visual pathway (retina, lateral geniculate nucleus, and striate cortex), although the loss is small relative to interindividual variability (Spear, 1993). In older adult rhesus monkeys, the visual sensory cortex exhibits a decline in the density of synapses and a thinning of the cortical layer (Peters et al., 2001). From human psychophysical studies it appears that changes at the neural level contribute significantly to the age differences in visual performance. Johnson et al. (1989) measured visual field sensitivity under test conditions that varied the potential contribution of preretinal factors (pupil size and lenticular transmission loss). The age-related decline in sensitivity across the visual field was independent of the test conditions, implying a contribution from the central nervous system level. Scialfa et al. (1999), for example, noted that age-related decline in the speed and accuracy of eye movements was consistent with changes in oculomotor neurons in the superior colliculus.

The age-related effects in the eye and visual pathways have clear implications for studies of aging and attention. Under comparable viewing conditions, the initial registration of the visual display is noisier for older adults than for younger adults, increasing the time that older adults require for the identification of individual display items (Scialfa, 1990; Madden and Allen, 1991). The relative importance of the sensory-level variables, however, depends on the viewing conditions for the task. When the task is resource-limited (Norman and Bobrow, 1975), in the sense that display duration is above threshold and participants' accuracy level is near ceiling, the sensory limitations may have minimal effects on performance. In a seminal study, for example, Plude and Doussard-Roosevelt (1989) demonstrated that under resource-limited conditions, RT in a feature search task (detection of a red X among a display of green Os) was independent of the number of items in the display for both younger and older adults, implying a very efficient search process for both age groups. In contrast, under data-limited conditions, in which display duration is near threshold and accuracy is below ceiling, the role of sensory variables is more critical. This role is clearly evident in investigations of visual masking and temporal integration, which have used the interference between successively presented visual displays to estimate the time course of visual feature extraction (Eriksen et al., 1970; Di Lollo et al., 1982; Walsh, 1982). These studies have consistently reported an age-related slowing in the rate of visual feature extraction.

Several investigations have focused specifically on visual search under data-limited conditions. The variation in accuracy associated with using a range of decision criteria (i.e. speed-accuracy trade-off functions) suggests that older adults are less efficient than younger adults in the early stages of visual feature identification (Madden and Allen, 1991). Zacks and Zacks (1993) used a forced-choice search task with briefly presented displays and found that the age-related slowing in the rate of search (i.e. display size effect) was replicable under these conditions. In addition, the rate of search estimated by Zacks and Zacks from the accuracy data was faster than that typically obtained from RT measures under resource-limited conditions, suggesting a contribution from decision-level processing to RT measures of search rate. Ellis et al. (1996) developed a model of search for limited-duration displays (40–240 ms) and found that an age-related deficit was evident in the model parameter representing display encoding speed but not in the parameter for decision speed. Davis et al. (2002) reported that when a feature search task (similar to that of Plude and Doussard-Roosevelt, 1989) was performed under data-limited conditions, the efficient visual search observed by Plude and Doussard-Roosevelt was no longer apparent. Instead, performance declined significantly as a function of an increase in the number of items in the display, and this display size effect was more pronounced for older adults than for younger adults.

These findings suggest that age-related changes in sensory physiology can contribute significantly to measures of age differences in visual attention, especially under data-limited conditions. This contribution does not imply, however, that the attentional effects can be explained completely on the basis of the sensory variables. It is important to note that investigations of younger adults have demonstrated that attention has an influence on sensory-level processing. Cameron et al. (2002), for example, examined changes in contrast sensitivity threshold, in an orientation discrimination task, as a function of whether the target location was attended (following the presentation of a spatial cue) or unattended. Attention led to improved performance across all locations in the visual field. Because the orientation target was presented without accompanying distractors (i.e. external noise was excluded), the authors concluded that the attentional benefit was the result of signal enhancement. Freeman et al. (2001) obtained similar findings regarding the psychophysical interactions among display items that were small patches of light and dark bands (Gabor patches). Participants performed a detection task for a centrally presented target patch concurrently with a spatial resolution task (Vernier offset) for a subset of flanker patches surrounding the target. Freeman et al. found that the contrast sensitivity threshold for the target was facilitated when the target and flanker bands were collinear, but only when the flankers were attended (i.e. included in the spatial resolution task).

This influence of attention on sensory-level processing also interacts with age differences in the sensory tasks. Sekuler and Bennett (2000) reported that age-related decline in the useful field of view, as assessed by a peripheral dot-detection task, was more pronounced when this task was performed under divided attention conditions (i.e. concurrently with a central letter detection task) than when dot-detection was performed in isolation. Thus, the sensory and attentional changes with age are not entirely separable and in fact may represent the effects of a common mechanism. An intriguing finding from psychometric investigations of higher-order cognitive abilities such as memory and reasoning is that a substantial proportion of the age-related variance in the cognitive measures (more than 0.90 in some instances) is shared with sensory measures of visual and auditory acuity (Lindenberger and Baltes, 1994). One plausible explanation for these results is that both sensory and cognitive measures reflect a common mechanism of age-related changes occurring throughout the brain and central nervous system during aging (Salthouse et al., 1996; Baltes and Lindenberger, 1997; Schneider and Pichora-Fuller, 2000).

3. General vs. specific effects of attention

Before attributing an age-related change in performance on a particular cognitive task to attentional processing, it is important to determine whether age differences in attention can in principle be distinguished from other explanations. As we noted in our discussion of sensory variables, the correlations among sensory threshold and cognitive ability measures suggest that age-related changes in perceptual and cognitive functioning are the effects of a general mechanism operating throughout the brain and nervous system. What is that mechanism, and how is it established that age differences in task performance are due to the specific effects of attention rather than to the more general mechanism?

There is substantial evidence, and a long-standing theoretical perspective, identifying speed of processing as the general mechanism of age-related cognitive change (Salthouse, 1985a,b, 1996; Cerella, 1990; Bashore, 1993; Madden, 2001). Birren and Fisher (1995) observed that data consistent with a generalized slowing mechanism appeared as early as Koga and Morant's (1923) analysis of Galton's (1885) data. Galton had collected a series of sensory and RT measures from over 9000 individuals between 5 and 80 years of age, and Koga and Morant analyzed the data for 3379 male participants in this sample. As Birren and Fisher noted, the correlations between visual RT and auditory RT in the Koga and Morant data were higher than the correlations of the RT measures with their corresponding sensory acuity measures. This pattern suggests that even simple RT measures reflect information processing beyond the level of a sensory threshold. Birren et al. (1962) developed a more explicit theory of age-related slowing, based on a factor analysis of 22 RT tasks, and found that a general factor relating to the processing speed accounted for more variance in the older adults' data than in the younger adults' data. Birren et al. proposed that a "lower speed of mediation of behavior by the nervous system" (p. 15), among other sources, was responsible for age-related slowing in task performance.

Brinley (1965) introduced a new method of analyzing age differences in cognitive performance that has had a significant impact on current views of age-related slowing. Brinley compared younger and older adults' performance of 18 speeded

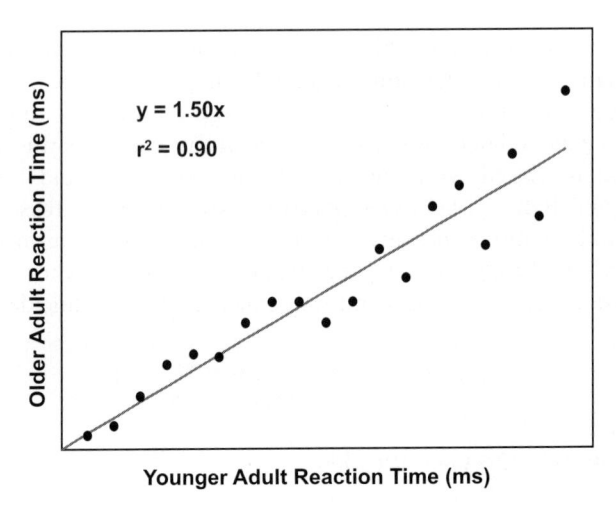

Fig. 2. A Brinley plot, in which the older adults' mean RTs are plotted as a function of the younger adults' values. Each point represents the mean value for a particular task condition, averaged across participants. The function is typically highly monotonic, with a slope between 1.50 and 2.0, representing the fact that the absolute value of the age difference in RT tends to be higher in the more difficult task conditions. Note that a slope of 1.0 would represent a pattern in which the age difference in RT is constant across task conditions.

tasks comprising verbal, arithmetic, and perceptual content areas. Within each content category, three of the tasks required shifting an attentional set across trials (e.g. selecting either a synonym, antonym, or rhyme response), and three tasks did not require a shift (e.g. selecting a synonym response consistently). Brinley found that the proportional increase in RT for the shift tasks, relative to the non-shift conditions, was greater for older adults than for younger adults, suggesting the possibility that older adults exhibit a specific difficulty with tasks that require shifting attention. But Brinley also found that when he plotted the 18 task condition mean RTs of the older adults as a function of the corresponding means of the younger adults, the result was a highly linear function ($r = 0.99$). This result led him to conclude that "response times for both groups and for each type of task variation may be conceived as varying along a single dimension which might be termed 'task difficulty'" (p. 131).

This type of analysis, which has come to be known as a Brinley plot, is illustrated with a simulated data set in Fig. 2. (The methodology is also referred to as a task complexity analysis, Cerella et al. (1980), and as the method of systematic relations, Salthouse, 1992b.) Typically, the slope of the function is between 1.5 and 2.0 (it was 1.68 in Brinley's data), and the intercept is negative. The overadditive interaction between age group and task condition that is frequently observed in analysis of mean or median RT (i.e. the increase in RT associated with task difficulty being more pronounced for older adults than for younger adults) can yield a highly monotonic Brinley plot. The implication of the Brinley methodology is that as long as the task condition mean RTs of the two age groups are related monotonically, there may be little reason to develop explanations based on the specific requirements (e.g. the attentional demands) of the task conditions. The degree of age-related slowing may vary in magnitude, with higher slope values reflecting relatively greater slowing, but the individual task conditions would not require specific interpretation.

The type of analysis devised by Brinley (1965) has been extremely influential in the interpretation of age differences in RT. Although the relation between younger and older adults' RT values has been consistently found to be monotonic, some variation in the Brinley function has also been observed. Multiple regression techniques can be used to determine whether this variation is greater than would be expected by chance (Myerson et al., 1992). At some level, task demands appear to have an important role in determining the Brinley plot slope. Lima et al. (1991) claimed that the critical dimension was task domain, with non-lexical tasks leading to higher Brinley plot slopes (i.e. a greater degree of slowing) than lexical tasks. Cerella (1985) proposed that the Brinley plot slope was higher for task conditions requiring some form of mental transformation (central processing) than for sensorimotor control conditions (peripheral processing). In contrast to Cerella's proposal, however, several analysis of Brinley plot functions in word identification tasks suggest that age-related slowing has a greater influence on peripheral processes (e.g. as defined by visual degradation effects) than on central processes such as lexical access (Madden, 1988, 1992a; Allen et al., 1993).

The Brinley plot slope has also varied reliably across participant groups. Individuals with Alzheimer's disease, for example, exhibit higher Brinley slopes than age-matched healthy older adults (Nebes and Madden, 1988; Nebes and Brady, 1992; Madden et al., 1999b), implying an acceleration of the generalized slowing effect. The regression analysis can, in addition, be extended from the group level to the individual participant level, allowing the prediction of an individual's speed of processing for diverse tasks (Hale and Jansen, 1994). The form of the Brinley plot is not always observed to be linear, however, and especially in the non-lexical domain, the data may be fit better by a positively accelerated power function rather than a linear one (Hale et al., 1987). Myerson et al. (1990) used a power function analysis of Brinley plots to derive an information-loss model of age-related slowing. The model assumes that the duration of a processing step is inversely proportional to the information available, and age-related deficits are accounted for in terms of the loss of information between steps. Nevertheless, the information-loss model retains the central assumption that age-related slowing is general rather specific to individual tasks or cognitive functions.

Another methodology that has been widely used to establish the existence of generalized age-related slowing relies on the statistical control of an independent measure of information processing speed. This approach can thus be considered an out-of-context assessment of generalized slowing, in that it uses information obtained outside the context of the behavioral task of interest, to assess the contribution of generalized slowing. The Brinley plot analysis, in contrast, represents a within-context assessment that uses the data within the task of interest to assess slowing (Salthouse, 1990).

The statistical control approach to generalized slowing (or shared influence analysis; Salthouse, 2000) has included a variety of specific statistical approaches and measures of processing speed. The assumptions and issues involved in this research area have been discussed by Salthouse (1985a, 1992a, 2000). It is important, for example, that the measure of processing speed be sufficiently complex that it elicits some information processing abilities beyond the sensorimotor level, but not so complex that it overlaps substantially with the behavioral task being assessed. Most frequently, some form of substitution coding task, similar to the Digit Symbol Substitution subtest of the Wechsler Adult Intelligence Scale, has been used as the control variable representing elementary perceptual speed. Linear regression procedures, such as the analysis of covariance, hierarchical regression, or structural equation modeling are then applied to the data to estimate the unique age-related variance in task performance that remains after the age-related variance associated with the processing speed measure is controlled. Alternatively, as a mixture of within-context and out-of-context approaches, the fastest set of responses from the complete RT distribution can be used as the speed measure to be controlled (Salthouse, 1998). Across all of these approaches, the assumption is that the contribution of generalized slowing can be estimated from the degree of attenuation in the age-related variance in the primary task that is provided by controlling statistically for the effects of the more elementary measure of speed.

Empirical studies using statistical control procedures have demonstrated that elementary perceptual speed accounts for a substantial proportion of age-related variance in cognitive performance measures. Salthouse (1993b) noted that across an extensive series of published studies, approximately 80% of the age-related variance in RT measures of cognitive functioning is shared with an elementary speed of processing dimension. This pattern has been observed when the outcome measure involves some form of memory recall (Bryan and Luszcz, 1996; Park et al., 1996), but has also been reported for tasks related specifically to attentional functions. Salthouse and Meinz (1995) investigated working memory as an outcome measure, controlling for variables representing attentional inhibition (from Stroop tasks) and perceptual speed. Although the attentional measures led to a substantial attenuation of the age-related variance in working memory, the attenuation was just as great when the mediating variable was an elementary perceptual speed measure. Similarly, Salthouse et al. (1998) reported that one type of attentional measure (task-switching ability) was related to age-related changes in memory and reasoning ability, but this relation was mediated primarily by speed. In analyses of RT distributions, Salthouse (1993a, 1998) concluded that the age-related variance in the slowest RTs was mediated almost entirely by the variance in the fastest RTs. This pattern suggested that age-related changes in performance were related more to a general mechanism operating throughout the entire RT distribution than to a specific process such as a lapse of attention, which would lead to independent age-related effects in the slowest RTs.

Naturally, objections have been raised to the idea that age differences in a wide array of cognitive functions, including those related to attention, can be attributed almost entirely to elementary perceptual processing speed. The debate regarding the analysis of Brinley functions has been reviewed cogently by Bashore (1994). One category of objection is that the plot of older vs. younger adult task condition means is not sensitive to local (task-specific) effects. Perfect (1994), for example, used computer simulated data sets to demonstrate that when data from different tasks with markedly different slowing functions were aggregated, the result was a single, highly linear Brinley function. In an empirical exploration of a similar point, Sliwinski and Hall (1998) proposed that ordinary least squares regression, which is typically used in Brinley plot analysis, is in fact inappropriate for this purpose. These authors used an alternative approach, hierarchical linear models, in a meta-analysis of RT data from 21 cognitive tasks. This alternative approach yielded evidence of task-dependent slowing that was not apparent from ordinary least squares regression. Specifically, the degree of age-related slowing associated with visual search and mental rotation tasks was greater than that associated with memory search tasks. Verhaeghen (2002) examined the difference between memory search and visual search within subjects, using accuracy measures, and confirmed the pattern observed by Sliwinski and Hall in a meta-analysis: age-related slowing of encoding processes was greater for visual search than for memory search.

Limitations to the statistical control approach to generalized slowing have also been noted. In some cognitive tasks (e.g. mental imagery), working memory is a more influential mediator of age-related variance than perceptual speed (Briggs et al., 1999). Piccinin and Rabbitt (1999) cautioned against using substitution coding tasks (e.g. Digit Symbol Substitution subtest) as an index of perceptual processing speed, because such tasks may themselves require higher-order cognitive processes such as learning and memory. Allen et al. (2001) used structural equation modeling to analyze the RT data from several previously published large-scale data sets, and proposed that although the best-fitting model for each data set usually included a common factor (e.g. processing speed), there were also direct effects of age across component cognitive, sensory, and physiological factors.

In view of the substantial amount of variance shared between measures of elementary processing speed and cognitive performance, what is the best method for identifying age-related changes related specifically to attention? There is no single answer, but several different approaches can be helpful. As Salthouse (2000) and Madden (2001) have noted, it is an oversimplification to view generalized slowing and task-specific interpretations as mutually exclusive theories of age-related performance change. Many tasks will include both a contribution from generalized slowing and some task-specific component.

A more constructive approach is to attempt to determine the relative contributions of the general and task-specific components. Madden et al. (1996), for example, using hierarchical regression, found that although perceptual speed accounted for the majority of age-related variance in performance on a visual search task, there were unique effects of age that reflected the attentional demands of specific task conditions. In analyses of RT distributions, Anderson et al. (1999) obtained evidence for age effects in the attentional demands of memory encoding and retrieval as well as for a generalized slowing effect. Another approach is to use the Brinley plot of task condition means as a null hypothesis (Madden et al.,

1992; Salthouse and Kersten, 1993). In this latter method, the effects of the independent variables are tested in an analysis of variance with the younger adults' data transformed by the Brinley plot function. Thus, Age Group × Task Condition interactions that remain significant following this transformation are viewed as being age effects that are independent of generalized slowing. Faust et al. (1999) developed a related method in which the transformation was defined at the level of the individual participant. None of these analytic methods provides a definitive solution, but the methods are useful in distinguishing age-related effects of attention from more general changes in performance.

4. Spatial attention, selection, and inhibition

As noted in the "Introduction," the ability to select some perceptual events rather than others is an important component of attention. Identifying age-related changes in visual selective attention has been a central concern in research on adult development. Many of the issues being investigated currently were anticipated in Rabbitt's (1964, 1965) studies of visual discrimination performance. Rabbitt (1964) reported the results of an experiment in which participants made a letter/digit response regarding a single, visually presented item. A cue, presented between 200 ms and 1500 ms before the display, indicated with 95% validity the category of the display item. In a control condition, a cue was presented with the same time course but did not provide any task-relevant information. Relative to the control condition, the valid cues led to a significant decrease in RT (i.e. a performance benefit) for younger adults, but not for older adults. Both age groups, however, exhibited an increase in RT in response to invalid cues (i.e. a performance cost), so even though older adults did not use the cues effectively they were attending to them. Rabbitt (1965) found that the display size effect in a card-sorting task was greater for older adults than for younger adults. Rabbitt's findings thus suggested that an age-related decline exists in some aspects of attention related to the use of advance cues and in selecting relevant display information. Rabbitt (1965) concluded that the underlying age-related change involved a "difficulty in ignoring irrelevant or redundant information."

These initial findings raised a variety of issues. Because, for example, in the Rabbitt (1964) study the two stimulus categories mapped directly onto two responses, the age difference in the use of advance information could reflect a limitation in either the categorization of the display item or the translation of this categorization into a motor response. Similarly, in the Rabbitt (1965) experiment all of the display items were task-relevant in the sense that any one of them could have been the target letter. Thus, the age difference obtained may represent a general age-related slowing of visual search performance rather than a specific deficit in the ability to ignore irrelevant information. Subsequent research has been devoted to defining more precisely which components of selective attention are vulnerable to age-related decline.

4.1. Selection by display dimensions

Investigating the ability to discriminate relevant and irrelevant information requires that the perceptual task includes some additional cue that defines a particular subset of the features of the display as being task-relevant. A straightforward method of doing this is to indicate that the relevant display information has a particular color or spatial location. When the perceptual task is defined in this manner, older adults have demonstrated a surprising degree of preservation of the ability to attend selectively to relevant information. This preservation has been reported in several investigations of search through multi-element displays. When participants have advance information regarding either the color (Nebes and Madden, 1983) or spatial location (Madden, 1983; Plude and Hoyer, 1986; Allen et al., 1994) of the target item, the improvement in search relative to a non-informative control condition is often at least as great for older adults as for younger adults. In fact, experiments using this type of design have tended to exhibit interactions between age group and task condition reflecting larger selective attention effects for older adults than for younger adults. This pattern occurs because the age-related deficits are usually more pronounced in the control condition, which does not provide target-relevant advance information. Thus an age-related decline in the identification of individual display items is magnified as the number of items requiring comparison is increased.

Several other spatial properties of multi-element displays have been investigated, confirming the trend of an age-related preservation of selective attention. Two of these properties are the movement of the display elements and the apparent depth at which they occur. Kramer et al. (1996), for example, reported the results from a search task in which the target was defined by a combination of features in the non-target items (i.e. conjunction search), and in which the target and one-half of the non-target items were in motion, among stationary non-targets (e.g. a moving O among moving Xs and stationary Os). Search was very efficient for both younger and older adults, approximately 10–14 ms per display item. This finding indicates that both age groups were able to use a movement filter to effectively inhibit or ignore the stationary items (e.g. the Os), thus reducing the task to a feature search in which the target O stood out visually from the non-target Xs.

Atchley and Kramer (1998, 2000) devised a technique, using stereoscopic vision, that allowed them to present visual displays at two different planes of apparent depth. Atchley and Kramer (1998) demonstrated that the change in RT associated with switching between display items at different apparent depths was similar for younger and older adults. Atchley and Kramer (2000) found that both age groups could restrict search to a single depth plane and attenuate the influence of distracting information at other depth locations. In these experiments, the authors used a visual cue (a red outline rectangle) to indicate the depth plane most likely to contain a search target (a red tilted line among gray tilted lines). For both younger and older adults, the disruptive influence of a distracting display item (a red vertical line) was less when it occurred at a different depth from the target, relative to distractors located at the same depth. Thus older adults appear to retain the ability to control attention in depth.

4.2. Vigilance

Research on the ability to sustain attention over time, or vigilance, has also suggested some degree of constancy as a function of age. Relatively few investigations have been conducted in this area, the majority by Parasuraman and colleagues (Parasuraman et al., 1989; Parasuraman and Giambra, 1991; Berardi et al., 2001). Vigilance tasks typically require participants to detect the presence of a pre-defined target event over an extended period of time. Performance is characterized in terms of measures of detectability and bias, derived from signal detection theory. Analogous to the display size effect in visual search, vigilance tasks typically exhibit a vigilance decrement effect, representing a decline in target detection ability as a function of increasing time on task. Parasuraman et al. (1989) found that the vigilance decrement was similar for younger and older adults, although target detectability was relatively lower overall for older adults. Parasuraman and Giambra (1991) reported that extensive practice (20 sessions) could eliminate the vigilance decrement for younger adults but not for middle-aged or older adults. Berardi et al. (2001), however, have emphasized the potential contribution of age-related health problems to apparent age differences in sustained attention ability. These authors conducted extensive screening for optimal health and found that the vigilance decrement, as well as overall detectability, were comparable for younger, middle-aged, and older adults.

4.3. Movement and distribution of attention

Most of the research on age-related changes in visual search assumes that attention is focused around a single spatial location, either as a spatially limited but variable power spotlight (Eriksen and Yeh, 1985), or as a more continuous gradient (Henderson, 1991). Several experiments have been concerned with how attention is shifted across spatial locations. One important issue is whether the shift represents voluntary or involuntary changes in the attentional focus. Folk and Hoyer (1992) separated these types of attentional processes on the basis of the validity and location of the cue. For example, any RT costs associated with cues that participants knew to be 100% invalid would be assumed to be the result of involuntary shifts of attention, because attending to the cues would be of no benefit to task performance. Folk and Hoyer found that the RT costs for these involuntary shifts of attention were similar in magnitude for younger and older adults, as were the RT changes associated with more voluntary attentional shifts (i.e. cues having less than 100% validity). Madden (1992b) reported that the allocation of attention to a probabilistic spatial cue (in terms of the estimated proportion of trials on which participants attended to the cued location) was similar for younger and older adults, although the time required to identify the cued item and shift attention across display locations was relatively greater for the older adults.

Hahn and Kramer (1995) constructed a search task that encouraged observers to split their attention between two spatially non-contiguous locations. The task required the comparison of two target letters for a match/mismatch response. Two distractor letters were located between the targets, and the distractors were either matched or mismatched, thus priming a particular response to the targets. Hahn and Kramer found that the distractors influenced performance (e.g. by priming a response incompatible with the correct response to the targets), but only when the distractors were presented as onset stimuli, that is, as new items in an otherwise blank display. This influence of the distractors was comparable for younger and older adults. More importantly, when the distractors were presented as non-onset stimuli, by the removal of lines from figure-eight characters, then the distractors did not influence target matching for either age group. In this latter condition both groups were able to divide their attention between the two target locations and successfully ignore the intervening distractors.

The Hahn and Kramer (1995) findings of an age preservation in the splitting of attention between non-contiguous locations raise the more general question of how attention is distributed across the visual field. As noted previously, there is no complete agreement, even in studies concerned only with younger adults, regarding the distribution of spatial attention. A useful starting point may be to consider the difference between relatively focused and relatively distributed attention, a distinction that can be defined empirically, though open to interpretation by different theoretical frameworks. One method for investigating the difference between focused and distributed attention was introduced by LaBerge (1983). Participants view two successively presented displays and respond overtly to the second display on the basis of some property of the first display. Thus, if the interval between the two displays is sufficiently brief, the distribution of attention during participants' processing of the second display can be inferred from the type of decision required to the first display.

Hartley and McKenzie (1991) used the LaBerge paradigm to investigate adult age differences in the spatial distribution of attention. In a focused attention condition, the task was to make a choice response to a single-target second display (7 vs. Z), if the first display (a row of alternating 8s and 5s) contained a S in the central position. In an unfocused attention condition, the entire row in the first display was either Ss or 8s. Hartley and McKenzie found that an effect of target eccentricity (an increase in errors as a function of the distance of the second display target from the central fixation point) was greater for older adults than for younger adults in the focused condition but not in the unfocused condition, suggesting that older adults maintained a more spatially limited distribution of attention, in the focused condition, than did younger adults.

Madden and Gottlob (1997) obtained related findings in a similar paradigm that required participants to make a choice response to a second display (a row of letters containing one target), on the basis of the identity of the central character in the first display. These authors examined changes in RT response compatibility effects, among the target and non-target letters of the second display, as a function of target location. For younger adults, the increase in RT associated with response-incompatibility was greater when second-display target location was unpredictable, as compared to when the target occurred consistently in the center of the row of letters. For older adults, in contrast, the RT response compatibility effect was similar to that of younger adults when the second-display target was presented consistently at fixation, and the older adults' response compatibility effect did not increase when the location of the second-display target was unpredictable. Thus, as in the Hartley and McKenzie (1991) data, there was evidence that the focus of spatial attention was more narrow for older adults than for younger adults (but cf. Greenwood and Parasuraman, 1999).

In research on selective attention there is currently a debate not only regarding the properties of the spatial distribution of attention, but also regarding the more fundamental issue of whether the appropriate metric is inherently spatial. That is, attention may be allocated selectively on the basis of objects in the visual environment, rather than on the basis of spatial location (Duncan, 1984). Kramer and Weber (1999) illustrated this distinction in a task in which younger and older adults viewed pictures of two overlapping wrenches. This was a conjunction search task that required a "yes" response if two properties, an open end and hexagonal end, were both present on the wrenches, and a "no" response if only one or neither of these types of ends were present. The critical finding was that, for both age groups, the "yes" responses were faster when both properties were located on the same wrench than when they were on different wrenches, even though the spatial separation between the two target properties was greater for the same-object properties than for the different-object properties. These results support object-based models of selective attention and suggest that object-based selection is resistant to age-related decline.

4.4. Time course effects

Selective attention also includes a dynamic component, in terms of the time required to adjust an attentional focus. This issue has been investigated in a wide range of studies, the most frequent approach being variation in the stimulus onset asynchrony (SOA), which is the interval between the onsets of two events, in this case a task-relevant cue and a visual display. Investigations of younger adults have demonstrated that RT decreases as a function of increasing SOA, up to some asymptote, as the information provided by the cue accumulates and primes a particular response (Eriksen and Schultz, 1979). Surprisingly, a general trend from the studies of adult age differences has been that the time course of attentional cuing is very similar for younger and older adults, especially when the visual display is limited to a single item (Nissen and Corkin, 1985; Folk and Hoyer, 1992; but cf. Lincourt et al., 1997).

Hartley et al. (1990) reported a thorough analysis of SOA effects across six experiments that examined different forms of cuing. These authors emphasized a distinction between cues, which provide probabilistic information regarding the upcoming target, and prompts, which provide an instruction regarding which aspect of the target requires a response. For both types of advance information, the pattern observed by Hartley et al. was similar to that of Nissen and Corkin (1985) and Folk and Hoyer (1992): Responses were slower for older adults than for younger adults, but the pattern of RT costs and benefits associated with both cues and prompts, and their change in relation to SOA, were relatively constant as a function of age. Hartley et al. concluded that age-related slowing may be primarily the result of response-related processes. Thus, from this perspective, the age-related decrement in the categorization process discussed by Rabbitt (1964, 1965) would be due primarily to the selection of a correct response rather than the selection of the target-relevant display information.

The age constancy in the time course of cuing effects is surprising because, as Hartley et al. (1990) noted, most theories of age-related decrease in attentional processing, especially those assuming an age-related slowing in the allocation of attention, would predict that cuing effects would emerge at a later SOA for older adults than for younger adults. The majority of the SOA experiments, however, have used single-target RT tasks, and some age differences in time course have been observed in the context of multi-element search. Madden (1990) reported that a bar-marker cue regarding the location of a target letter led to a decrease in RT at a later SOA for older adults than for younger adults, when the target was accompanied by distractor letters. When the target letter was presented in isolation, however, the cue had a minimal effect on RT for both age groups. Madden and Gottlob (1997) found that the decrease in RT associated with increasing SOA between two successively presented displays, in a LaBerge paradigm, was well fit by an exponential decay function for both younger and older adults (cf. Myerson et al., 1992). Using the parameters of this function, Madden and Gottlob defined SOA' (SOA-prime) as the point at which the SOA function approaches the asymptote to within some arbitrary value. Estimates of SOA' were in fact higher for older adults than for younger adults, consistent with an age-related slowing of attentional allocation.

4.5. Attentional inhibition

Investigations that are concerned with the spatial distribution and time course of attention do not necessarily address the issue of the nature of the processing occurring at an attended display location. As mentioned previously in the "Introduction" section, the concept of selective attention refers not only to the ability to focus on relevant information, but also the ability to inhibit irrelevant or distracting information. These different components of attention are difficult to isolate completely, but tasks that emphasize the inhibitory aspect of selective attention have been found to yield significant evidence of age-related decline. This topic has led to an extensive research literature, however, and not all of the results are consistent. Hasher, Zacks, and colleagues have conducted a programmatic series of studies on this topic, primarily in the context of memory tasks (Hasher and Zacks, 1988; May et al., 1995). These authors propose that aging is associated with a decrease in the efficiency of inhibitory processing, which would lead to an increase in task-irrelevant information being maintained in working memory. As a result, the capacity of working memory would be reduced, and the quality of older adults' encoding, retrieval, and comprehension processes would suffer (but cf. Burke, 1997; McDowd, 1997).

Evidence for age-related decline in inhibitory processing is not restricted to memory tasks and has also been obtained in the context of visual search and comparison. The main conclusion that emerges from this research is that inhibition is not a unitary construct (Kramer et al., 1994, 1999b). Age-related deficits in inhibition reflect specific task demands rather than a general ability. Several different types of RT tasks have been used to measure age differences in inhibitory function. The Stroop task has arguably been the most consistent source of support for the concept of an age-related decline in inhibitory functioning. In this task, participants attempt to name the color in which a word is printed, and on interference trials the word is a color name that conflicts with the printed color (i.e. "red" printed in blue). Thus, increased RT on interference trials relative to control trials suggests a difficulty in inhibiting the meaning of the word to be named. An age-related increase in the Stroop interference effect has been observed in several investigations, suggesting an age-related decline in the ability to inhibit word meaning, although not all of the studies have performed the types of analysis necessary to distinguish the age-related interference effect from generalized slowing (Verhaeghen and De Meersman, 1998). Brink and McDowd (1999), Hartley (1993), and Spieler et al. (1996) have performed the requisite analysis and have demonstrated that the age-related increase in Stroop interference is greater than would be expected on the basis of generalized slowing.

The Hartley (1993) investigation additionally demonstrated an interesting interaction between Stroop interference and selective attention to spatial location. In the typical version of the Stroop task, the color to be named and the interfering word (a color name) are presented as an integrated unit. Hartley separated these items by presenting a color name (printed in a neutral color), and a block of color, at separate but adjacent display locations. This manipulation virtually eliminated the age differences observed in the typical Stroop task, indicating that older adults can successfully inhibit the conflicting information when a spatial dimension is available for selecting the relevant information. Brink and McDowd (1999) replicated this interaction between spatial selection and Stroop interference.

The stop-signal paradigm, in which participants are given a signal, on some proportion of trials, to inhibit the primary task response (e.g. refrain from responding to a visual display when a tone is presented) has also yielded evidence suggesting an age-related decline in inhibitory functioning. This paradigm has the interesting feature of allowing the estimation of the time required to inhibit a prepared response. Kramer et al. (1994) and Bedard et al. (2002) have reported an age-related increase, beyond that attributable to generalized slowing, in the time required to inhibit a primary task response.

Experiments investigating negative priming and inhibition of return effects have provided less consistent support for the inhibitory deficit model. Negative priming refers to a slowing of target identification on a current trial when the target item was defined as a distractor on a recently preceding trial. Some studies of negative priming effect have found that younger adults demonstrate this effect whereas older adults do not (Hasher et al., 1991; Kane et al., 1994). This pattern may reflect an age-related decline in the inhibition of distractor items, thus reducing the interference for the older adults when the previous distractors appeared subsequently as targets. Later research, however, found that measurable negative priming was evident for both younger and older adults (Kramer et al., 1994; Kieley and Hartley, 1997; Little and Hartley, 2000). The different findings across studies may be the result of subtle differences in task difficulty and the variability of older adults' responses (Kramer et al., 1999b).

The inhibition of return effect refers to the slowing of the allocation of attention to a previously cued spatial location. The interpretations of this effect have proposed that it reflects a useful mechanism for facilitating overall performance, by preventing display locations that were recently inspected from being searched again, at least within some time interval. The investigations of inhibition of return have generally yielded little support for specific age-related deficits in inhibition, in that the slowing of target identification at a recently cued location (following an initial 300–400 ms period of facilitation) is relatively constant as a function of age (Hartley and Kieley, 1995). A related finding is that of Kramer et al. (1999b), who reported that distraction from a sudden onset in the display led to a comparable disruption of the pattern of eye movements for younger and older adults.

Maylor and Lavie (1998) demonstrated an important interaction between age-related deficits in inhibitory functioning and the perceptual load of visual search. These authors found that when the search task required participants to ignore a distractor presented outside the display, the magnitude of the distraction (in terms of response slowing) for response-incompatible distractors, relative to neutral distractors, decreased as the number of items in the display (perceptual load) increased. That is, selective attention was actually more efficient when the processing demands of the task were high, at the larger display sizes, because little excess attentional capacity was available to be engaged by the peripheral distractor. This perceptual load effect was more pronounced for younger adults than for older adults and appeared to represent age-related declines in both selective attention and attentional capacity. At the lower values of display size (i.e. lower perceptual load), the interference from the response-incompatible distractor was greater for older adults than for younger adults, reflecting an age-related decline in selective attention (inhibitory control). There was a greater improvement in attentional selectivity as a function of increasing display size for older adults than for younger adults, which Maylor and Lavie attributed to the older adults' relatively lower level of attentional capacity. That is, the older adults' processing limits were reached with a relatively smaller number of display items.

Madden and Langley (2003) replicated the effects of perceptual load on selective attention reported by Maylor and Lavie (1998), but found that the age differences were evident primarily when display duration was brief and the error rate was relatively high (i.e. data-limited conditions). Under data-limited viewing conditions, failure of selective attention (interference from a response-incompatible distractor) was greater for older adults than for younger adults, and this age difference was evident only at the lower display sizes, as reported by Maylor and Lavie. One departure in the Madden and Langley data from that of Maylor and Lavie, however, was that the increase in display size necessary to eliminate distractor interference was the same for the two age groups, which suggests that the age difference in selective attention was not attributable to an attentional capacity limitation as proposed by Maylor and Lavie. In addition, Madden and Langley found that under resource-limited viewing conditions (i.e. longer display duration and lower error rates) the disruptive influence of the distractor was not due entirely to response competition, but also included a more general inhibitory function, arising from internal recognition responses to display items. Both the general and response-specific forms of inhibition, under resource-limited viewing conditions, were similar in magnitude for younger and older adults. Thus, variables such as task difficulty, the structure of the display (e.g. whether the distractor is presented within or external to the display) and display duration interact to determine the degree of age-related decline in attentional inhibition.

5. Practice and the development of automaticity

The majority of research conducted on age-related changes in attention provides participants with low or moderate amounts of practice in unfamiliar, laboratory-specific cognitive tasks. This is an appropriate approach for the goal of obtaining measures of cognitive performance that are not dependent on highly overlearned strategies, and for minimizing individual differences in task-relevant experience. In cognitive tasks performed outside the laboratory, however, practice is an extremely important determinant of both the level of performance and the attention demands of the task. One of the most valuable consequences of practice is that an initially difficult and attention demanding task can (ideally) be transformed into a highly skilled and effortless performance. This transformation is often referred to as the development of automaticity, reflecting the distinction between controlled or attention-demanding performance, and automatic or attention-free performance, introduced by Schneider and Shiffrin (1977).

The effects of practice, especially in real-world tasks, pose a critical challenge for theoretical accounts of age-related changes in attention, because some findings are difficult to integrate into the explanations developed for age-related changes in laboratory tests of visual search and comparison. Charness (1981a,b), for example, found that, in a sample of chess players representing a range of skill and age, the ability to solve chess problems was related more closely to skill than to age. In fact, within a decision tree for a particular chess problem, older adults appeared to locate an acceptable move with a less extensive search, and they searched at approximately the same rate as younger players. The older chess players, however, were vulnerable to age-related cognitive decline, as evident in measures of the incidental recall of the chess positions following the problem-solving protocol. Salthouse (1984) reported similar findings in a study of skilled typists. Older adults who were experienced typists were slower than their younger adult counterparts on laboratory measures of perceptual-motor speed, but the older typists were able to maintain a typing speed comparable to the younger adults, apparently by being more sensitive to characters farther in advance of the currently typed character. Thus, although as we discussed previously (in the section on "General vs. specific effects of attention"), age-related slowing is a prominent feature of age differences in cognitive performance, the development of expertise from specific practice can provide some compensation for age-related decline in basic mechanisms of information processing.

In these investigations of chess and typing skill, the expertise was acquired before the research assessments were conducted, and the role of pre-existing individual differences is difficult to determine. An alternative approach is to investigate expertise from the assessment of practice with unfamiliar tasks, a method that has been adopted in several studies of age-related changes in visual attention. A critical variable in this research is the mapping of the task elements to responses (Schneider and Shiffrin, 1977). In a consistent mapping condition, for example, the same items remain consistently assigned as targets (i.e. those requiring a response indicating their presence in the memory set or display). With practice, consistent mapping leads to a decrease in the attentional demands of the task as reflected in reduction in the magnitude of the RT effects for memory set size or display size. The practice-related reductions in the RT effects are less pronounced with varied mapping, in which individual items occur as both targets and non-targets across trials. Madden and Nebes (1980) compared younger and older adults' performance in a consistently mapped search task, across a moderate amount of practice (2592 trials), and found that the decline in the RT effect for memory set size was similar for the two age groups. Salthouse and Somberg (1982) reported that, across approximately 5000 trials of practice with a consistently mapped memory search task, the magnitude of improvement was at least as great for older adults as for younger adults. In both of these experiments, age-related performance deficits remained significant at the end of practice. The two age groups were similar in their ability to use the task-relevant experience to reduce the attentional demands of the task, but practice did not entirely eliminate the age difference in performance.

In contrast, Fisk, Rogers, and their colleagues have proposed that practice in consistent mapping search tasks reveals significant age differences in attentional processing (e.g. Fisk and Rogers, 1991; Rogers et al., 1994). In this research, the task of interest was frequently a semantic search task in which a variable number of categories are specified as a memory set (e.g. fruits, musical instruments, animals). On each trial participants decided whether display of one or more category exemplars contained an item from one of the memory set categories. Fisk and Rogers have found that over the course of extensive practice in this and related tasks (using letters and digits), consistent mapping does not lead to the development of automaticity as readily for older adults as for younger adults. Both the amount of practice-related improvement and the disruption from transfer to new target sets were greater for younger adults than for older adults. This pattern was interpreted as an age-related deficit in priority learning, the ability to regulate the attention-attracting strength of display items, on the basis of perceived similarity to a search target. Consistent with this hypothesis of an age-related decline in priority learning, Jenkins and Hoyer (2000) reported that younger adults reached asymptotic performance at an earlier level of practice than did older adults, in a target enumeration task (i.e. press a key corresponding to the number of targets in a display).

Scialfa et al. (2000) and Ho and Scialfa (2002) obtained a different pattern of results in several experiments comparing younger and older adults' practice effects in consistent mapping search tasks (e.g. search for a white vertical line among white horizontal lines and black vertical lines). These authors found that several aspects of the data were similar for the two age groups, which would not be predicted by an age-related deficit in priority learning: The improvement in search with consistent mapping practice, the disruption of search from reversing the target-distractor mapping following practice, and the tendency to visually fixate target-relevant display items, were all comparable for younger and older adults. Scialfa et al. suggested that, for both younger and older adults, the practice-related improvement in these search tasks more likely reflected a general perceptual mechanism related to the efficient use of visual cues rather than the development of specific attentional processes as defined by priority learning.

The Scialfa et al. account is in many respects similar to a priority learning explanation, but Scialfa et al. emphasize that evidence from the eye movement and fixation data indicate that the use of visual cues mediates performance at the initial stages of practice, before the priority learning mechanisms would have had time to become established. The Scialfa et al. results differ from previous studies of age differences in visual search, in that there were minimal age-related changes in the display size effect (e.g. a tendency for the older adults' display size effects to be increased differentially on the target-absent trials). It will thus be useful to test the priority-learning deficit hypothesis further, under conditions that elicit an age-related increase in the display size effect at the early stages of practice.

6. Varieties of attentional control

A visual search task requires that attention be directed specifically to the target item rather than to the distractor items. How is this accomplished? The research discussed in this chapter shows that attentional control in visual search is multiply determined. The type and quality of information in a visual display, the mapping of targets to responses, and the amount of experience that the observer brings to the task, are all important influences on performance. In current models of visual search, these influences are often categorized as bottom–up and top–down forms of attentional control (Treisman and Sato, 1990; Wolfe, 1994, 1998). These models often share the assumption that an observer possesses a cognitive representation of the display (i.e. an activation map), in which the various features of the display are activated to a greater or lesser degree, on the basis of their similarity to the target's features. Attention is directed to the features within the map by the magnitude of the activations, thus leading to a perceptual decision and response. Bottom–up processes are those that guide the allocation of attention within the feature map on the basis of local changes in the physical properties of the display. When, for example, the target is black and all of the distractors are white (e.g. the feature task in Fig. 1), attention is drawn to the target in a bottom–up manner. Top–down processes influence attention by means of the observer's knowledge and experience with the task. The latter processes are valuable in conjunction search tasks, in which there is no single feature in the activation map denoting the presence of the target (e.g. the conjunction search task in Fig. 1). In this instance top–down processes can guide attention to the subset of display items most likely to contain the target (e.g. the black items).

The majority of search tasks represent a combination of bottom–up and top–down attentional processes, which are difficult to isolate completely. The way in which adult age interacts with these processes is an active area of investigation. Scialfa and colleagues have conducted an extensive series of experiments that have focused primarily on bottom–up processes related to the visual similarity of the target and distractor items (Scialfa and Harpur, 1994; Scialfa and Thomas, 1994; Scialfa et al., 1998). A consistent theme in this research is that increasing target-distractor similarity, which impairs target identification performance of both younger and older adults, has a more pronounced impact on older adults. This pattern would be expected from the age-related decline in visual sensory processing, and generalized slowing, discussed previously in this chapter. The results also suggest, however, that aging affects some task-dependent processes, such as shifts in response criterion (Scialfa and Harpur, 1994; Scialfa et al., 2000) that would not necessarily be predicted from the assumption of a generalized age-related decline in visual information processing.

The experiments on the effects of the color and spatial location of the display items, discussed previously in the section on "Spatial attention, selection, and inhibition" can also be considered as a form of selective attention driven by bottom–up processing. As noted in that section, there is an age constancy in many of these experiments for attentional guidance from the display properties. As an additional example, Plude and Doussard-Roosevelt (1989) reported that, in a conjunction search task (e.g. red X target among an equal number of red Os and green Xs) search rate improved dramatically for both age groups when a subset of the display items shared the target's color (e.g. a red X and two red Os among 22 green Xs), demonstrating that both age groups were able to use color as a basis for guiding attention to a subset of the display items. Madden et al. (1999a) obtained a similar pattern of results using accuracy rather than RT as the performance measure. However, variation in the spatial structure of the distractors (e.g. a homogeneous set of rotated Ls in the same orientation vs. a heterogeneous set rotated in different directions), has yielded some evidence of age-related decline in attentional guidance (Madden et al., 1996). Over the course of learning in a visual search task, the presence of covariation between the identities of the items in an individual display and the spatial location of the target leads to comparable improvements in performance for younger and older adults, even though participants are not aware that such covariation exists (Schmitter-Edgecombe and Nissley, 2002).

Tasks that depend more on top–down attentional control have also exhibited age constancy. Humphrey and Kramer (1997), for example, varied the visual features of the display in a way that was intended to isolate top–down guidance. These authors confirmed previous findings indicating that search for a target representing the conjunction of three features (e.g. red, small, and vertical) was easier than the typical conjunction search involving two features (e.g. red and vertical). As in the double conjunction case, the features defining the triple conjunction targets were distributed equally across all of the distractor items, and thus the activation map provided little guidance from bottom–up processing. The triple conjunction targets, however, differed from each individual distractor on two features (rather than one), and there was thus additional opportunity for top–down processing to either enhance the target features or inhibit the non-target features in the activation map. The advantage in search performance for the triple conjunctions was similar for younger and older adults, consistent with a preservation of top–down attentional control.

In other studies, top–down guidance has been driven by memory processes. Madden (1987) reported that younger and older adults showed a comparable performance advantage in letter search when the display formed a word, relative to when the display was a pronounceable non-word, suggesting that long-term memory information can guide attention in this task in a similar manner for both age groups. Kramer and Atchley (2000) examined top–down control in a search task relying on very short-term memory for display items. On each trial in the critical condition of this search task, one-half of the distractor items appeared first (for 1 s), and then the remaining distractors (plus the target, if present) were added. Participants knew that the target could only appear among the second distractor set. Search performance in this condition was markedly better, for both younger and older adults, than in a condition in which all of the display items were presented simultaneously. Kramer and Atchley proposed that the improvement associated with the successively presented displays represented the top–down inhibition of the first set of distractors, a phenomenon termed visual marking. That is, once the display locations of the first set of distractors are marked (within the activation map), search can be restricted to the remaining display items. Kramer and Atchley concluded that this type of attentional control was equally effective for younger and older adults, although other aspects of the RT data suggested that using this form of top–down control required more effort on the part of older adults.

Folk and Lincourt (1996) reported evidence indicating some age-related decline in top–down attentional control. Folk and Lincourt used a paradigm similar to the Kramer and Atchley (2000) investigation of visual marking, but reached a different conclusion. In the Folk and Lincourt experiment all of the display items appeared simultaneously, but each one oscillated in a particular direction (e.g. a vertically oscillating X among vertically oscillating Os and horizontally oscillating Xs). The critical manipulation was the phase of the distractor oscillation. Folk and Lincourt found that search for the vertically oscillating X target was more efficient when the display items exhibiting non-target (horizontal) motion oscillated coherently (in phase), whereas search was unaffected by whether the items sharing the target (vertical) motion oscillated coherently or incoherently. The specific association of the coherence effect to the motion of the non-targets indicates that a top–down inhibition of the non-targets is involved. Although both age groups exhibited this effect of non-target motion coherence in search RT, it was proportionately greater for younger adults, suggesting some age-related decline in this form of attentional guidance.

The experiments on age-related changes in top–down attentional control have typically used difficult search tasks, in which the target item is a conjunction of features of different non-target items. This is a logical context in which to expect a prominent contribution from top–down attentional processes, because conjunction searches are designed so that the contribution of local feature differences (i.e. bottom–up processing) to target identification is minimal. There is also evidence, however, that top–down attention can influence search performance even when the comparison process itself is highly efficient and determined primarily by bottom–up processes.

Search for a target singleton, for example, in which the target differs from all of the distractors on the same feature dimension, can be performed efficiently (i.e. with minimal effects of display size on RT). Wolfe et al. (2003) have demonstrated that younger adults' performance in a singleton search task could be influenced by top–down processing. The Wolfe et al. task required a yes/no response regarding the presence of a singleton target (e.g. a red bar among green bars). Mean RT for a color singleton was faster during blocks of trials in which the participants knew that the singleton would be a specific color, as compared to trial blocks in which the singleton feature would be color on some trials and orientation or size on other trials. In each type of trial block, however, the display size effects were minimal. Thus, this singleton search was a highly efficient, bottom–up process that could nevertheless be influenced by top–down control, in terms of knowledge of the singleton feature.

In an experiment that is currently in progress, we are using a modification of the Wolfe et al. (2003) paradigm to investigate adult age differences in this type of top–down attentional guidance. Each trial requires a yes/no response regarding the presence of a singleton. Examples of target-present displays are presented in Fig. 3. In the Feature condition, participants know that the singleton, if present, will have a particular feature value (e.g. a black bar among white bars). In the Dimension condition, participants know that the target will differ from the distractors in a particular feature dimension, but the particular value will vary randomly across trials (e.g. a black bar among white bars vs. a white bar among black bars). In the Mixed condition, the singleton feature dimension also varies randomly (i.e. the singleton may differ from the distractors in either color, size, or orientation). A useful aspect of this design is that the comparison among the conditions can be restricted to displays that have exactly the same physical properties (e.g. black targets in the Feature condition vs. blacks targets in the Mixed condition), thus equating the contribution of bottom–up processing. Our preliminary results replicate

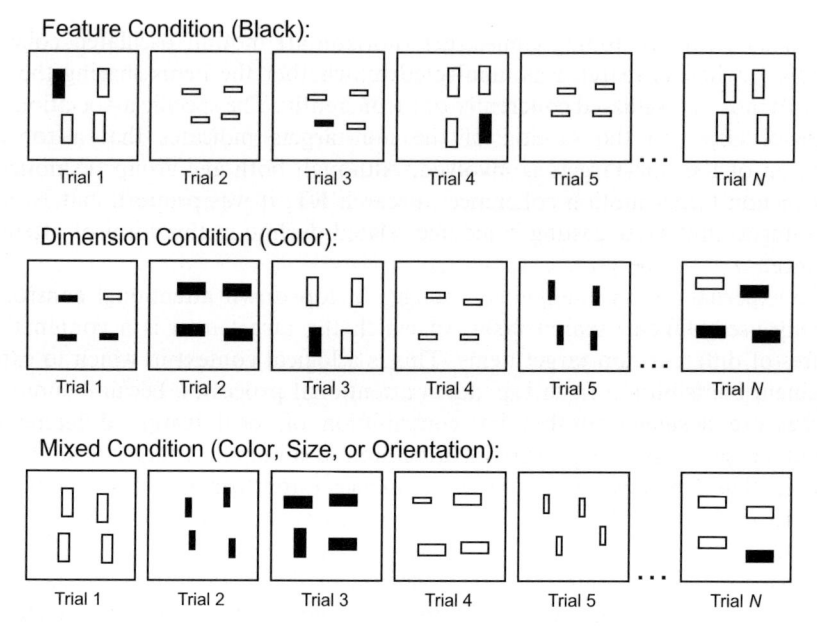

Fig. 3. A search task for investigating top–down attentional control. This is a singleton search task that requires a yes/no response to each display, regarding whether an individual target (bar) is present that differs from other display items on some feature dimension (e.g. a black bar among white bars). For the purpose of illustration, display size is constant at four items but in practice would vary. In the Feature condition, the singleton target feature is constant (e.g. the target is always a black bar). In the Dimension condition, the particular feature that distinguishes the target varies across trials, but the dimension remains constant (e.g. the target always differs from the distractors in color, but the particular target color varies). In the Mixed condition, the dimension that distinguishes the target varies across trials (e.g. the target can differ from the distractors in either color, orientation, or size). Thus, the influence of top–down attentional guidance in the Feature and Dimension conditions, relative to the Mixed condition (which does not provide any opportunity for top–down control), can be estimated for the displays (e.g. black bar targets) that have exactly the same physical properties in each condition.

the observation of Wolfe et al. that the display size effects are minimal in all of the conditions, consistent with an efficient, bottom–up search. There is also a substantial top–down influence, however, and mean RT is approximately 150 ms lower in the Feature condition than in the Mixed condition. The Dimension condition yields a smaller (50 ms) but significant advantage relative to the Mixed condition. In our preliminary analysis this pattern is very similar for younger and older adults, implying that this form of top–down attentional control is preserved as a function of adult age.

7. Divided attention

In many of the cognitive tasks performed outside the laboratory, the ability to divide attention is critical. Even though age-related decline may be minimal for some individual tasks or component processes, a decline in the ability to divide attention between tasks may disproportionately impair older adults' performance. For example, higher accident rates among older drivers have been attributed to older adults' decreased ability to efficiently co-ordinate the many functions required while driving. Simulated driving studies have found that, relative to younger adults, older adults have more difficulty keeping the simulated vehicle in its lane of traffic when performing an additional task (Ponds et al., 1988; Brouwer et al., 1991). It is difficult, however, to simulate a real-life divided attention (DA) driving experience in the laboratory setting, because real-life driving requires the co-ordination of a variety of complex abilities. Most studies have, instead, focused on whether older adults can co-ordinate two measurable cognitive tasks.

Whether older adults are truly less efficient in dividing their attention is a matter of some debate. Most of this debate centers not around whether age differences are *present* in DA tasks, but whether such differences are largely the result of age differences in single task performance where each task is performed separately, in isolation. Further, age differences in the costs of dividing attention are present in some studies (e.g. Salthouse et al., 1984), but not in others (e.g. Somberg and Salthouse, 1982). The presence of age differences in DA depends largely on one's definition of DA and the cognitive tasks and methodologies used to measure this complex construct. This section will discuss some of the methodological concerns associated with DA and aging research and will review the literature relevant to the question of whether the ability to divide attention declines with age.

7.1. Different design methodologies

The number and variety of studies on aging and DA has become quite large (see Hartley, 1992; McDowd and Shaw, 2000, for reviews). One way of categorizing these studies is in terms of two classes of task design methodologies, or paradigms. One paradigm uses the DA, or dual-task, paradigm to assess the amount of attentional resources that are required to perform a specific task – here, the DA paradigm is used as a tool to assess whether age differences in some cognitive task are the result of declining attentional resources with age. This approach investigates the intensive aspect of attention, as a limited resource that the observer must allocate among ongoing task demands (Kahneman, 1973; Lavie and Tsal, 1994). For example, Craik and McDowd (1987) examined whether age-related declines in word recall performance could be explained in terms of attentional resources. In their study, participants performed a secondary task (four-choice RT) while simultaneously recalling a list of words. Both word recall and RT task performance were compared to a condition in which each respective task was performed without distraction. For each task, the difference in performance between divided and single task conditions is the "cost" of dividing attention. Older adults showed greater DA costs both in terms of recall performance and increased RTs, leading Craik and McDowd to conclude that age-related declines in memory recall were, in part, the result of declining processing resources.

The second type of DA study questions whether older adults have a greater difficulty dividing their existing resources, regardless of whether the magnitude of these resources varies as a function of age. The distinction between these two camps may seem subtle, but they are asking very different questions. The former being, "Is older adults' lower performance on a task (e.g. memory retrieval) due to their limited attentional resources?" and the latter being, "Do older adults have greater difficulty sharing the resources they do have between two tasks?" Studies of the latter type may assume that older adults have more limited resources and that these limitations are, in part, responsible for age-related declines on cognitive tasks. What is central to this latter paradigm is the idea that older adults may have greater difficulty dividing, sharing, or co-ordinating what resources they do have relative to younger adults. Declines in such functions would point to an age-related change in what has been referred to as executive control. Here we use a definition of executive control that encompasses processes such as updating and maintaining information in working memory, shifting between mental sets, and intentionally inhibiting irrelevant information (Miyake et al., 2000).

Regardless of which of the two fundamental above questions are being asked, the most precise way to measure the ability to divide or share existing resources is to obtain an aggregate measure of DA performance reflecting performance on both tasks as well as any performance trade-offs between the two tasks. Typically, when two tasks are measured simultaneously in a DA paradigm, the result is two performance scores for each participant. Thus, one does not have a combined measure of simultaneous performance, but two separate measures. If age differences are present in one measure (e.g. word recall) but not the other (e.g. choice RT), one cannot rule out the possibility that the younger adults prioritized the recall task whereas the older adults did not. One way to control for this potential confound is to instruct participants to prioritize Task A, Task B, or both tasks, in separate conditions under DA. Performance on Tasks A and B is plotted along the x and y-axes, respectively, for each participant with single task performance being the intercept of each respective axis. The resulting functions are termed Attention Operating Characteristics (AOCs) and provide a single measure of DA difficulty, which can be expressed either as the cost of dividing attention (area above the AOC) or the amount of resources allocated (area under the AOC).

The debate regarding whether older adults are less able to divide their *existing* resources was sparked by two studies by Salthouse and colleagues (Somberg and Salthouse, 1982; Salthouse et al., 1984) that used AOCs to assess DA performance. In the first of these two carefully controlled studies, Somberg and Salthouse noted several important issues that are often not addressed, such as the interpretation of secondary task performance. Somberg and Salthouse suggested that age differences in DA performance may result because differences already exist when comparing age groups on each task in isolation. Thus age effects on DA performance may not be due to difficulties in dividing resources, but instead, reflect age differences in single task performance (see also Wright, 1981). In their experiment, Somberg and Salthouse required participants to detect a visual stimulus in two separate but simultaneously presented displays (DA condition). To control for potential age differences in single task performance, the detection tasks were presented separately, and display duration was varied until both age groups attained similar levels of accuracy under these single task conditions. Thus, any age differences under DA conditions could not be attributed to single task performance. With this methodology there were no age differences in DA costs, leading the authors to conclude that older and younger adults are equally capable of processing the additional information in the DA condition.

In a later study, Salthouse et al. (1984) proposed that the previous lack of an age effect in Somberg and Salthouse (1982) might have been due to the relatively low attentional demands required by the task in that study. Consequently, Salthouse et al. (1984) had participants remember strings of letters and digits simultaneously, assuming that this task might demand more attentional resources. As with the previous study, the two age groups were equated on single task performance. This time, however, age differences in DA costs were obtained. Older adults exhibited greater performance declines between DA and single task conditions relative to younger adults. The authors argued that the discrepancy between the two studies was likely due to the increased complexity and memory demands of the tasks used in the later study.

McDowd and Craik (1988) and Salthouse et al. (1995) provided additional evidence in support of a task complexity account of age differences in DA. McDowd and Craik plotted older adults' RTs for each task at each level of complexity, in both divided and full attention conditions, against younger adults' RTs (i.e. a Brinley plot). When age differences were plotted in this way, linear relationships between age and divided and full attention performance were present at all levels of complexity. Assuming that the same processes were required for each complexity level, these results suggest that performance under low and high levels of complexity was qualitatively similar for the two age groups. Similarly, with hierarchical regression procedures, Salthouse et al. (1995) used single task measures as well as simple processing speed to predict age-related differences in DA conditions. Few age-related differences in DA ability remained after partialling out these variables, leading Salthouse et al. to conclude that much of the age-related variance in DA ability is mediated by more basic processing resources. Thus, converging evidence suggests that task complexity contributes significantly to age differences in DA performance and that more fundamental (single task) processing resources may better account for age-related declines in DA than executive processes unique to DA such as sharing, co-ordinating, or shifting between tasks. Nonetheless, executive control processes specific to DA situations may play some role in age differences in DA given that single task processing is unable to account for all of the age-related variance in DA scores.

7.2. Divided attention and memory

Given that noticeable memory declines are a common complaint among older adults, many researchers have posited that attentional resource limitations might be, in part, responsible for these age-related declines. Studies of DA and episodic (context-dependent) memory have typically examined the encoding (study phase) and/or retrieval stages of memory. A consistent finding is that dividing attention during encoding is significantly detrimental to later memory recall while dividing attention during retrieval has little effect on recall performance (e.g. Park et al., 1989; Craik et al., 1996; Anderson et al., 1998; Whiting, 2003). Although word retrieval appears to be less sensitive to DA relative to encoding for both younger and older adults, older adults typically exhibit greater secondary task DA costs relative to younger adults when attention is divided at retrieval (Whiting and Smith, 1997; Anderson et al., 1998; Whiting, 2003). It is unclear whether age differences in these studies are greater at encoding or retrieval, because most studies used only single task analysis that fail to fully incorporate the DA costs of the other task. Nonetheless, these findings suggest that retrieving information may be particularly attentionally demanding for older adults.

The pattern of results from the above-mentioned studies illustrates the challenge of assessing encoding and retrieval differences by measuring primary and secondary task costs separately. That is, larger DA costs in the word recall task are often found during encoding, but secondary task costs are often greater during retrieval. In a recent study using the AOC methodology described previously in this section, Whiting (2003) found that encoding processes demanded more attentional resources than retrieval for both age groups. Older adults also were found to have more difficulty dividing their existing resources compared to younger adults, replicating the findings of Salthouse et al. (1984) and indicating that single task performance may not fully account for age differences in DA. These age differences, however, did not interact with encoding/retrieval, suggesting that age-related declines in DA were not related to specific memory processes. The Salthouse et al. and Whiting studies are consistent with the idea that age differences in DA are the result of declining executive processes, because younger and older participants were equated on single task performance.

7.3. Time sharing effects

One of the assumptions in the interpretation of DA performance is that participants are performing both primary and secondary tasks simultaneously, and this assumption can be questioned. Consider, for example, the task of walking through a lighted tunnel while reading a book. One would expect that the time to get through the tunnel and/or the amount read would be negatively affected relative to doing either task alone. The assumption is that for at least some duration of task time, both tasks are being performed in concert and that both tasks are competing for the same pool of resources. An alternative interpretation is that participants spend little or no time processing the tasks simultaneously, but instead parse the tasks in a serial fashion. That is, one could run half way through the tunnel, stop and read very quickly, then run out the other end. In this scenario the amount read and travel time through the tunnel may have been the same as the first scenario, except that in the latter there is no DA or time sharing of the two tasks. The core of this issue is not just whether tasks are processed only in parallel or only serially, but also whether which aspects of each task are *capable* of being performed in parallel (Pashler, 1998). So, one may be able to hold the book and see the words on the page while jogging or walking, but comprehension or maintaining one's place on the page may be impaired.

Allen et al. (1998) tested younger and older adults' time sharing ability for two tasks (e.g. Task 1 = dot location, Task 2 = letter matching) presented in closely overlapping moments in time (e.g. an SOA between tasks ranging from 150 to 1100 ms). Their hypothesis was that a response selection bottleneck might better account for age differences in dual-task processing as opposed to general processing resource limitations (Kahneman, 1973). According to Pashler's (1994) response-selection bottleneck model, in DA conditions, a response for Task 2 cannot be given until the completion of the response to Task 1. Thus, RTs to Task 2 should be longer when the Task 2 onset occurs shortly after Task 1 because responding to Task 1 delays the response to Task 2. Allen et al. found that the increase in Task 2 RT across decreasing SOA was greater for older adults than for younger adults. The authors argued that older adults have greater time-sharing difficulties than younger adults and that the locus of these difficulties occurs during response selection processes. Hartley (2001) has generally corroborated these results but proposed in addition that the time sharing bottleneck is not response selection, but rather the later process of generating the motor response.

7.4. Task switching

A relatively new line of research has proposed that some of these age-related declines in DA may be due to declines in the ability to effectively switch mental sets as required in a DA paradigm. That is, most DA tasks require the participant to respond in some alternating fashion to two tasks. Given that each task requires a different mental strategy, one possibility is that the executive control process of switching between strategies in a DA paradigm poses an additional load on attentional resources.

Some studies have mimicked such patterns of responding using task switching paradigms. Typically participants will respond to Task A for two or more consecutive trials, and then have to switch their mental set to accommodate Task B. In their simplest form, these designs follow an $A_1 A_2 B_3 B_4 A_5 A_6 B_7 B_8$ design (e.g. Kray and Lindenberger, 2000). In some studies, a cue stimulus will precede the switch between tasks to warn of a task switch (e.g. Kramer et al., 1999a), whereas in other experiments the switch will occur every n trials, and to prepare for the switch participants must monitor the number of trials since the last switch (e.g. Kray and Lindenberger, 2000). The RT difference between A_2 and B_3 is generally found to be larger than between A_1 and A_2 (Rogers and Monsell, 1995). This discrepancy is often termed the *local switch cost*. Several studies have investigated whether this switch cost might be more pronounced for older adults given age-related declines in executive function (West, 1996). The findings, however, have been mixed with some studies showing reliable age differences in local switch costs (Kramer et al., 1999a; Cepeda et al., 2001; Mayr, 2001; Meiran et al., 2001) whereas others have not (Kray and Lindenberger, 2000; Mayr and Liebscher, 2001).

A more consistent finding in task switching studies is that the mean RT for A_2 and A_6 trials is often larger in switch conditions relative to analogous non-switch/single task conditions (i.e. all trials involve the same task). This difference is considered to represent a *global switch cost*, because if task switching effects were localized only to local switches (e.g. B_3 or A_5), then RTs to non-switch trials would be the same regardless of whether they occurred in a switch or single task condition. Further, this global switch cost is typically greater than the local switch cost, and age effects are typically larger with respect to global switch costs (Mayr, 2001; Mayr and Liebscher, 2001; Meiran et al., 2001). These age-related declines have been proposed to be the result of declines in executive processes that are required under switch conditions (e.g. Kramer et al., 1999a).

As with DA studies, though single task performance accounts for a significant proportion of age-related declines in switching, significant age-related variance remains after controlling for single task performance, suggesting that there is some type of age-sensitive executive processing that appears to be distinct from executive and/or speed-related processing required by the single tasks (Kramer et al., 1999a; Cepeda et al., 2001). In fact, Cepeda et al. have argued that executive processes become more differentiated with age, as component processes (processing speed, working memory, and single task RT) accounted for less switch cost variance in older adults (47%) relative to younger adults (89%).

To conclude, evidence from DA, time sharing, and task switching studies suggests that older adults are less able to divide or co-ordinate attentional resources across multiple tasks. This type of dual-task processing places large demands on executive processing, which is proposed to be sensitive to the effects of aging. This notwithstanding, the fact that much of the age-related variance in DA and task switching can be attributable to single task performance suggests that more basic processing resources (e.g. speed of processing) may explain much of the age-related variance in these tasks. There is, however, age-related variance in these tasks that cannot be explained by general slowing in terms of single task performance. Identifying these processes, be they response conflicts or specific forms of executive processing, will need to be examined further in future research.

8. Cognitive neuroscience of aging and attention

In this chapter, we have been concerned primarily with the behavioral evidence relevant to age-related changes in visual attention, but naturally the age-related changes in the brain and central nervous system are an important determinant of the behavioral changes. Although investigation of the age-related changes in the neural systems mediating cognitive performance has a long past, it has a short history as an identifiable category of research. A landmark in this research area was the volume "Behavior, Aging, and the Nervous System," edited by Welford and Birren (1965). This perspective was also emphasized in Hartley's (1992) review of age-related changes in attention, which concluded with a section titled "Toward a Cognitive Neuroscience of Aging and Attention." The research methods and findings in this area span a variety of disciplines, including the clinical neuropsychology of aging and research in Alzheimer's disease and related dementias. Arguably the most important impetus to the emergence of the cognitive neuroscience of aging, however, has been the rapid development in neuroimaging methods, such as event-related brain potentials (ERPs), positron emission tomography (PET), and functional magnetic resonance imaging (fMRI), which have led to a series of findings with implications for age-related changes in attention.

Neuroimaging methods can be categorized into structural measures (such as structural MRI), which yield information regarding the static, physical properties of neural tissue, and functional measures (such as ERPs, fMRI, and PET), which reveal changes in some aspect of brain metabolic activity, during the performance of perceptual and cognitive tasks. Reviews of the application of these neuroimaging techniques to age-related cognitive changes have been provided by Raz (2000), Cabeza (2001), Bashore and Ridderinkhof (2002), and Madden et al. (in press). Each of the functional neuroimaging methods has characteristics that provide an advantage in a particular research context. The ERP measures have relatively coarse spatial localization for brain activity, because they are measured from the placement of electrodes on the scalp, but they have a high level of temporal resolution (on the order of milliseconds). The PET measures have relatively coarse temporal resolution (on the order of minutes), but PET yields a three-dimensional localization of brain activity within several millimeters, as well as a quantitative measure of regional cerebral blood flow (when arterial sampling is conducted). An even higher level of spatial resolution can be obtained from fMRI, and temporal resolution is on the order of seconds, but the metabolic measure is blood oxygenation rather than blood flow.

Measures from ERP have provided evidence on two issues of particular concern to understanding aging and attention. First, the ERP data support the response-bottleneck models discussed previously (Allen et al., 1998; Hartley, 2001). Bashore et al. (1989), for example, reported an important meta-analysis of studies that included both RT and the P300 component of the ERP. The latency of this ERP component is widely regarded as an index of stimulus identification time, independent of response processing. When Bashore et al. performed Brinley plot analysis on these data (see General vs. specific effects of attention), they found that the Brinley plot slope for the P300 latencies was near 1.0, whereas the slope for the RT values was above 1.0 as is typically observed. Because the P300 latency is affected minimally by response-related variables, these results suggest that response processing may contribute disproportionately to the age-related slowing depicted in Brinley plots of RT data.

The second issue on which ERP measures have been informative is the comparison between older adults and brain damaged patients. Bashore and Ridderinkhof (2002), applying Brinley plot methodology to meta-analysis of data from brain damaged patients, found that, as in the case of older adults, the slowing exhibited by brain damaged individuals, relative to age-matched controls, was disproportionately influenced by response processing. The slowing related to stimulus identification processes, however, was greater than in the case of aging. In addition, the response slowing associated with brain damage appeared to represent a reduced activation of the response system, whereas for healthy older adults response slowing appeared to result from an increased activation of the response system. Thus, although the results from PET and fMRI investigations provide important information regarding the regional changes in brain function associated with aging, it is also important to bear in mind that aging is not equivalent to brain damage.

Hartley (1992) noted that age-related changes in attention can be interpreted in the context of anterior and posterior attention systems defined on the basis of neuroimaging studies. The anterior system, involving the anterior cingulate and basal ganglia, mediates attention to cognitive operations, whereas the posterior system, involving the superior parietal cortex, pulvinar, and superior colliculus, mediates selective attention to individual objects or spatial locations, as well as shifting attention between stimuli (Posner and Dehaene, 1994). In view of the behavioral evidence reviewed in this chapter, a logical prediction would be that age-related changes in brain function would be more clearly evident for tasks relying on the anterior attention system (e.g. dual-task performance) than for tasks relying on the posterior system (e.g. selective attention to spatial location; Hartley, 1993). This type of prediction has been developed more explicitly in the frontal lobe hypothesis of cognitive aging, which proposes that a differential decline in the structure and function of the frontal lobe leads to the observed pattern of age-related decline in behavioral measures of memory and attention. Dempster (1992) discussed this hypothesis with regard to the specific function of inhibitory control. West (1996) outlined a comprehensive theory of age-related change in frontal lobe functioning in relation to several aspects of memory and attention.

Although, relatively few neuroimaging studies of age-related changes in attention have been conducted, the results are suggestive of a prominent role for frontal cortical regions. Johannsen et al. (1997) used PET to measure regional cerebral blood flow (rCBF) while older adult participants performed either a sustained attention task (monitoring a repeating stimulus in either the visual or tactile modalities for a change in frequency) or a divided attention task (monitoring both modalities simultaneously). Relative to control conditions that included comparable stimuli without the monitoring requirement, rCBF was increased in the middle frontal gyrus of the right hemisphere during both tasks, with more prominent activation during divided attention. Activation in the right inferior parietal lobule was more evident during the sustained attention condition. All of the participants in the Johannsen et al. study were between 51 and 73 years of age, however, and age-related changes were not assessed. Madden et al. (1997) examined age differences in selective and divided attention using PET. Participants searched through series of nine-letter displays for the presence of a target letter that either occurred predictably in the central location (the selective attention condition) or could appear in any of

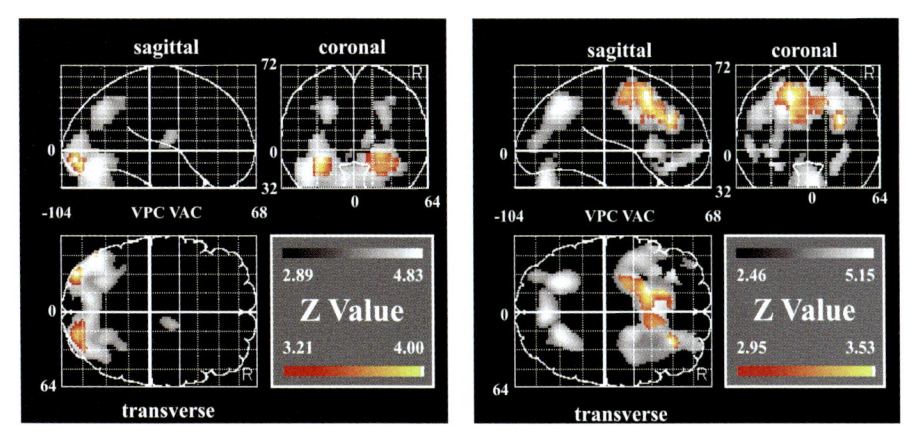

Fig. 4. Changes in regional cerebral blood flow associated with dividing attention during visual search performance (reprinted with permission from Madden et al., 1997). Measurement of cerebral blood flow was obtained by PET during a two-choice search task in which, on each of a series of trials, participants pressed one of two response keys according to which of two pre-assigned target letters was present in a 3×3 letter display. In the Central condition, the target was always presented in the central display location. In the Divided condition, the target could occur at any of the nine locations. The images are normalized voxel maps representing the average increase in blood flow associated with the Divided condition, relative to the Central condition. The images are presented in standard neurologic orientation, so that the left half of the coronal image and the upper half of the transverse image correspond to the subject's left hemisphere. The increases in cerebral blood flow for each age group are presented in the gray-scale values. Within each age group, those voxels that differed significantly from those of the other age group are presented in the color-scale values. The figure illustrates activation in occipital cortex that was relatively greater for younger adults, and activation in prefrontal cortex that was relatively greater for older adults.

the nine display positions (the divided attention condition). Age differences in the RT and accuracy of search performance, as well as in rCBF activation, were greater in the divided attention condition than in the selective attention condition. In the divided attention condition, activation in the occipital cortex was greater in magnitude for younger adults than for older adults, whereas activation in prefrontal cortex was relatively greater in magnitude, and more extensive spatially, for older adults (Fig. 4).

In view of West's (1996) hypothesis of an age-related decline in prefrontal functioning, the finding of an age-related increase in prefrontal activation is surprising. If this pattern of prefrontal activation is viewed as increased effort, however, then the Madden et al. data may be consistent with the West model. That is, some search processes that rely on divided attention may require a minimum level of executive control for younger adults and can be completed efficiently by letter recognition processes mediated by the occipital cortex. For older adults, however, these same processes require the recruitment of additional attentional functions mediated by prefrontal cortical regions. A similar pattern of age-related increase in prefrontal activation has been noted in several PET studies of memory tasks and has led to the proposal that the older adults' activation represents a compensatory recruitment of prefrontal processing (Cabeza et al., 1997; Grady and Craik, 2000).

Studies using fMRI have suggested that the age-related increase in prefrontal activation is related to specific forms of attentional control. DiGirolamo et al. (2001) emphasized the role of executive processing. These authors compared younger and older adults' fMRI activation and behavioral performance associated with switching between two tasks (judging either the identity or number of items in a visual display), relative to a non-switch (single task) baseline and fixation control conditions. Older adults exhibited both greater switch costs and a different pattern of prefrontal activation than younger adults. Specifically, both age groups exhibited activation in dorsolateral and medial prefrontal cortex during the task switching condition, relative to the fixation control. For the younger adults, however, activation in the non-switch, single task condition was at a low level, comparable to the fixation control, whereas the older adults exhibited a higher level of prefrontal activation in the non-switch condition relative to the fixation condition. Thus, the level of task switching activation relative to the non-switch condition was actually smaller for older adults than for younger adults, because the older adults, and not the younger adults, were engaging prefrontal regions during non-switch condition. The spatial extent of the prefrontal activation was also relatively greater for the older adults. DiGirolamo et al. suggested that the older adults recruited prefrontal regions in a compensatory manner to engage executive attentional control processes that were not required by younger adults.

Nielson et al. (2002) characterized age-related increases in prefrontal activation, obtained from fMRI, in terms of the inhibitory control aspect of attention. Four groups from 18 to 78 years of age performed a conditional go/no-go task that required monitoring a series of individually presented letters for X and Y targets. Participants responded manually when the current target was an alternation (e.g. respond to a current Y when the most recent target was an X), but withheld a response when the target was a repetition (e.g. do not respond to the current Y when the most recent target was another Y). Analysis of fMRI activation indicated that right prefrontal and parietal regions were activated generally across the age groups. Older adults, especially those who were less successful at response inhibition, activated additional areas within the right hemisphere, as well as in left prefrontal and parietal areas, which Nielson et al. interpreted in terms of compensatory recruitment. Milham et al. (2002) performed an fMRI analysis of the Stroop task and reported that the presence of irrelevant information (i.e. the presence of either a congruent or incongruent color word, relative to a neutral word) was associated with age-related decreases in dorsolateral, prefrontal, and parietal activation. The conflicting information represented by incongruent trials, however, led to age-related increases in anterior inferior regions of prefrontal cortex, as well as in the anterior cingulate. Milham et al. discussed this pattern of age differences in terms of attentional control rather than recruitment. Because older adults' attentional control of the competing sources of task information was less efficient than that of younger adults, additional irrelevant information entered working memory, resulting in additional activation.

Although an age-related increase in the magnitude and extent of prefrontal activation is one type of result suggesting a compensatory mechanism, other patterns of brain activation may also fulfill this role. Madden et al. (2002) compared younger and older adults' search performance (detection of an upright L among rotated Ls), using PET, and found that very similar regions of activation in the anterior and posterior attentional systems were evident for the two age groups. Activation in the occipital and temporal cortical regions associated with visual processing was more prominent for younger adults than for older adults, which appeared to result from older adults' maintaining a higher level of activation (relative to younger adults) in the easier task conditions, a pattern also noted by DiGirolamo et al. (2001). Thus, age-related compensation may involve an adjustment of the level of activation within a region, rather than the recruitment of additional prefrontal regions. In addition, age-related increases in the spatial extent of activation, while compensatory, may represent a more general principle related to a reduction in hemispheric asymmetry of function (Cabeza, 2002).

Current applications of neuroimaging to age differences in cognitive performance have been particularly concerned with the prefrontal regions, because both the structural and metabolic changes that occur in these cortical regions, as a function of age, are greater than in other brain regions. Age-related changes occur throughout the brain, however, and as this research progresses the potential contribution of other cortical and subcortical brain regions, functioning in concert with prefrontal systems, should become more clear. Rubin (1999), for example, has emphasized that prefrontal cortical regions function in the context of neural pathways to subcortical nuclei (basal ganglia) and that it may be counterproductive to focus exclusively on prefrontal regions in isolation from this larger context. Rubin pointed out that many of the age-related cognitive changes attributed to the frontal lobe are also consistent with the known functions of components of the basal ganglia, such as the caudate nucleus. Because the speed of information processing depends on the integrity of the caudate and related subcortical structures (Hicks and Birren, 1970), neuroimaging of cortical-subcortical circuits may prove useful in addressing the important theoretical issue of whether specific attentional functions such as inhibition and selection can be distinguished from the more general resource of processing speed.

A fundamental assumption of functional neuroimaging is that the metabolic activity of gray matter (nerve cells) represents sensory and cognitive processing, and it is thus natural that this research has focused primarily on the structural and functional properties of gray matter. The white matter (axon) tracts may also be an important source of age-related change, however, because these tracts mediate the transmission of neural signals among cortical regions. Among healthy older adults 84–95 years of age, the reduction in prefrontal white matter volume is greater than the reduction in prefrontal gray matter volume, compared to individuals 65–76 years of age (Salat et al., 1999). Subclinical pathology of white matter in otherwise healthy adults, evident on structural MRI scans as white matter hyperintensities, increases with age and correlates with performance declines on psychometric tests of processing speed, attention, and memory (Gunning-Dixon and Raz, 2000).

A recently developed imaging modality, diffusion tensor MRI, provides a measure of the integrity of white matter in terms of fractional anisotropy (FA), the directionality of water diffusion. Increasing FA represents greater integrity of white matter tracts, with axons oriented in the same direction. Pfefferbaum et al. (2000) reported an age-related decline in FA within the corpus callosum, which was more pronounced for the anterior segment (genu) than for the posterior segment (splenium). This finding is consistent with the frontal lobe hypothesis discussed previously. Similarly, O'Sullivan et al. (2001) found that the FA value of selected anterior brain regions, but not posterior regions, declined significantly as a function of adult age, even when white matter volume was taken into account. These authors also reported that, within the older group, declining FA was correlated with declining performance on a psychometric test of attention (Trail Making). Further studies of diffusion tensor MRI will thus complement other measures of structural and functional neuroimaging in providing a more comprehensive account of the neural systems mediating age-related changes in attention.

9. Conclusion

The research reviewed in this chapter illustrates the multifaceted aspect of attention and the wide range of influences on age-related changes in attentional functioning. A major focus of this research has been the attempt to isolate different aspects or components of attention, such as selection, effort, and vigilance. Developments in cognitive neuroscience and neuroimaging have, in addition, made it possible to investigate age-related changes in the components of attention within the context of the cognitive neuroscience of aging. Although considerable progress has been made, this research also leads to the recognition that, at least in the visual modality, the various influences on attention operate interactively rather than in isolation.

Investigations of sensory-level processing have documented a significant contribution from age-related decline in sensory processes (e.g. visual feature extraction) to performance in visual search and attention tasks. The sensory decline is most clearly evident in data-limited tasks (e.g. with extremely brief display duration) and is not sufficient as an explanation for all age-related attentional effects, because performance in psychophysical sensory tasks is itself influenced by attention. The age-related sensory changes are highly correlated with age-related effects in higher-order cognitive functions such as memory and reasoning, however, and this relation, as well as the substantial proportion of age-related variance that nearly all cognitive tasks share with elementary measures of perceptual-motor speed, indicates that a generalized slowing of the speed of information processing in the central nervous system is a fundamental aspect of age-related changes in measures of visual attention. In visual search tasks, for example, age-related slowing, combined with the requirement to discriminate relevant and irrelevant information (i.e. separate the target item from surrounding distractors), typically leads to an age-related increase in the display size effect. Similarly, dividing attention among simultaneously competing tasks is often more difficult for older adults than for younger adults, which suggests that age differences in the efficiency of executive control processes, especially those related to response selection, make a unique contribution to age-related changes in cognitive performance.

This evidence of age-related decline is balanced by a preservation of several attentional functions. In the domain of highly skilled tasks, performance is often more closely related to the level of expertise than to age. The rate of improvement in some search tasks is also comparable for younger and older adults, implying some preservation of the attentional control processes related to learning. An age constancy has been frequently observed in the ability to improve performance from advance cuing of the relevant display information (i.e. selective attention). These selective attention effects can be driven either from the physical properties of the display (bottom–up) or the observer's knowledge of the task (top–down). The line between these various forms of attentional guidance, which are relatively preserved as a function of age, and executive control processes, which are relatively impaired, has not yet been established.

The attentional processes that exhibit age-related decline, as well as those that exhibit a preserved level of function, are properties of the brain and central nervous system, and findings from neuroimaging and related techniques are leading to the development of a cognitive neuroscience of aging. One theme emerging from this research area is that age-related changes in the structure and functions of the prefrontal cortical region mediate many of the declines in attentional and cognitive performance exhibited by older adults. The neuroimaging evidence highlighting this central role for prefrontal regions often includes an age-related increase in prefrontal activation during cognitive performance, which may represent a compensatory recruitment of prefrontal regions not typically used by younger adults for a particular task. Other patterns of age-related change in cortical activation, however, such as a differential activation within the same neural pathway activated by younger adults, may also represent a compensatory mechanism. As this work in cognitive neuroscience progresses, we expect that the focus will not be limited to specific brain regions, but will include neural systems distributed throughout the brain. Because speed of processing is a fundamental aspect of age-related change in attention, the properties of subcortical structures such as the basal ganglia, as well as the integrity of the white matter pathways connecting cortical regions, are also promising avenues of investigation.

Acknowledgments

Preparation of this chapter was supported by research grants R37 AG02163 and R01 AG11622 from the National Institute on Aging. We are grateful to Susanne Harris and Leslie Crandell for technical assistance.

References

Allen, P.A., Hall, R.J., Druley, J.A., Smith, A.F., Sanders, R.E., Murphy, M.D., 2001. How shared are age-related influences on cognitive and non-cognitive variables? Psychol. Aging 16, 532–549.

Allen, P.A., Madden, D.J., Weber, T.A., Groth, K.E., 1993. Influence of age and processing stage on visual word recognition. Psychol. Aging 8, 274–282.

Allen, P.A., Smith, A.F., Vires-Collins, H., Sperry, S., 1998. The psychological refractory period: Evidence for age differences in attentional time-sharing. Psychol. Aging 13, 218–229.

Allen, P.A., Weber, T.A., Madden, D.J., 1994. Adult age differences in attention: filtering or selection? J. Gerontol. Psychol. Sci. 49, P213–P222.

Anderson, N.D., Craik, F.I.M., Naveh-Benjamin, M., 1998. The attentional demands of encoding and retrieval in younger and older adults: 1. Evidence from divided attention costs. Psychol. Aging 13, 405–423.

Anderson, N.D., Craik, F.I.M., Naveh-Benjamin, M., 1999. The attentional demands of encoding and retrieval in younger and older adults: 2. Evidence from secondary task reaction time distributions. Psychol. Aging 14, 645–655.

Atchley, P., Kramer, A.F., 1998. Spatial cuing in a stereoscopic display: Attention remains "depth-aware" with age. J. Gerontol. Psychol. Sci. 53B, P318–P323.

Atchley, P., Kramer, A.F., 2000. Age-related changes in the control of attention in depth. Psychol. Aging 15, 78–87.

Baddeley, A., 1993. Working memory or working attention? In: Baddeley, A., Weiskrantz, L. (Eds.), Attention: Selection, Awareness, and Control, Clarendon Press, Oxford, pp. 152–170.

Ball, K.K., Beard, B.L., Roenker, D.L., Miller, R.L., Griggs, D.S., 1988. Age and visual search: Expanding the useful field of view. J. Opt. Soc. Am. A-Opt. Image. Sci. 5, 2210–2219.

Baltes, P.B., Lindenberger, U., 1997. Emergence of a powerful connection between sensory and cognitive functions across adult life span: A new window to the study of cognitive aging? Psychol. Aging 12, 12–21.

Bashore, T.R., 1993. Differential effects of aging on the neurocognitive functions subserving speeded mental processing. In: Cerella, J., Rybash, J., Hoyer, W., Commons, M.L. (Eds.) Adult Information Processing: Limits on Loss, Academic Press, San Diego, pp. 37–76.

Bashore, T.R., 1994. Some thoughts on neurocognitive slowing. Acta Psychol. 86, 295–325.

Bashore, T.R., Osman, A., Heffley, E.F., 1989. Mental slowing in elderly persons: A cognitive psychophysiological analysis. Psychol. Aging 4, 235–244.

Bashore, T.R., Ridderinkhof, K.R., 2002. Older age, traumatic brain injury, and cognitive slowing: Some convergent and divergent findings. Psychol. Bull. 128, 151–198.

Bedard, A.-C., Nichols, S., Barbosa, J.A., Schachar, R., Logan, G.D., Tannock, R., 2002. The development of selective inhibitory control across the life span. Dev. Neuropsychol. 21, 93–111.

Berardi, A., Parasuraman, R., Haxby, J.V., 2001. Overall vigilance and sustained attention decrements in healthy aging. Exp. Aging Res. 27, 19–39.

Birren, J.E., Fisher, L.M., 1995. Aging and speed of behavior: Possible consequences for psychological functioning. Annu. Rev. Psychol. 46, 329–353.

Birren, J.E., Riegel, K.F., Morrison, D.F., 1962. Age differences in response speed as a function of controlled variations of stimulus conditions: Evidence of a general speed factor. Gerontol. 6, 1–18.

Briggs, S.D., Raz, N., Marks, W., 1999. Age-related deficits in generation and manipulation of mental images: I. The role of sensorimotor speed and working memory. Psychol. Aging 14, 427–435.

Brink, J.M., McDowd, J.M., 1999. Aging and selective attention: An issue of complexity or multiple mechanisms? J. Gerontol. Psychol. Sci. 54B, P30–P33.

Brinley, J.F., 1965. Cognitive sets, speed and accuracy of performance in the elderly. In: Welford, A.T., Birren, J.E. (Eds.), Behavior, Aging, and the Nervous System, Charles C. Thomas, Springfield, IL, pp. 114–149.

Brouwer, W.H., Waterink, W., Van Wolffelaar, P.C., Rothengatter, T., 1991. Divided attention in experienced young and older drivers: Lane tracking and visual analysis in a dynamic driving simulator. Hum. Factors 33, 573–582.

Bryan, J., Luszcz, M., 1996. Speed of processing as a mediator between age and free recall performance. Psychol. Aging 11, 3–9.

Burke, D.M., 1997. Language, aging, and inhibitory deficits: Evaluation of a theory. J. Gerontol. Psychol. Sci. 52B, P254–P264.

Cabeza, R., 2001. Functional neuroimaging of cognitive aging. In: Cabeza, R., Kingstone, A. (Eds.), Handbook of Functional Neuroimaging of Cognition, MIT Press, Cambridge, MA, pp. 331–377.

Cabeza, R., 2002. Hemispheric asymmetry reduction in old adults: The HAROLD model. Psychol. Aging 17, 85–100.

Cabeza, R., Grady, C.L., Nyberg, L., McIntosh, A.R., Tulving, E., Kapur, S., Jennings, J.M., Houle, S., Craik, F.I.M., 1997. Age-related differences in neural activity during memory encoding and retrieval: A positron emission tomography study. J. Neurosci. 17, 391–400.

Cameron, E.L., Tai, J.C., Carrasco, M., 2002. Covert attention affects the psychometric function of contrast sensitivity. Vision Res. 42, 949–967.

Carrasco, M., Penpepci-Talgar, C., Eckstein, M., 2000. Spatial covert attention increases contrast sensitivity along the CSF: Support for signal enhancement. Vision Res. 40, 1203–1215.

Cepeda, N.J., Kramer, A.F., Gonzalez de Sather, J.C., 2001. Changes in executive control across the life span: Examination of task-switching performance. Dev. Psychol. 37, 715–730.

Cerella, J., 1985. Information processing rates in the elderly. Psychol. Bull. 98, 67–83.

Cerella, J., 1990. Aging and information-processing rate. In: Birren, J.E., Schaie, K.W. (Eds.), Handbook of the Psychology of Aging, 3rd ed. Academic Press, San Diego, pp. 201–221.

Cerella, J., Poon, L.W., Williams, D.M., 1980. Age and the complexity hypothesis. In: Poon, L.W. (Ed.), Aging in the 1980s: Psychological Issues, American Psychological Association, Washington, DC, pp. 332–340.

Charness, N., 1981a. Aging and skilled problem solving. J. Exp. Psychol. Gen. 110, 21–38.

Charness, N., 1981b. Search in chess: Age and skill differences. J. Exp. Psychol. Hum. Percept. Perform. 7, 467–476.

Craik, F.I.M., Govoni, R., Naveh-Benjamin, M., Anderson, N.D., 1996. The effects of divided attention on encoding and retrieval processes in human memory. J. Exp. Psychol. Gen. 125, 159–180.

Craik, F.I.M., McDowd, J.M., 1987. Age differences in recall and recognition. J. Exp. Psychol. Learn. Mem. Cogn. 13, 474–479.

Craik, F.I.M., Naveh-Benjamin, M., Ishaik, G., Anderson, N.D., 2000. Divided attention during encoding and retrieval: Differential control effects? J. Exp. Psychol. Learn. Mem. Cogn. 26, 1744–1749.

Davis, E.T., Fujawa, G., Shikano, T., 2002. Perceptual processing and search efficiency of young and older adults in a simple-feature search task: A staircase approach. J. Gerontol. Psychol. Sci. 57B, P324–P337.

Dempster, F.N., 1992. The rise and fall of the inhibitory mechanism: Toward a unified theory of cognitive development and aging. Dev. Rev. 12, 45–75.

DiGirolamo, G.J., Kramer, A.F., Barad, V., Cepeda, N.J., Weissman, D.H., Milham, M.P., Wszalek, T.M., Cohen, N.J., Banich, M.T., Webb, A., Belopolsky, A.V., McAuley, E., 2001. General and task-specific frontal lobe recruitment in older adults during executive processes: A fMRI investigation of task-switching. NeuroReport 12, 2065–2071.

Di Lollo, V., Arnett, J.L., Kruk, R.V., 1982. Age-related changes in rate of visual information processing. J. Exp. Psychol. Hum. Percept. Perform. 8, 225–237.

Dosher, B.A., Lu, Z., 2000. Mechanisms of perceptual attention in precuing of location. Vision Res. 40, 1269–1292.

Duncan, J., 1984. Selective attention and the organization of visual information. J. Exp. Psychol. Gen. 113, 501–517.

Duncan, J., 1993. Selection of input and goal in the control of behavior. In: Baddeley, A., Weiskrantz, L. (Eds.), Attention: Selection, Awareness, and Control, Clarendon Press, Oxford, pp. 53–71.

Eckstein, M.P., Thomas, J.P., Palmer, J., Shimozaki, S.S., 2000. A signal detection model predicts the effects of set size on visual search accuracy for feature, conjunction, triple conjunction, and disjunction displays. Percept. Psychophys. 62, 425–451.

Ellis, R.D., Goldberg, J.H., Detweiler, M.C., 1996. Predicting age-related differences in visual information processing using a two-stage queuing model. J. Gerontol. Psychol. Sci. 51B, P155–P165.

Eriksen, C.W., 1990. Attentional search of the visual field. In: Brogan, D. (Ed.), Visual Search, Taylor & Francis, London, pp. 3–19.

Eriksen, C.W., Hamlin, R.M., Breitmeyer, R.G., 1970. Temporal factors in visual perception as related to aging. Percept. Psychophys. 7, 354–356.

Eriksen, C.W., Schultz, D.W., 1979. Information processing in visual search: A continuous flow conception and experimental results. Percept. Psychophys. 25, 249–263.

Eriksen, C.W., Yeh, Y.-Y., 1985. Allocation of attention in the visual field. J. Exp. Psychol. Hum. Percept. Perform. 11, 583–597.

Faust, M.E., Balota, D.A., Spieler, D.H., Ferraro, F.R., 1999. Individual differences in information processing rate and amount: Implications for group differences in response latency. Psychol. Bull. 125, 777–799.

Fisk, A.D., Rogers, W.A., 1991. Toward an understanding of age-related memory and visual search effects. J. Exp. Psychol. Gen. 120, 131–149.

Folk, C.L., Hoyer, W.J., 1992. Aging and shifts of visual spatial attention. Psychol. Aging 7, 453–465.

Folk, C.L., Lincourt, A.E., 1996. The effects of age on guided conjunction search. Exp. Aging Res. 22, 99–118.

Fozard, J.K., Gordon-Salant, S., 2001. Changes in vision and hearing with aging. In: Birren, J.E., Schaie, K.W. (Eds.), Handbook of the Psychology of Aging, 5th ed. Academic Press, San Diego, pp. 241–266.

Freeman, E., Sagi, D., Driver, J., 2001. Lateral interactions between targets and flankers in low-level vision depend on attention to flankers. Nat. Neurosci. 4, 1032–1036.

Galton, F., 1885. On the anthropometric laboratory at the late International Health Exhibition. J. Anthropol. Inst. 14, 205–218.

Glasser, A., Campbell, M.C.W., 1999. Biometric, optical and physical changes in isolated human crystalline lens with age in relation to presbyopia. Vision Res. 39, 1991–2015.

Grady, C.L., Craik, F.I.M., 2000. Changes in memory processing with age. Curr. Opin. Neurobiol. 10, 224–231.

Greene, H.A., Madden, D.J., 1987. Adult age differences in visual acuity, stereopsis, and contrast sensitivity. Am. J. Optom. Physiol. Opt. 64, 749–753.

Greenwood, P.M., Parasuraman, R., 1999. Scale of attentional focus in visual search. Percept. Psychophys. 61, 837–859.

Groth, K.E., Allen, P.A., 2000. Visual attention and aging. Front. Biosci. 5, d284–d297.

Gunning-Dixon, F.M., Raz, N., 2000. The cognitive correlates of white matter abnormalities in normal aging: A quantitative review. Neuropsychology 14, 224–232.

Haegerstrom-Portnoy, G., Schneck, M.E., Brabyn, J.A., 1999. Seeing into old age: Vision function beyond acuity. Optom. Vis. Sci. 76, 141–158.

Hahn, S., Kramer, A.F., 1995. Attentional flexibility and aging: You don't need to be 20 years of age to split the beam. Psychol. Aging 10, 597–609.

Hale, S., Jansen, J., 1994. Global processing-time coefficients characterize individual and group differences in cognitive speed. Psychol. Sci. 5, 384–389.

Hale, S., Myerson, J., Wagstaff, D., 1987. General slowing of nonverbal information processing: Evidence for a power law. J. Gerontol. 42, 132–136.

Hartley, A.A., 1992. Attention. In: Craik, F.I.M., Salthouse, T.A. (Eds.), The Handbook of Aging and Cognition, Erlbaum, Hillsdale, NJ, pp. 3–50.

Hartley, A.A., 1993. Evidence for the selective preservation of spatial selective attention in old age. Psychol. Aging 8, 371–379.

Hartley, A.A., 2001. Age differences in dual-task interference are localized to response-generation processes. Psychol. Aging 16, 47–54.

Hartley, A.A., Kieley, J.M., 1995. Adult age differences in the inhibition of return of visual attention. Psychol. Aging 10, 670–683.

Hartley, A.A., Kieley, J.M., Slabach, E.H., 1990. Age differences and similarities in the effects of cues and prompts. J. Exp. Psychol. Hum. Percept. Perform. 16, 523–537.

Hartley, A.A., McKenzie, C.R.M., 1991. Attentional and perceptual contributions to the identification of extrafoveal stimuli: Adult age comparisons. J. Gerontol. Psychol. Sci. 46, P202–P206.

Hasher, L., Stoltzfus, E.R., Zacks, R.T., Rypma, B., 1991. Age and inhibition. J. Exp. Psychol. Learn. Mem. Cog. 17, 163–169.

Hasher, L., Zacks, R.T., 1988. Working memory, comprehension, and aging: A review and a new review. In: Bower, G.H. (Ed.), The Psychology of Learning and Motivation, Vol. 22. Academic Press, Orlando, pp. 193–225.

Henderson, J.M., 1991. Stimulus discrimination following covert attentional orienting to an exogenous cue. J. Exp. Psychol. Hum. Percept. Perform. 17, 91–106.

Hicks, L.H., Birren, J.E., 1970. Aging, brain damage, and psychomotor slowing. Psychol. Bull. 74, 377–396.

Ho, G., Scialfa, C.T., 2002. Age, skill transfer, and conjunction search. J. Gerontol. Psychol. Sci. 57B, P277–P287.

Humphrey, D.G., Kramer, A.F., 1997. Age differences in visual search for feature, conjunction, and triple-conjunction targets. Psychol. Aging 12, 704–717.

Jenkins, L., Hoyer, W.J., 2000. Instance-based automaticity and aging: Acquisition, reacquisition, and long-term retention. Psychol. Aging 15, 551–565.

Johannsen, P., Jakobsen, J., Bruhn, P., Hansen, S.B., Gee, A., Stodkilde-Jorgensen, H., Gjedde, A., 1997. Cortical sites of sustained and divided attention in normal elderly humans. NeuroImage 6, 145–155.

Johnson, C.A., Adams, A.J., Lewis, R.A., 1989. Evidence for a neural basis of age-related visual field loss in normal observers. Invest. Ophthal. Vis. Sci. 30, 2056–2064.

Kahn, H.A., 1977. The Framingham eye study. 1. Outline and major prevalence findings. Amer. J. Epidemiol. 106, 17–41.

Kahneman, D., 1973. Attention and Effort, Prentice-Hall, Englewood Cliffs, NJ.

Kane, M.J., Hasher, L., Stoltzfus, E.R., Zacks, R.T., Connelly, S.L., 1994. Inhibitory attentional mechanisms and aging. Psychol. Aging 9, 103–112.

Kieley, J.M., Hartley, A.A., 1997. Age-related equivalence of identity suppression in the Stroop color-word task. Psychol. Aging 12, 22–29.

Kline, D.W., Scialfa, C.T., 1996. Visual and auditory aging. In: Birren, J.W., Schaie, K.W. (Eds.), Handbook of the Psychology of Aging, 4th ed. Academic Press, San Diego, pp. 181–203.

Koga, Y., Morant, G.M., 1923. On the degree of association between reaction times in the case of different senses. Biometrika 15, 346–372.

Kramer, A.F., Atchley, P., 2000. Age-related effects in the marking of old objects in visual search. Psychol. Aging 15, 286–296.

Kramer, A.F., Hahn, S., Gopher, D., 1999a. Task coordination and aging: Explorations of executive control processes in the task switching paradigm. Acta. Psychol. 101, 339–378.

Kramer, A.F., Hahn, S., Irwin, D.E., Theeuwes, J., 1999b. Attentional capture and aging: Implications for visual search performance and oculomotor control. Psychol. Aging 14, 135–154.

Kramer, A.F., Humphrey, D.G., Larish, J.F., Logan, G.D., Strayer, D.L., 1994. Aging and inhibition: Beyond a unitary view of inhibitory processing in attention. Psychol. Aging 9, 491–512.

Kramer, A.F., Martin-Emerson, R., Larish, J.F., Andersen, G.J., 1996. Aging and filtering by movement in visual search. J. Gerontol. Psychol. Sci. 51B, P201–P216.

Kramer, A.F., Weber, T.A., 1999. Object-based attentional selection and aging. Psychol. Aging 14, 99–107.

Kray, J., Lindenberger, U., 2000. Adult age differences in task switching. Psychol. Aging 15, 126–147.

LaBerge, D., 1983. Spatial extent of attention to letters and words. J. Exp. Psychol. Hum. Percept. Perform. 9, 371–379.

Lavie, N., Tsal, Y., 1994. Perceptual load as a major determinant of the locus of selection in visual attention. Percept. Psychophys. 56, 183–197.

Lima, S.D., Hale, S., Myerson, J., 1991. How general is general slowing? Evidence from the lexical domain. Psychol. Aging 6, 416–425.

Lincourt, A.E., Folk, C.L., Hoyer, W.J., 1997. Effects of aging on voluntary and involuntary shifts of attention. Aging Neuropsychol. Cog. 4, 290–303.

Lindenberger, U., Baltes, P.B., 1994. Sensory functioning and intelligence in old age: A strong connection. Psychol. Aging 9, 339–355.

Little, D.M., Hartley, A.A., 2000. Further evidence that negative priming in the Stroop color-word task is equivalent in older and younger adults. Psychol. Aging 15, 9–17.

Madden, D.J., 1983. Aging and distraction by highly familiar stimuli during visual search. Dev. Psychol. 19, 499–507.

Madden, D.J., 1987. Aging, attention, and the use of meaning during visual search. Cog. Dev. 2, 201–216.

Madden, D.J., 1988. Adult age differences in the effects of sentence context and stimulus degradation during visual word recognition. Psychol. Aging 3, 167–172.

Madden, D.J., 1990. Adult age differences in the time course of visual attention. J. Gerontol. Psychol. Sci. 45, P9–P16.

Madden, D.J., 1992a. Four to ten milliseconds per year: Age-related slowing of visual word identification. J. Gerontol. Psychol. Sci. 47, P59–P68.

Madden, D.J., 1992b. Selective attention and visual search: Revision of an allocation model and application to age differences. J. Exp. Psychol. Hum. Percept. Perform. 18, 821–836.

Madden, D.J., 2001. Speed and timing of behavioral processes. In: Birren, J.E., Schaie, K.W. (Eds.), Handbook of the Psychology of Aging, 5th ed. Academic Press, San Diego, pp. 288–312.

Madden, D.J., Allen, P.A., 1991. Adult age differences in the rate of information extraction during visual search. J. Gerontol. Psychol. Sci. 46, P124–P126.

Madden, D.J., Gottlob, L.R., 1997. Adult age differences in strategic and dynamic components of focusing visual attention. Aging Neuropsychol. Cog. 4, 185–210.

Madden, D.J., Gottlob, L.R., Allen, P.A., 1999a. Adult age differences in visual search accuracy: Attentional guidance and target detectability. Psychol. Aging 14, 683–694.

Madden, D.J., Langley, L.K., 2003. Age-related changes in selective attention and perceptual load during visual search. Psychol. Aging 18, 54–67.

Madden, D.J., Nebes, R.D., 1980. Aging and the development of automaticity in visual search. Dev. Psychol. 16, 377–384.

Madden, D.J., Pierce, T.W., Allen, P.A., 1992. Adult age differences in attentional allocation during memory search. Psychol. Aging 7, 594–601.

Madden, D.J., Pierce, T.W., Allen, P.A., 1996. Adult age differences in the use of distractor homogeneity during visual search. Psychol. Aging 11, 454–474.

Madden, D.J., Plude D.J., 1993. Selective preservation of selective attention. In: Cerella, J., Rybash, W., Hoyer, Commons, M.L. (Eds.), Adult Information Processing: Limits on Loss. Academic Press, San Diego, CA, pp. 273–300.

Madden, D.J., Turkington, T.G., Provenzale, J.M., Denny, L.L., Langley, L.K., Hawk, T.C., Coleman, R.E., 2002. Aging and attentional guidance during visual search: Functional neuroanatomy by positron emission tomography. Psychol. Aging 17, 24–43.

Madden, D.J., Turkington, T.G., Provenzale, J.M., Hawk, T.C., Hoffman, J.M., Coleman, R.E., 1997. Selective and divided visual attention: Age-related changes in regional cerebral blood flow measured by $H_2^{15}O$ PET. Hum. Brain Mapp. 5, 389–409.

Madden, D.J., Welsh-Bohmer, K.A., Tupler, L.A., 1999b. Task complexity and signal detection analyses of lexical decision performance in Alzheimer's disease. Dev. Neuropsychol. 16, 1–18.

Madden, D.J., Whiting, W.L., Huettel, S.A., in press. Age-related changes in neural activity during visual perception and attention. In: Cabeza, R., Nyberg, L., Park, D.C. (Eds.), Cognitive Neuroscience of Aging: Linking Cognitive and Cerebral Aging. Oxford University Press, New York.

May, C.P., Kane, M.J., Hasher, L., 1995. Determinants of negative priming. Psychol. Bull. 118, 35–54.

Maylor, E.A., Lavie, N., 1998. The influence of perceptual load on age differences in selective attention. Psychol. Aging 13, 563–573.

Mayr, U., 2001. Age differences in selection of mental sets: The role of inhibition, stimulus ambiguity, and response-set overlap. Psychol. Aging 16, 96–109.

Mayr, U., Liebscher, T., 2001. Is there an age deficit in the selection of mental sets? Eur. J. Cogn. Psychol. 13, 47–69.

McDowd, J.M., 1997. Inhibition in attention and aging. J. Gerontol. Psychol. Sci. 52B, P265–P273.

McDowd, J.M., Craik, F.I.M., 1988. Effects of aging and task difficulty on divided attention performance. J. Exp. Psychol. Hum. Percept. Perform. 14, 267–280.

McDowd, J.M., Shaw, R.J., 2000. Attention and aging: A functional perspective. In: Craik, F.I.M., Salthouse, T.A. (Eds.), The Handbook of Aging and Cognition, 2nd ed. Erlbaum, Hillsdale, NJ, pp. 221–292.

Meiran, N., Gotler, A., Perlman, A., 2001. Old age is associated with a pattern of relatively intact and relatively impaired task-set switching abilities. J. Gerontol. Psychol. Sci. 56B, P88–P102.

Milham, M.P., Erickson, K.I., Banich, M.T., Kramer, A.F., Webb, A., Wszalek, T., Cohen, N.J., 2002. Attentional control in the aging brain: Insights from an fMRI study of the Stroop task. Brain Cogn. 49, 277–296.

Miliken, B., Tipper, S.P., 1998. Attention and inhibition. In: Pashler, H. (Ed.), Attention, Psychology Press, East Sussex, UK, pp. 191–221.

Miyake, A., Friedman, N.P., Emerson, M.J., Witzki, A.H., Howerter, A., Wager, T.D., 2000. The unity and diversity of executive functions and their contributions to complex "frontal lobe" tasks: A latent variable analysis. Cog. Psychol. 41, 49–100.

Myerson, J., Ferraro, F.R., Hale, S., Lima, S.D., 1992. General slowing in semantic priming and word recognition. Psychol. Aging 7, 257–270.

Myerson, J., Hale, S., Wagstaff, D., Poon, L.W., Smith, G.A., 1990. The information loss model: A mathematical theory of age-related cognitive slowing. Psychol. Rev. 97, 475–487.

Nebes, R.D., Brady, C.B., 1992. Generalized cognitive slowing and severity of dementia in Alzheimer's disease: Implications for the interpretation of response-time data. J. Clin. Exp. Neuropsychol. 14, 317–326.

Nebes, R.D., Madden, D.J., 1983. The use of focused attention in visual search by young and old adults. Exp. Aging Res. 9, 139–143.

Nebes, R.D., Madden, D.J., 1988. Different patterns of cognitive slowing produced by Alzheimer's disease and normal aging. Psychol. Aging 3, 102–104.

Nielson, K.A., Langenecker, S.A., Garavan, H., 2002. Differences in the functional neuroanatomy of inhibitory control across the adult life span. Psychol. Aging 17, 56–71.

Nissen, M.J., Corkin, S., 1985. Effectiveness of attentional cueing in older and younger adults. J. Gerontol. 40, 185–191.

Norman, D.A., Bobrow, D.G., 1975. On data-limited and resource-limited processes. Cog. Psychol. 7, 44–64.

O'Sullivan, M., Jones, D.K., Summers, P.E., Morris, R.G., Williams, S.C.R., Markus, H.S., 2001. Evidence for cortical disconnection as a mechanism of age-related cognitive decline. Neurology 57, 632–638.

Parasuraman, R., 1984. Sustained attention in detection and discrimination. In: Parasuraman, R., Davies, D.R. (Eds.), Varieties of Attention, Academic Press, Orlando, FL, pp. 234–271.

Parasuraman, R., Giambra, L., 1991. Skill development in vigilance: Effects of event rate and age. Psychol. Aging 6, 155–169.

Parasuraman, R., Nestor, P., Greenwood, P., 1989. Sustained-attention capacity in young and older adults. Psychol. Aging 4, 339–345.

Park, D.C., Smith, A.D., Dudley, W.N., Lafronza, V.N., 1989. Effects of age and a divided attention task presented during encoding and retrieval on memory. J. Exp. Psychol. Learn. Mem. Cogn. 15, 1185–1191.

Park, D.C., Smith, A.D., Lautenschlager, G., Earles, J.L., Frieske, D., Zwahr, M., Gaines, C.L., 1996. Mediators of long-term memory performance across the life span. Psychol. Aging 11, 621–637.

Pashler, H., 1994. Dual-task interference in simple tasks: Data and theory. Psychol. Bull. 116, 220–244.

Pashler, H.E., 1998. The Psychology of Attention, MIT Press, Cambridge, MA.

Perfect, T.J., 1994. What can Brinley plots tell us about cognitive aging? J. Gerontol. Psychol. Sci. 49, P60–P64.

Peters, A., Moss, M.B., Sethares, C., 2001. The effects of aging on layer 1 of primary visual cortex in the rhesus monkey. Cereb. Cortex 11, 93–103.

Pfefferbaum, A., Sullivan, E.V., Hedehus, M., Lim, K.O., Adalsteinsson, E., Moseley, M., 2000. Age-related decline in brain white matter anisotropy measured with spatially corrected echo-planar diffusion tensor imaging. Magn. Reson. Med. 44, 259–268.

Piccinin, A.M., Rabbitt, P.M.A., 1999. Contribution of cognitive abilities to performance and improvement on a substitution coding task. Psychol. Aging 14, 539–551.

Pitts, D.G., 1982. The effects of aging on selected visual functions: Dark adaptation, visual acuity, stereopsis, and brightness contrast. In: Sekuler, R., Kline, D., Dismukes, K. (Eds.) Aging and Human Visual Function, Alan R. Liss, Inc., New York, pp. 131–159.

Plude, D.J., Doussard-Roosevelt, J.A., 1989. Aging, selective attention, and feature integration. Psychol. Aging 4, 98–105.

Plude, D.J., Hoyer, W.J., 1986. Age and the selectivity of visual information processing. Psychol. Aging 1, 4–10.

Ponds, R.W.H., Brouwer, W.H., van Wolffelaar, P.C., 1988. Age differences in divided attention in a simulated driving task. J. Gerontol. Psychol. Sci. 43, P151–P156.

Posner, M.I., 1980. Orienting of attention. Quart. J. Exp. Psychol. 32, 3–25.

Posner, M.I., Dehaene, S., 1994. Attentional networks. Trends Neurosci. 17, 75–79.

Rabbitt, P.M.A., 1964. Set and age in a choice-response task. J. Gerontol. 19, 301–306.

Rabbitt, P.M.A., 1965. Age and discrimination between complex stimuli. In: Welford, A.T., Birren, J.E. (Eds.), Behavior, Aging, and the Nervous System, Charles C. Thomas, Springfield, IL, pp. 35–53.

Rabbitt, P., 1984. The control of attention in visual search. In: Parasuraman, R., Davies, D.R. (Eds.), Varieties of Attention, Academic Press, Orlando, FL, pp. 273–291.

Raz, N., 2000. Aging of the brain and its impact on cognitive performance: Integration of structural and functional findings. In: Craik, F.I.M., Salthouse, T.A. (Eds.), Handbook of Aging and Cognition, 2nd ed. Erlbaum, Mahwah, NJ, pp. 1–90.

Rogers, R.D., Monsell, S., 1995. Costs of a predictable switch between simple cognitive tasks. J. Exp. Psychol. Gen. 124, 207–231.

Rogers, W.A., Fisk, A.D., Hertzog, C., 1994. Do ability-performance relationships differentiate age and practice effects in visual search? J. Exp. Psychol. Learn. Mem. Cogn. 20, 710–738.

Rubin, D.C., 1999. Frontal-striatal circuits in cognitive aging: Evidence for caudate involvement. Aging Neuropsychol. Cog. 6, 241–259.

Salat, D.H., Kaye, J.A., Janowsky, J.S., 1999. Prefrontal gray and white matter volumes in healthy aging and Alzheimer's disease. Arch. Neurol. 56, 338–344.

Salthouse, T.A., 1984. Effects of age and skill in typing. J. Exp. Psychol. Gen. 113, 345–371.

Salthouse, T.A., 1985a. A Theory of Cognitive Aging, Elsevier, Amsterdam.

Salthouse, T.A., 1985b. Speed of behavior and its implications for cognition. In: Birren, J.E., Schaie, K.W. (Eds.), Handbook of the Psychology of Aging, 2nd ed. Van Nostrand Reinhold, New York, pp. 400–426.

Salthouse, T.A., 1990. Working memory as a processing resource in cognitive aging. Dev. Rev. 10, 101–124.

Salthouse, T.A., 1992a. Mechanisms of Age-Cognition Relations in Adulthood, Erlbaum, Hillsdale, NJ.

Salthouse, T.A., 1992b. Shifting levels of analysis in the investigation of cognitive aging. Hum. Dev. 35, 321–342.

Salthouse, T.A., 1993a. Attentional blocks are not responsible for age-related slowing. J. Gerontol. Psychol. Sci. 48, P263–P270.

Salthouse, T.A., 1993b. Speed mediation of adult age differences in cognition. Dev. Psychol. 29, 722–738.

Salthouse, T.A., 1996. The processing-speed theory of adult age differences in cognition. Psychol. Rev. 103, 403–428.

Salthouse, T.A., 1998. Relation of successive percentiles of reaction time distributions to cognitive variables and adult age. Intelligence 26, 153–166.

Salthouse, T.A., 2000. Aging and measures of processing speed. Biol. Psychol. 54, 35–54.

Salthouse, T.A., Fristoe, N., McGuthry, K.E., Hambrick, D.Z., 1998. Relation of task switching to speed, age, and fluid intelligence. Psychol. Aging 13, 445–461.
Salthouse, T.A., Fristoe, N.M., Lineweaver, T.T., Coon, V.E., 1995. Aging of attention: Does the ability to divide decline? Mem. Cognit. 23, 59–71.
Salthouse, T.A., Hancock, H.E., Meinz, E.J., Hambrick, D.Z., 1996. Interrelations of age, visual acuity, and cognitive functioning. J. Gerontol. Psychol. Sci. 51B, P317–P330.
Salthouse, T.A., Kersten, A.W., 1993. Decomposing adult age differences in symbol arithmetic. Mem. Cogni. 21, 699–710.
Salthouse, T.A., Meinz, E.J., 1995. Aging, inhibition, working memory, and speed. J. Gerontol. Psychol. Sci. 50B, P297–P306.
Salthouse, T.A., Rogan, J.D., Prill, K.A., 1984. Division of attention: Age differences on a visually presented memory task. Mem. Cogni. 12, 613–620.
Salthouse, T.A., Somberg, B.L., 1982. Skilled performance: Effects of adult age and experience on elementary processes. J. Exp. Psychol. Gen. 111, 176–207.
Schmitter-Edgecombe, M., Nissley, H.M., 2002. Effects of aging on implicit covariation learning. Aging Neuropsychol. Cog. 9, 61–75.
Schneider, B.A., Pichora-Fuller, M.K., 2000. Implication of perceptual deterioration for cognitive aging research. In: Craik, F.I.M., Salthouse, T.A. (Eds.), The Handbook of Aging and Cognition, 2nd ed. Erlbaum, Mahwah, NJ, pp. 155–219.
Schneider, W., Shiffrin, R.M., 1977. Controlled and automatic human information processing: I. Detection, search, and attention. Psychol. Rev. 84, 1–66.
Scialfa, C.T., 1990. Adult age differences in visual search: The role of non-attentional processes. In: Enns, J.T. (Ed.), The Development of Attention: Research and Theory, Elsevier, Amsterdam, pp. 509–526.
Scialfa, C.T., Esau, S.P., Joffe, K.M., 1998. Age, target-distractor similarity, and visual search. Exp. Aging Res. 24, 337–358.
Scialfa, C.T., Hamaluck, E., Skaloud, P., Pratt, J., 1999. Age differences in saccadic averaging. Psychol. Aging 14, 695–699.
Scialfa, C.T., Harpur, L.L., 1994. Effects of similarity and duration on age differences in visual search. Can. J. Aging 13, 51–65.
Scialfa, C.T., Jenkins, L., Hamaluk, E., Skaloud, P., 2000. Aging and the development of automaticity in conjunction search. J. Gerontol. Psychol. Sci. 55B, 27–46.
Scialfa, C.T., Kline, D.W., 1996. Vision. In: Birren, J.E. (Ed.), Encyclopedia of Gerontology, Academic Press, San Diego, pp. 605–612.
Scialfa, C.T., Kline, D.W., Lyman, B.J., 1987. Age differences in target identification as a function of retinal location and noise level: Examination of the useful field of view. Psychol. Aging 2, 14–19.
Scialfa, C.T., Thomas, D.M., 1994. Age differences in same-different judgments as a function of multidimensional similarity. J. Gerontol. Psychol. Sci. 49, P173–P178.
Sekuler, A.B., Bennett, P.J., 2000. Effects of aging on the useful field of view. Exp. Aging Res. 26, 103–120.
Sliwinski, M.J., Hall, C.B., 1998. Constraints on general slowing: A meta-analysis using hierarchical linear models with random coefficients. Psychol. Aging 13, 164–175.
Somberg, B.L., Salthouse, T.A., 1982. Divided attention abilities in young and old adults. J. Exp. Psychol. Hum. Percept. Perform. 8, 651–663.
Spear, P.D., 1993. Neural basis of visual deficits during aging. Vision Res. 33, 2589–2609.
Spieler, D.H., Balota, D.A., Faust, M.E., 1996. Stroop performance in healthy younger and older adults and in individuals with dementia of the Alzheimer's type. J. Exp. Psychol. Hum. Percept. Perform. 22, 461–479.
Treisman, A., Sato, S., 1990. Conjunction search revisited. J. Exp. Psychol. Hum. Percept. Perform. 16, 459–478.
Verhaeghen, P., 2002. Age differences in efficiency and effectiveness of encoding for visual search and memory search: A time-accuracy study. Aging Neuropsychol. Cog. 9, 114–126.
Verhaeghen, P., De Meersman, L., 1998. Aging and the Stroop effect: A meta-analysis. Psychol. Aging 13, 120–126.

Walsh, D.A., 1982. The development of visual information processes in adulthood and old age. In: Sekuler, R., Kline, D., Dismukes, K. (Eds.) Aging and Human Visual Function, Alan R. Liss, Inc., New York, pp. 203–230.

Weale, R.A., 1961. Retinal illumination and age. Trans. Illumin. Eng. Soc. 26, 95–100.

Welford, A.T., Birren, J.E. (Eds.), 1965. Behavior, Aging, and the Nervous System. Charles C. Thomas, Springfield, IL.

West, R.L., 1996. An application of prefrontal cortex function theory to cognitive aging. Psychol. Bull. 120, 272–292.

Whiting, W.L., 2003. Adult age differences in divided attention: Effects of elaboration during memory encoding. Aging Neuropsychol. Cog. 10, 141–157.

Whiting, W.L., Smith, A.D., 1997. Differential age-related processing limitations in recall and recognition tasks. Psychol. Aging 12, 216–224.

Wolfe, J.M., 1994. Guided search 2.0 A revised model of visual search. Psychonomic Bull. Rev. 1, 202–238.

Wolfe, J.M., 1998. Visual search. In: Pashler, H. (Ed.), Attention, Psychology Press, East Sussex, UK, pp. 13–73.

Wolfe, J.M., Butcher, S.J., Lee, C., Hyle, M., 2003. Changing your mind: On the contributions of top-down and bottom-up guidance in visual search for feature singletons. J. Exp. Psychol. Hum. Percept. Perform. 29, 483–502.

Wright, R.E., 1981. Aging, divided attention, and processing capacity. J. Gerontol. 36, 605–614.

Zacks, J.L., Zacks, R.T., 1993. Visual search times assessed without reaction times: A new method and an application to aging. J. Exp. Psychol. Hum. Percept. Perform. 19, 798–813.

Advances in
Cell Aging and
Gerontology

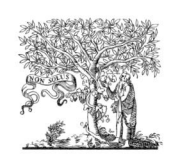

Studies of aging, hypertension and cognitive functioning: With contributions from the Maine-Syracuse study

Merrill F. Elias[1,2,*], Michael A. Robbins[1], Marc M. Budge[3], Penelope K. Elias[2], Barbara A. Hermann[1] and Gregory A. Dore[1]

[1]*University of Maine;* [2]*Boston University;* [3]*Australian National University Medical School*

Contents

1. Introduction — *90*
2. Hypertension: an age relevant health concern — *91*
   2.1. Prevalence and incidence — *91*
   2.2. Health consequences — *92*
   2.3. Catastrophic deficit — *92*
3. From episodic to longitudinal studies — *93*
   3.1. Lessons from episodic studies — *93*
     3.1.1. Cognitive deficit: general or specific? — *93*
     3.1.2. Education — *94*
     3.1.3. Blood pressure — *94*
     3.1.4. Treatment — *95*
4. Hypertension in a dynamic context — *96*
   4.1. The Maine-Syracuse study: basic design — *96*
   4.2. Cross-sectional studies — *97*
     4.2.1. Overview — *97*
     4.2.2. Replication of earlier cross-sectional study: factor scores — *98*
     4.2.3. Cross-sectional findings with comment — *98*
     4.2.4. Consistency across the life span? — *100*
     4.2.5. Biological feasibility? — *100*
     4.2.6. Alternative explanations — *102*
     4.2.7. Skepticism prevails — *102*
     4.2.8. Cross-sectional design limitations: Conclusions — *103*
   4.3. Prospective designs: issues of causality — *103*

*Corresponding author. Department of Psychology, 5742 Little Hall (Room 301), University of Maine, Orono, ME 04469-5742, USA. Tel.: 207-581-2097; fax: 207-581-6128.
E-mail address: mfelias@aol.com (M.F. Elias).

Advances in Cell Aging and Gerontology, vol. 15, 89–131
ISSN: 1566-3124   DOI: 10.1016/S1566-3124(03)15004-3
© 2004 Elsevier Science BV.
All rights reserved

    4.4. Longitudinal studies   *104*
         4.4.1. Two measurement points   *104*
         4.4.2. Three times of measurement   *104*
         4.4.3. Wider age range and a larger sample   *116*
         4.4.4. Continuing work   *117*
         4.4.5. Decline in BP over time   *117*
5. Unresolved issues in hypertension and cognitive function research   *117*
    5.1. Identifying abilities related to hypertension   *118*
         5.1.1. Predictions from the biology of hypertension   *118*
         5.1.2. Factor analysis studies   *118*
         5.1.3. Information processing studies   *119*
         5.1.4. Theoretical issues   *119*
         5.1.5. Is antihypertensive treatment an effective intervention and if so, for whom?   *120*
         5.1.6. Summary   *121*
6. What are the clinical and population implications of high blood pressure?   *121*
    6.1. Individuals vs. groups   *121*
    6.2. The population and risk estimates   *122*
    6.3. Treatment   *124*
7. Where do we go from here?   *124*
    Acknowledgments   *125*
    References   *125*

1. Introduction

The interactive effects of hypertension and age on cognitive functioning have been a major focus of research in life span developmental psychology for three decades. Thirty-two years after the initial longitudinal studies of hypertension and intelligence test performance by Wilkie and Eisdorfer (1971), it has become clear, as a result of further longitudinal studies, that hypertension is indeed a risk factor for subtle, but progressive, acceleration of decline in fluid abilities over the adult life span (Wilkie and Eisdorfer, 1971; Elias et al., 1986, 1989, 1998a,b) and may be a precursor of stroke-related cognitive deficit and dementia in subsets of individuals (Hansson et al., 1999). This chapter provides a history of the progression of studies leading to our current understanding of the association between hypertension and decline in normal cognitive functioning.

We had five goals in writing this chapter: (1) to discuss the importance of studies of hypertension and cognitive function to aging research; (2) to review some of the major methodological issues that must be addressed by these studies; (3) to summarize the contributions of cross-sectional vs. longitudinal studies to our current understanding of the associations of hypertension, aging, and cognitive function; (4) to discuss the significance of these studies from a patient-treatment and population perspective; and (5) to place these findings in the broader context of the relation of total cardiovascular risk to the preservation of cognitive functioning with advancing age. Our focus is primarily on normal cognitive functioning across the adult life span, although we briefly review the literature pertaining to more major deviations associated with dementia. The hypertension literature relative to the elderly, and demented adults is discussed briefly in order to provide a context for investigations of hypertension and aging across a segment of life that could be characterized as marked by young adulthood and young-elderly status at its opposite poles.

In this review and discussion we emphasize findings based on our 28-year study of hypertension and cognitive function, the Maine-Syracuse Longitudinal Study of Hypertension and Cognitive Function. To place these studies in context we relate them to the literature in general, and particularly to our cognitive studies with the Framingham Heart Study population.

It is important to emphasize that the study of hypertension in relation to aging provides a model for the study of cardiovascular disease, aging, and cognition in general. Hypertension is a diagnostic category. As such, it is not a disease process but rather a categorization based on an arbitrary cut-off of a conveniently available clinical measurement. More broadly, it is a single manifestation of a genetic, environmental, and metabolically determined multi-faceted hypertensive cardiovascular syndrome. In fact, as we emphasize at the end of this chapter, the impact of hypertension on cognitive function can only be fully understood in the context of the other major cardiovascular risk factors.

2. Hypertension: an age relevant health concern

Hypertension is relevant to aging for three major reasons: (1) Fifty-million individuals (one in four adults) in the United States are hypertensive (American Heart Association, 1998); (2) hypertension is an insidious destructive developmental process that increases in prevalence and incidence with advancing age, and, it is important to note that the population, as a whole, is aging; and (3) hypertension is a not only a well-established risk factor for major causes of disability and death, such as myocardial infarction and stroke, but an emerging body of evidence suggests that it is a risk factor for Alzheimer's Disease as well as vascular dementia.

2.1. Prevalence and incidence

Approximately one in four adults in the United States is hypertensive (American Heart Association, 1998). Of these 50 million hypertensive individuals, approximately 90%–95% are classified as essential hypertensive, a term that designates that no endocrine or remediable cause has been established. In white Americans, the 9.5-year incidence of hypertension (new cases) increases from 8% between 25 and 34 years of age to 47% over 65 years of age (LaCroix, 1993). These figures are doubled for African Americans. Despite emphasis on aggressive detection and treatment of hypertension, both remain problematic, as does adherence with prescribed treatment regimens (Izzo and Black, 1993; Sixth Report, JNC, 1997; Meissner et al., 1999; Prisant and Moser, 2000).

2.2. Health consequences

Arterial hypertension is associated with cerebral vascular disease and its complications, e.g. cerebral infarction, hemorrhage, transient ischemic attack, and multi-infarct dementia (Kannel et al., 1970, 1976; Wolf, 1993), and with alterations in brain structure and function (Gifford, 1989; Phillips and Whisnant, 1992), including white matter lesions in the brain (Schmidt et al., 1991; Salerno, et al., 1992; Manolio et al., 1994; Patoni and Garcia, 1995; Liao et al., 1996; Fazekus et al., 1988; Carmelli et al., 1998; Kuller et al., 1998), and disturbed cerebral perfusion and impaired brain cell metabolism (Waldstein, 1995). Thus it is not surprising to find that hypertension is associated with lower levels of cognitive functioning of all ages. See reviews by Elias et al. (1987a), Elias and Robbins (1991a), Waldstein et al. (1991a), and Waldstein (1995).

2.3. Catastrophic deficit

Hypertension may be a risk factor for dementia, but this is not the only major reason why it is important to track hypertension-related deficits from young adulthood to old age. We found over 400 citations to papers relating hypertension to dementia in an unsystematic review (Medline, 1990 to 2003). The two most common types of dementia are vascular dementia and Alzheimer's disease (AD). Mixed forms are not uncommon and often distinctions among the classes of dementia defy even the most sophisticated diagnostic expertise. It is clear that cardiovascular risk factors, including hypertension, play a role in vascular dementia (Hansson et al., 1999) and that studies relating BP level to dementia are important. Both hypotension and hypertension are more prevalent in AD (Hansson et al., 1999).

It has been suggested that hypertension may be the result, not the cause of AD or other forms of dementia. Reports of prospective associations between elevated BP years before the development of dementia (Skoog et al., 1996; Peila et al., 2001) weaken this argument as do data from the Syst-Eur trial. Here patients who were randomized to active antihypertensive drug therapy evidenced significantly lower incidence of dementia (Forette et al., 2002).

The Maine-Syracuse Studies provide a center-piece for the chapter. Consequently, we do not focus on dementia as an outcome variable. At least one more wave of data collection, following our current effort, will be necessary in order for significant numbers of our participants to reach ages where they will be at high risk for dementia. Nevertheless, we touch on this literature to emphasize the importance of hypertension as a health concern but also to emphasize the fact that studies relating blood pressure to changes in normal cognitive functioning over time are essential to an understanding of the pathways from normal cognitive decline to dementia.

3. From episodic to longitudinal studies

What we have learned about relations among hypertension, aging, and cognition in the past 30 years has been based on four fundamental designs: (1) episodic; (2) prospective; (3) cross-sectional; and (4) longitudinal. Combinations of these designs can be very effective in separating age differences from age changes. Thus we find it convenient to organize our consideration of the literature by study design.

3.1. Lessons from episodic studies

The term "episodic" is applied to studies "at a point in time." By definition they do not involve stratification by age-cohort nor do they follow study participants longitudinally. Episodic data on hypertension and cognitive function are abundant. Studies with younger adults were predominant in the early episodic literature, but more recently the focus has been on studies of the elderly. Episodic studies at various segments of the life span indicate that hypertension has an adverse affect on cognitive functioning throughout the adult years (Waldstein et al., 1991a; Waldstein, 1995; Waldstein and Katzel, 2001).

Four major issues have been addressed in episodic studies: (1) determination of which cognitive abilities are more vulnerable to effects of hypertension; (2) consideration of the possible protective role of education; (3) delineation of the role of continuous blood pressure as opposed to diagnostic cut points; and (4) separation of the effects of treatment for hypertension from those of hypertension per se. Investigation of each of these issues has helped to advance the conceptual and methodological quality of research on hypertension and cognitive aging, in part by providing a better understanding of the controls necessary when conducting cross-sectional and longitudinal studies.

3.1.1. Cognitive deficit: general or specific?

Many cognitive domains (e.g. psychomotor speed, visual-constructive ability, episodic learning, memory, selective attention, and speed of performance) are adversely affected by hypertension and increments in BP (Elias and Robbins, 1991a; Waldstein et al., 1991a; Waldstein, 1995, 2000). Waldstein (1995) has noted that crystallized-verbal abilities appear to be less affected by hypertension than other abilities. We find this to be true with respect to longitudinal decline in cognitive functioning (Elias et al., 1998a,b). This finding may be related to the fact that crystallized-verbal abilities (e.g. information and vocabulary subtests of the Wechsler Adult Intelligence Scale (WAIS)) are less vulnerable to aging and benefit from cognitive reserve due to a lifetime of use. Generally, however, the literature indicates an association between hypertension and abilities in multiple cognitive domains when performance level at one point in time is considered (Elias and Robbins, 1991a; Waldstein, 1995). This generalized rather than domain-specific lowering of performance level is consistent with the fact that high BP is associated with morphologic changes and physiological events which are diffuse and involve multiple brain areas (Carmelli et al., 1998), including all the watershed areas of the cerebral arteries (Baumbach and Heistad, 1997).

Recently executive functioning has received attention as a "hypertension-vulnerable ability." The argument is "biologically plausible." There is some evidence that relatively greater damage to frontal–subcortical neuronal circuits (i.e. a higher prevalence of white matter lesions) may lead to selective impairment of frontally mediated abilities, i.e. executive functioning (De Carli et al., 1995; Longstreth et al., 1996). Many tests of fluid ability make heavy demands on executive function (planned, organized, integrated, purposeful, and volitional action). This may be why we have seen no significant change in crystallized-verbal ability in relationship to hypertension or high BP, but have observed significant decline in visual-constructive and speed performance tests which place demands on executive functioning (Elias et al., 1998a,b). At this point, it is not clear whether the failure to clearly identify more cognitive-specific deficits in cognitive function is related to the fact that effects of hypertension on the brain are generalized and diffuse or to the fact that clinical tests, widely employed in these studies, lack specificity. This problem is discussed more fully at the end of this chapter.

3.1.2. Education

Several studies, including the Maine-Syracuse study, indicate that high levels of education are protective with regard to the effect of hypertension on cognitive functioning (Elias et al., 1987b; Stewart et al., 2001). The high correlation between education and crystallized-verbal abilities may be one reason why the crystallized-verbal abilities appear to "resist" the effects of hypertension.

3.1.3. Blood pressure

Unfortunately, investigators were very slow to focus on relations between blood pressure and cognitive functioning, despite the fact that demonstration of this relationship is essential if one is to entertain any notion that there may be causal associations between high blood pressure (hypertension) and cognitive function.

It is well recognized that demonstration of a "dose–response" relationship is particularly important with regard to issues of causality. It is thus surprising that blood pressure level received such little attention prior to 1990. Up to that time the preponderance of studies employed designs in which hypertensive individuals were compared with normotensive individuals. In a chapter considering mechanisms linking hypertension to cognitive function, our group (Elias et al., 1987a) argued that diagnosed hypertensive individuals differed in so many respects (other than possible hypertension-related pathophysiology) from normotensive individuals that these case-control designs were not persuasive with regard to the argument that under-lying physiological processes associated with hypertension were responsible for differences in cognitive functioning between hypertensive and normotensive individuals. The argument was that BP is positively and continuously related to cardiovascular morbidity and mortality (Kannel et al., 1970, 1976; Wilson, 1993; Wolf, 1993) and to white matter lesions, silent stroke, and related events (Manolio et al., 1994), and therefore it was necessary to the pathophysiological mechanism argument to show that BP was related to cognitive functioning in the same way. The argument was buttressed by a cross-sectional study with the Maine-Syracuse participants. Using multiple regression methods, data from this study indicated that BP level, diastolic and systolic, was inversely related to cognitive functioning (Elias et al., 1990a) despite adjustment for many possible confounding variables. It is most important to note that linear associations between BP and cognitive function were observed in this study even when the sample was restricted to individuals with no history of antihypertensive treatment and BP values within normal to high normal, traditionally untreated BP ranges (systolic BP from 83 to 139 mmHg and diastolic BP from 58 to 89 mmHg).

3.1.4. Treatment

It is still not clear whether antihypertensive treatment has a positive, negative, or null effect on cognitive functioning. Major reviews of the literature indicate that the findings are mixed (Muldoon et al., 1995; Jonas et al., 2001). Clearly some well-controlled clinical trials have indicated modest positive effects of treatment on cognition (Croog et al., 1986; Dimsdale and Newton, 1992), while others have indicated null effects (Applegate et al., 1994; Croog et al., 1994). Treatment for hypertension is a risk factor for stroke in the Framingham Stroke Risk profile, but it is obvious that treatment lowers the risk of stroke (Wolf et al., 1991; D'Agostino et al., 1994). Negative effects of treatment may merely reflect the fact that treatment for hypertension is a proxy for hypertension. In other words, where treatment is highly prevalent in a study sample, treatment and hypertension are confounded. Controlling for treatment under these circumstances may attenuate or even remove effects of hypertension.

A number of studies have avoided the problems inherent to statistical adjustment for antihypertensive treatment where treatment prevalence is high in a study sample. A study by Waldstein et al. (1991b), and recent reviews (Waldstein, 2000) indicate that effects of hypertension on cognitive function are observed in never-treated subjects. The Maine-Syracuse group contributed several studies to this literature using data collected in connection with a clinical drug trial (Croog et al., 1994) sponsored by Glaxo Pharmaceutical Company and data from the Framingham Heart Study.

In the Glaxo study, we were able to analyze data obtained in a large drug trial with cognitive functioning as the outcome measure (Robbins et al., 1994). We examined data for 315 elderly hypertensive women, age range 60 to 80 years, who were removed from their antihypertensive drugs in the run-in phase of a clinical trial. Cognitive measures were obtained after BP had become established at hypertensive levels for all women. With this hypertensive group of women, diastolic BP was inversely and significantly related to Trails A, Digit Span Forward, Digit Span Backward, and Digit Symbol Substitution performance measures.

Our collaboration with Framingham investigators made it possible for us to examine associations between BP and cognitive performance for a large group of Framingham Study participants ($N=1702$) for whom only 13% were taking antihypertensive medications. Diastolic and systolic BP were inversely, but modestly, related to measures of verbal and visual-spatial memory, and digit-span memory measured 12 to 14 years after the BP assessment window (Elias et al., 1993). The same results were obtained when analyses were repeated for a subset of individuals ($N = 1038$) who were untreated for hypertension for 26 years (Elias et al., 1993).

It is quite clear from the literature that the adverse effects of drugs on cognitive functioning, presuming some drugs act in this way, do not explain the effects of hypertension on cognitive performance. And, our reading of the literature suggests that proper drug treatment, with new generation drugs, can attenuate the effects of hypertension on cognitive functioning via the reduction in BP level.

4. Hypertension in a dynamic context

Obviously the major limitation of episodic studies is that hypertension does not stand still. It is a progressively destructive process and its impact on the brain is cumulative. It must be studied in a developmental context. We now turn to a description of the Maine-Syracuse study so that its major features will be better understood when we report Maine-Syracuse data in the next sections of the chapter.

4.1. The Maine-Syracuse study: basic design

The Maine-Syracuse Longitudinal Study of Hypertension and Cognitive Functioning (Maine-Syracuse study) began in Syracuse, NY in 1974 as the result of collaboration between M.F. Elias and D.H.P. Streeten (Professor of Medicine). It has benefited from continuous support from the National Institute on Aging for 25 years. It was designed to characterize the effects of hypertension, and hypertension-related diseases, on cognitive functioning. With support from a new research grant from the National Heart, Lung and Blood Institute the goals of the study were expanded in 2001 so as to include examination of multiple risk factors such as diabetes, obesity, lipids, homocysteine, and ApoE4 genotype, in relation to cognitive function.

It is essentially a time-lagged cross-sectional and prospective longitudinal study (Dwyer and Feinleib, 1991). Presently, there are five cohorts defined by the fact that they entered the study at different points in time (time lag) and have thus completed different numbers of longitudinal examinations.

The study involves a comprehensive battery of tests including tests from the Halstead-Reitan Neuropsychological Test Battery (Reitan and Wolfson, 1993), the original Wechsler Adult Intelligence Scale, and tests from the Wechsler Memory Scale. Recently updated subtests from the WAIS and WMS have been added to the battery as well as test measures allowing us to duplicate the battery of tests presently being used with the Framingham Heart Study offspring.

In addition, various measures of mood state and other psychosocial and demographic variables are included on the data set. Information on the sample with respect to demographic, cardiovascular risk factor, and co-existing disease characteristics has been published previously (Elias et al., 1990a; Elias and Robbins, 1991b; Elias et al., 1998a). Medical data have been obtained from clinic visits and physician examination, where necessary, as well as medical interview and hospital and treatment records. A supplementary award from the National Institute on Aging has permitted us to analyze data from the Framingham Heart Study. Support from Glaxo Pharmaceutical Company (to M.F. Elias) has allowed us to analyze a subset of data from a large clinical trial. No conflicts with Glaxo exist and the study has enjoyed continued approval from the Institutional Review Boards for the Protection of Human Subjects of all institutions involved.

It is possible to include a significant number of covariates in statistical analyses. Unless otherwise specified, our basic models for data reported in the next sections include adjustment for age, sex, education, occupation, and treatment with antihypertensive drugs. Given change in criteria for hypertension over the years of the study, 35% of the hypertensive longitudinal subjects were untreated at some time during the study, allowing us to control for treatment (yes/no) or number of antihypertensive drugs. We now turn to the literature on cross-sectional and then longitudinal studies.

4.2. Cross-sectional studies

4.2.1. Overview

Wilkie and Eisdorfer's (1971) longitudinal study of hypertension and performance on the Wechsler Adult Intelligence Scale (WAIS) has been given credit for sparking interest in aging and hypertension interactions in the aging literature. Paradoxically, the study stimulated a spate of cross-sectional studies in which Age Cohort by Hypertension interactions were examined. Many of the studies focusing on an age range from young adulthood to late middle age were case-control-type studies.

There have been several comprehensive reviews of this literature (Elias et al., 1987a; Elias and Robbins, 1991a; Starr and Whalley, 1992; Waldstein, 1995). The most interesting and unexpected finding was that the combination of older age and hypertension did not result in the lowest level of performance. Where interactions were observed, the neuropsychological test performance of younger adults was affected more by hypertension than the cognitive performance of their middle-aged counterparts. We will refer to this finding as the younger-adult-BP phenomenon. One of the earliest reports of this younger-adult-BP phenomenon came from our earliest cross-sectional study of the WAIS in Syracuse (Schultz et al., 1979). Despite replications of this work with other outcome variables and in other laboratories (Waldstein et al., 1996; Madden and Blumenthal, 1998), we were strongly motivated to replicate it with a substantially larger sample and with better controls for education. In the next section we report the results of analyses for 1138 participants of the Maine-Syracuse study. This study is still in progress and thus we will provide only a summary of the data currently available.

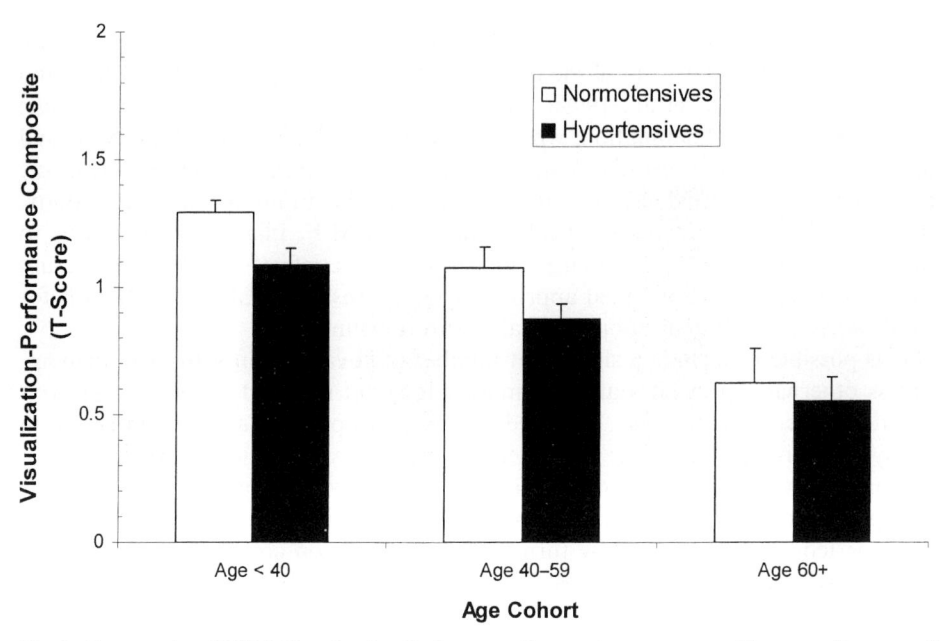

Fig. 1. Cross-sectional WAIS Visualization-Performance Composite mean scores (T-score = Z score + 1) and standard errors of the mean for Normotensive and Hypertensive Groups by Age Cohort ($n = 1138$).

4.2.2. Replication of earlier cross-sectional study: factor scores

The Schultz et al. (1979) study used the traditional WAIS Verbal and Performance scales. Our replication made use of composite scores resulting from extensive factor analytic studies with the WAIS (Horn and McArdle, 1980; Horn, 1985): Crystallized-Verbal (Comprehension, Similarities, Vocabulary, and Information); Visualization-Performance (Picture Completion, Picture Arrangement, Block Design, and Object Assembly); Memory-Span (Arithmetic, Digit Span Forward, and Digit Span Backward); and Psychomotor Speed (Digit Symbol Substitution). The Digit Symbol Substitution Test is largely a measure of psychomotor speed (Salthouse, 1992) that does not load highly with the other factors (Horn, 1985). Other factors have been developed, but these served our purpose relative to major issues in the literature. Following McArdle et al. (1991), we assign a percent correct score for each subtest of the WAIS and then average the subtest scores to form the composite score.

4.2.3. Cross-sectional findings with comment

We will focus on two variables that have been related to hypertension and BP in our cross-sectional replication and in our longitudinal studies that follow. Data for three age-cohorts, 20–39, 40–59, and 60–79 years old are presented in Figs. 1 and 2. The WAIS composite scores are expressed as t-scores for which a constant of 1 is added to the standardized (z) scores. Hypertension was defined as systolic BP of 140 mmHg or higher or diastolic BP of 90 mmHg or higher; normal blood pressure was defined as systolic BP less than 140 mmHg and diastolic BP less than

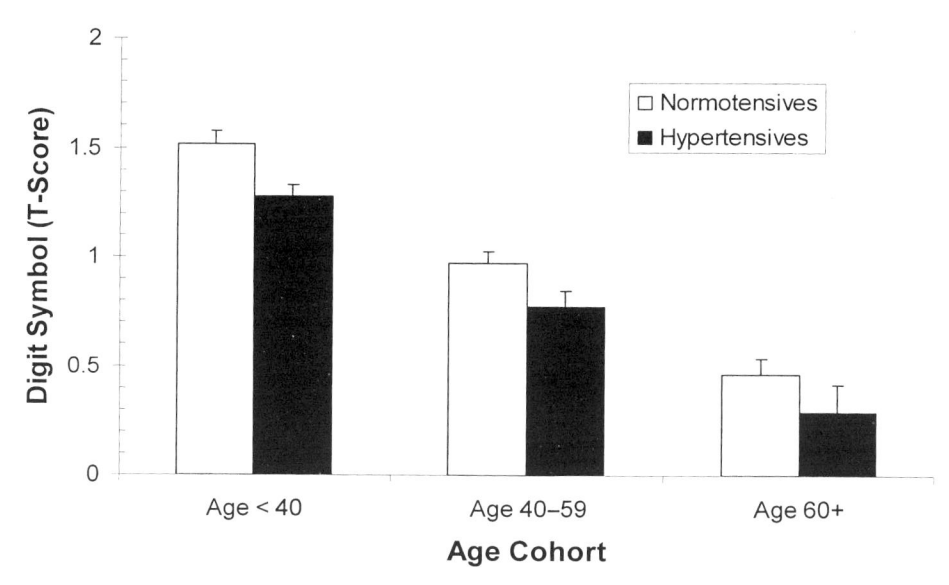

Fig. 2. Cross-sectional WAIS Digit Symbol Substitution (Psychomotor Speed) mean scores (T-score = Z score + 1) and standard errors of the mean for Normotensive and Hypertensive Groups by Age Cohort ($n = 1138$).

90 mmHg. The Hypertension by Age-Cohort interactions did not reach statistical significance ($p > 0.60$), rather there were Hypertension main effects ($p < 0.05$). However, for the Visualization-Performance composite score (Fig. 1), a priori tests of differences between the hypertensive and normotensive cohorts indicated a significant difference for the youngest group ($p < 0.05$), a marginal difference for the middle-aged group ($p < 0.06$), and no difference for the oldest group ($p > 0.30$). Corresponding a priori tests at each age for the Psychomotor Speed (Digit Symbol Substitution) scores indicated significant differences for the youngest and middle-aged groups ($p < 0.01$), but no difference for the oldest group ($p > 0.30$).

These findings were not unique to the WAIS. We observed the young adult-BP phenomenon when we examined data for a smaller sample of 301 individuals, age range 20–72 years, who were administered many of the tests employed in the Halstead-Reitan Battery (Elias et al., 1990a). Blood pressure was the major predictor in this study. Diastolic BP was related to significantly lower levels of performance on an overall index of performance, the Category Test, the Tactual Performance Test (TPT)-Memory, and the TPT-Location, with adjustment for age, education, gender, and antihypertension drug treatment. These results were replicated when all medicated hypertensives were excluded from the sample and analyses were repeated ($N = 182$). In this case, an Age by BP interaction was observed for Trails-B and for TPT-Location scores. Inspection of this interaction indicated that the combination of younger age and higher BP resulted in lower performance than the combination of older age and higher BP.

Thus we are confronted with an interesting set of studies in which younger hypertensive individuals, even those with uncomplicated essential hypertension, appear to be more vulnerable to the effects of hypertension on cognitive functioning than older hypertensive individuals (Schultz et al., 1979; Elias et al., 1990a).

4.2.4. Consistency across the life span?

The trend toward greater vulnerability to BP with decreasing age is not consistently observed in elderly individuals. In our own work with 1695 subjects of the Framingham Heart Study (Elias et al., 1995a, 1997, 2000; P.K. Elias et al., 1995), we found no BP (systolic or diastolic) by Age interactions for subjects ranging from 55 to 88 years of age when BP and age were considered as continuous variables or when three age cohorts were examined: (1) 55–64 years; (2) 65–74 years; (3) 75–88 years. However, averaging across age groups, diastolic BP was inversely associated with performance level on measures of verbal memory, visual-spatial memory, memory-span, and new learning and memory. On the other hand, Zelinski et al. (1998) found that very modest negative effects of high BP, diabetes, and lower health ratings were observed at the younger end of the continuum of old age (age range 70 to 103 years), but hypertension effects were either smaller or not existent for the oldest old.

4.2.5. Biological feasibility?

The importance of separating studies of the elderly from studies at the younger end of the life span is dictated by the fact that the mechanisms relating hypertension or BP to cognitive functioning may be very different for these two segments of the adult population. Diastolic BP rises until about age 45 and then reaches asymptote and declines while systolic BP continues to rise and systolic hypertension becomes increasingly prevalent in the elderly (Gavras and Gavras, 1983). Thus, for example, endothelial dysfunction is one of the mechanisms targeted as a link between hypertension and cognitive functioning in youth, while arterial stiffness is given more attention in old age (O'Rourke, 2000).

Candidate biological mechanisms with respect to the link between hypertension and deficits in cognitive function have been proposed in several reviews (Elias et al., 1987a, 1989, 1998a; Elias and Robbins, 1991a; Waldstein, 1995; Waldstein and Katzel, 2001). Several of these papers (Waldstein, 1995; Waldstein and Katzel, 2001) are especially helpful with respect to pathophysiological mechanisms that may link high BP and cognitive functioning at different segments of the life span. Table 1 attempts to capture this classification briefly.

While the categorization of mechanisms presented in Table 1 helps greatly in the recognition of possible biological mechanisms that may intervene between hypertension and cognitive functioning in young adults, it does not explain why the combined impact of hypertension and age does not play-out as a disproportionately greater difference in performance between hypertensive and normotensive individuals with advancing age. Briefly, hypertension begins as a risk factor and, with time, results in cerebral vascular endothelial dysfunction, atherosclerotic vascular wall-change, and the consequent potential for multi-infarct disease (Pessina and Pauletto, 1997; Suzuki et al., 1997). As noted previously the cerebral arteries and all watershed areas

Table 1
Potential vascular and neurological mechanisms underlying hypertension-related cognitive deficit in various age groups

Young adult	Young adult–middle age	Late midlife and old age

• Cerebral metabolism and neurochemistry
• Cellular function
• Pulsatile variations in cerebral blood flow
• Disturbances in autoregulation
• Alteration in cellular or neurochemical activity
	• Pathophysiologic changes
	  ⇒ Cerebral vasculature
	  ⇒ Cerebral metabolism
	  ⇒ Autoregulation[a]
	  ⇒ Neurochemistry[b]
	• Subtle, intermittent, or chronic disturbances in cerebral blood flow
	• Enhanced cardiovascular reactivity
	• Enhanced neuroendocrine activity[c]
	• Metabolic Syndrome[d]
		• White matter lesions[e]
		• Advanced atherosclerosis
		• Multi-infarct disease
		• Impaired cerebral blood flow
		• Brain matter atrophy

Note. This table is based on discussions by Waldstein and Katzel (2001), Waldstein (1995), and Elias (1998).

[a]Process by which blood flow to brain tissues is maintained at relatively constant levels despite variations in perfusion pressure. This occurs via sympathetic stimulation that causes changes in vascular resistance, accumulation of metabolites, and hormones.

[b]Neuronal functioning is dependent upon concentrations of potassium, calcium, magnesium, hydrogen, and other ions in the cerebral fluid. Additionally, decreases in oxygen tension and pH, as well as increases in carbon dioxide tension and osmolality, produce vasodilation via relaxation of arterioles and precapillary sphincters. Nitric oxide is an endothelium-derived relaxing factor (EDRF) that plays a key role in vasodilation and there is some evidence that EDRF deficiency can cause clinical hypertension and that EDRF may also be involved in the pathogenesis of artherosclerosis.

[c]Many circulatory hormones affect the brain's vascular system, including vasodilators such as kinins, VIP, and ANP, and vasoconstrictors including vasopressin, norepinephrine, epinephrine, and angiotensin II.

[d]May include insulin dysregulation, dyslipidemia, central adiposity, hematologic abnormalities, and abnormal renal regulation of fluid volume.

[e]Morphological abnormalities of the white matter without well-defined etiology. On CT, WML appear as ill-defined patchy or diffuse areas of hypodensity without cortical involvement, which contrasts the usually clear demarcation of lacunes and infarcts.

are, to a lesser or greater degree, affected, although there is some evidence that hypertension-associated microvascular lesions are more likely to occur in sub-cortical regions (brain stem, basal ganglia, and peri-ventricular white matter) and frontal association areas (De Carli et al., 1995; Longstreth et al., 1996). These areas may be more susceptible to ischemic insult given the cumulative effects of aging and hypertension on end-artery tortuosity and consequent local perfusion (Baumbach and Heistad, 1997).

In short, structural and functional changes in the brain seen in hypertension are progressive and cumulative and generally irreversible once they occur. Thus, the impact of hypertension on cognitive function should increase with advancing age. One should see accelerated decline in cognitive functioning, particularly in the absence of treatment and blood pressure control. Thus, in our view, disproportionately greater differences in the performance of younger hypertensive and normotensive individuals do not fit with the developmental progression of the disease.

4.2.6. Alternative explanations

We (Elias et al., 1987a; Elias and Robbins, 1991a) have offered several alternative explanations, including the possibility that in some case-control studies, differences between young adult hypertensive and normotensive cohorts may be related to the failure to control for anxiety, depression, and other psycho-social factors, or may simply be the result of being identified as "hypertensive." Our own attempts to establish these links between hypertension and cognitive function have not been successful (Elias et al., 1987a), although further attempts should not be discouraged.

We have also offered a "signal-to-noise" ratio explanation of shrinking differences between hypertensive and normotensive cohorts with advancing age. The argument by Elias is summarized by Siegler et al. (2002, p. 491):

"... In youth, hypertension occurs more against a background of relatively good health than it does in middle or advanced age. The prevalence of hypertension-related pathophysiology and comorbidity increases with age. Thus, as an individual ages, hypertension becomes a risk factor seen against a background of multiple diseases and other risk factors (e.g. diabetes, cardiovascular disease, pulmonary disorders, lipidemia, high homocysteine, B12 deficiency)."

This is a plausible explanation and a reason to control hypertension-related comorbidity. It is not clear, however, that it explains the Maine-Syracuse data because the young adult-BP/hypertension phenomenon was observed where hypertension-related comorbidity was controlled (Elias et al., 1990a). One could argue that occult morbidity was not controlled completely, and that is clearly a possibility as new risk factors for cardiovascular disease and stroke are being recognized with surprising frequency.

4.2.7. Skepticism prevails

While the biological (Waldstein, 1995) and the "signal-to-noise ratio" (Siegler et al., 2002) explanations of the "young adult phenomenon" deserve careful consideration, one must seriously consider the possibility that the vulnerability-of-young-adults to hypertension phenomenon is merely an artifact of the cross-sectional design.

Very simply those who survive into old age may be those with less severe hypertension and/or higher levels of cognitive functioning (Siegler, 1975; Schultz et al., 1979; Elias et al., 1990b; Waldstein, 1995; Zelinski et al., 1998). Survival effects offer an explanation of inconsistent findings for subjects in advanced age, but are more difficult to apply to middle-aged, uncomplicated, essential hypertensive individuals.

For subject samples ranging in age from young adult to late middle-age we strongly suspect that selective volunteering is probably the artifactual culprit. Persons with lower levels of cognitive functioning may not volunteer for studies involving cognitive functioning. We know from the Maine-Syracuse studies (McArdle et al., 1991), and from the work of Siegler and Botwinick (1979) that poorer performing subjects and subjects in ill health drop out of longitudinal studies at a disproportionately higher rate. We have every reason to believe that poorer performing subjects (where poor health may be more prevalent) may be less likely to volunteer for studies involving cognitive testing.

4.2.8. Cross-sectional design limitations: Conclusions

In our view, cross-sectional studies, although useful in many respects, can never adequately address the question of interactions of aging and blood pressure. There are two reasons. First, the methods available allow one to suspect, and partially evaluate survivor and volunteer effects, but they cannot be evaluated with the degree of sophistication possible with longitudinal studies. Second, effects of age are pitted against effects of hypertension and the two may be inseparable when looked at from this perspective. One must examine relations between hypertension, or better yet BP level, and cognitive change over time. In this respect, effects of chronological age and intra-individual change over time may be disentangled.

Before moving to our consideration of longitudinal studies it is important to consider the literature generated by prospective designs. Very often, but not of necessity, these designs are hybrid episodic and longitudinal designs. Thus, it is fitting that they be discussed prior to our discussion of longitudinal studies.

4.3. Prospective designs: issues of causality

As in any scientific study of relationships, it is important to obtain evidence with respect to the issue of causality. Prospective designs help to address this issue. They generally involve measuring the predictor variables (e.g. BP) at one point in time and the cognitive outcome variable after a significant amount of time has elapsed. They can be longitudinal with respect to either the predictor set or the outcome variables. These designs are very highly regarded and very common in epidemiological studies.

Episodic and cross-sectional studies of BP and cognitive functioning reported in the behavioral literature, including studies by our group, have measured BP and cognitive functioning concurrently (i.e. at points very near in time, at the same visit or the same day); thus raising a problem with respect to establishing a causal association between high BP and cognition. Fortunately, prospective associations between chronic hypertension and cognitive functioning and between BP level and cognitive functioning have been established. In our Framingham study analyses (Elias et al., 1993, 1995a), discussed previously, BP values were obtained 12–14 years before measures of cognitive functioning were obtained. Following our study, a number of papers using similar prospective designs appeared in the medical literature. We can provide only a few major examples.

The Honolulu Heart Study investigators reported that elevated systolic BP was related to cognitive functioning measured 9 to 18 years later (Launer et al., 1995). Swan et al. (1996) reported similar results when cognitive functioning was measured 25 to 30 years after the BP assessment window. In a study with 999 males from the Uppsala sample, Kilander et al. (1998) found that the lower the BP at age 50, the higher the level of cognitive function at age 70. Interestingly, other aspects of hypertension such as left ventricular hypertrophy and a non-dipping 24 hour BP profile, were also related to lower cognitive function. Recent prospective findings from the East Boston Study are reviewed in the section on longitudinal studies. It is our view that these prospective studies, with their large numbers of community-based subjects, were very important in convincing the medical community that this was an important research problem to pursue.

In a commentary on these studies, Glynn et al. (1999) note that several of these prospective studies failed to find BP–cognitive function relations for the episodic aspect of the analysis, i.e. for data from the examination at which BP was measured concurrently with cognitive functioning. However, many studies have shown relations between BP and cognitive function under these circumstances. Often where concurrent measurement is associated with negative results the fault lies with too few BP measurements at only one occasion. See a discussion of this issue by Elias et al. (1995b) and an example provided by a series of studies with the Framingham Heart Study sample (Farmer et al., 1987, 1990; Elias et al., 1993). Many of the prospective studies reported have utilized measurements of BP on multiple and widely spaced occasions, thus capturing magnitude and duration of BP effects (e.g. Elias et al., 1993). Longitudinal studies with the Maine-Syracuse sample clearly indicate that multiple measurements of BP over an extended period of time yield stronger associations between BP and cognitive function than do multiple measurements at a single occasion, although both are related to cognitive function.

4.4. Longitudinal studies

Given problems inherent in cross-sectional designs, longitudinal data is extremely valuable to the understanding of interactions between cognitive aging (change in cognitive functioning over time) and hypertension. It is the design of choice.

4.4.1. Two measurement points

Table 2 summarizes longitudinal studies, conducted since 1990, with only two measurement points. Because of space limitations, our brief review of longitudinal studies is limited to those with at least three measurement points, baseline plus two additional measurements (waves of cognitive data) over time. This is not an arbitrary decision. Two-measurement point studies provide limited information. One cannot evaluate the possibility of higher-order tends. More importantly, reliability for the estimation of longitudinal slopes goes up dramatically when one moves from two to three waves of measurement (Willett, 1988). This does not mean that every subject must have had at least two waves of longitudinal assessment after baseline, but it does mean that the information obtained is much more limited if the study is essentially a difference score study with two measurement points only for each subject.

4.4.2. Three times of measurement

The very few studies of hypertension and cognitive functioning that have involved baseline and at least two additional cognitive assessments are summarized in Table 3. Participants in all of these studies were middle-aged or older at baseline. One study

Table 2
A summary of major studies since 1990 of hypertension (or blood pressure) and cognitive functioning employing two assessments of cognitive function over time

Study name	Sample size	Baseline age range (years)	Cognitive follow-up (years)	Cognitive exams	Outcomes	Predictors	Synopsis of findings
Intergenerational Studies from the Institute of Human Development in Berkeley, California[a]	103	49–63 at Exam 2	Approx. 11	2	Digit Span (DS) forward & backward, Block Design, Object Assembly, and Digit Symbol (DSy)	Diastolic blood pressure (DBP), start of antihypertensive use between exams	Exam 1 and 2 DBP and change in hypertensive medication status significantly predicted Exam 2 DS forward
The Western Collaborative Group Study (WCGS)[b]	1173	39–59	25–30	2	Iowa Screening Battery for Mental Decline, Mini-Mental Status Examination (MMSE)	Systolic blood pressure (SBP), DBP	SBP and DBP in midlife were significant predictors of cognitive decline 25 to 30 years later
Healthy Old People in Edinburgh (HOPE)[c]	603	70–88	Median 4.2	2	Change in MMSE score	SBP, DBP	Higher baseline SBP significantly predicted decline in MMSE performance
The Kungsholmen Project[d]	1736	75–101	Mean 3.4	2	MMSE	SBP, DBP	SBP and DBP were positively related to exam 1 MMSE. SBP, but not DBP, was positively associated with MMSE at Exam 2
Healthy Old People in Edinburgh (HOPE)[e]	387	70–88	4	2	Raven's Progressive Matrices (RPM) & Logical Memory (LM) at Exam 2 only. NART	Hypertension, SBP, DBP	Both SBP and DBP related prospectively to RPM scores, but not to LM. Hypertensive subjects at follow-up had significantly lower RPM, but not LM. scores than disease-free unmedicated subjects with low/medium BP

(*Continued*)

Table 2
Continued

Study name	Sample size	Baseline age range (years)	Cognitive follow-up (years)	Cognitive exams	Outcomes	Predictors	Synopsis of findings
The Kungsholmen Project[f]	924	75 and older	Mean 3.4	2	MMSE	SBP, DBP	Neither baseline SBP nor DBP, at any level, predicted cognitive decline (defined as MMSE decline of >10%). Exam 1 to Exam 2 SBP reduction of ≥10 mmHg was related to higher risk of cognitive decline for women but not men
Medical Research Council (MRC) Treatment Trial of Hypertension in Older Adults[g]	387	Mean 70.2	9–12	2	MMSE	SBP, DBP	Less decline in SBP (i.e., Exam 1 SBP minus mean Exam 2 SBP) was associated with poorer cognitive outcome (log-transformed MMSE score)
The Atherosclerosis Risk in Communities (ARIC) study[h]	10,963	47–70	Mean 6.0	2	Delayed Word Recall (DWR), DSy, Word Fluency (WF)	Hypertension defined via SBP or DBP or use of antihypertensive medications, SBP	Exam 1 hypertension was associated with greater decline in DSy only for subjects ≥58 years. No U-shaped association between any cognitive test and stratified SBP using cut-off pts of Glynn et al. (1999) was found; subjects with lowest SBP had the least decline in DSy and WF

| The Atherosclerosis Risk in Communities (ARIC) study[j] | 8058 | 48–67 | 6 | 2 | DWR, DSy, WF (Change scores) | Hypertension defined via history, use of antihypertensive medications, SBP, or DBP | Uncontrolled or partially controlled hypertension was associated with negative change for DSy and WF. For DSy, adverse effects of uncontrolled hypertension were strongest for older subjects (>age 56 at exam 2) |
| Duke Established Populations for Epidemiologic Studies of the Elderly (EPESE)[j] | 4136 | 65–105 | 3 | 2 | Change in Short Portable Mental Status Questionnaire (SPMSQ) score | SBP, DBP, hypertension, use of antihypertensive medications | U-shaped relationship between SBP and change in SPMSQ score for older white subjects was found—extreme BP values were associated with cognitive decline. No significant relationship for African Americans was found. |

[a]Sands & Meredith (1992).
[b]Swan et al. (1996).
[c]Starr et al. (1997).
[d]Guo et al. (1997).
[e]Deary et al. (1998).
[f]Zhu et al. (1998).
[g]Cervilla et al. (2000).
[h]Knopman et al. (2001).
[i]Alves de Moraes et al. (2002).
[j]Bohannon et al. (2002).

Table 3
A summary of major studies since 1990 of hypertension (or blood pressure) and cognitive functioning employing three or more assessments of cognitive function over time

Study name	Sample size	Baseline age (years)	Cognitive follow-up (years)	Cognitive exams	Outcomes	Predictors	Synopsis of findings
Medical Research Council Elderly Hypertension Trial[a]	2,584	65–74	4.5	5	Paired Associates Learning Test (PALT), Trailmaking Test (TMT) part A	Systolic blood pressure (SBP), diastolic blood pressure (DBP), use of antihypertensive medications	No significant association between SBP or DBP at entry and change in PALT scores with time was found
The Seattle Longitudinal Study[b]	845	22–70	7–21	5	Extensive battery[c]	Hypertension, atherosclerosis	Atherosclerosis predicted greater decline on space and number but less decline on verbal meaning. Cerebrovascular disease was negatively associated with cognitive level and increased the risk of and amount of cognitive decline. Hypertensives with other CVD complications performed worse over time than uncomplicated hypertensives or normotensives
East Boston component of the Established Populations for the Epidemiologic Study of the Elderly (EPESE) and the Hypertension Detection and Follow-up Program (HDFP)[d]	3,657	65–102	6	3	East Boston Memory Test (EBMT), Short Portable Mental Status Questionnaire (SPMSQ)	SBP, DBP	Overall, no linear association between BP and cognition was found. Results indicated possibilities of more complex associations, (i.e. U-shaped relationship between BP and cognitive errors)
The Epidemiology of Vascular Aging (EVA) Study[e]	1,373	59–71	4	3	Mini-Mental Sate Examination (MMSE)	Hypertension defined via SBP or DBP or use of antihypertensive medications	High BP was associated with cognitive decline (defined as MMSE drop of ≥4pts from Exam 1 to Exam 3). The odds ratio (OR) was higher for subjects with high BP at Exam 1 & Exam 2 than for subjects with high BP at only 1 time point. The OR was highest for hypertensive subjects who were not taking antihypertensive medications. For subjects taking antihypertensive medications, ORs did not differ on the basis of normal vs. high BP.

The Cardiovascular Health Study (CHS)[f]	5,888	65 and older	5 or 7	3	MMSE, DSy	SBP, ankle-arm BP	SBP predicted declines in both MMSE and DSy
The Maine-Syracuse Study[g]	140	40–70	Mean 18.8	2 for 86 subjects, 3 for 26 subjects, and 5 for 28 subjects	4 cognitive factor scores based on factor analyses with 12 WAIS subtests[h]	SBP, DBP, hypertension	Higher all-exam DBP was associated with longitudinal decline for Visualization-Performance (VP) ability and Speed, with average BP over examinations being a stronger predictor than initial BP level. Hypertension was a weaker predictor of VP and was unrelated to Speed
Washington Heights-Inwood Columbia Aging Project[i]	1,259	65 and older	7	2	Extensive battery[j]	Categories of SBP and DBP, hypertension, hypertension history	Hypertension history was associated with an increased risk for VaD but not AD. Hypertension was not associated with changes in memory, language, or general cognitive functions over time
The Maine-Syracuse Study[k]	529	18–83	Mean 18.9	2 for 286 subjects, 3–5 for 239 subjects	4 cognitive factor scores based on factor analyses with 12 WAIS subtests[h]	SBP, DBP, Hypertension	BP indices predicted longitudinal decline in Visualization-Fluid-Performance factor scores, but not Crystallized-Verbal, Memory, or Speed of Performance factor, over time

[a] Prince et al. (1996).
[b] Schaie (1996).
[c] Letter series, number series, and word series, object and alphanumeric rotation, cube comparison, addition, subtraction, and multiplication, ETS vocabulary V-2 and V-4, PMA word fluency, identical pictures, finding As, number comparison, immediate and delayed recall.
[d] Glynn et al. (1999).
[e] Tzourio et al. (1999).
[f] Haan et al. (1999).
[g] Elias et al. (1998).
[h] Four cognitive factors: 1. Crystallized-Verbal factor from Information, Comprehension, Similarities, and Vocabulary subtests. 2. Visualization-Performance factor from Picture Completion, Block Design, Picture Arrangement, and Object Assembly subtests. 3. Memory-Span factor from Digit Span Forward, Digit Span Backward, and Arithmetic subtests. 4. Psychomotor Speed factor from Digit Symbol Substitution subtest.
[i] Posner et al. (2002).
[j] MMSE, Boston Naming Test, Controlled Word Association test, category naming, Complex Ideational Material & Phrase Repetition subtests of Boston Diagnostic Aphasia Evaluation, Abstract Reasoning, Similarities, nonverbal Identities and Oddities of the Mattis Dementia Rating Scale, the Rosen Drawing Test, Benton Visual Retention Test, and seven subtests of the Selective Reminding Test.
[k] Robbins et al. (2002).

that did not report associations between BP and cognitive decline (four assessments of Paired Associates Learning Test performance over a 54-month period) was conducted with participants who were hypertensive (systolic BP > 160 mmHg) at baseline (Prince et al., 1996). Another study with participants 65 years of age or older found that hypertension was associated with increased risk of vascular dementia, but not with cognitive decline over a seven year period (Posner et al., 2002).

In the East Boston Study, Glynn et al. (1999) reported prospective associations of BP with performance level and change over a 6-year period for a measure of mental status but not a memory measure. Elevated systolic BP (160 mmHg or higher) was related to an increase in error rate on the mental status measure. However, they also reported null results and curvilinear relations for other indices of BP with mental status change and level. For the curvilinear relations both elevated BP and low BP were associated with poorer performance.

Linear associations relating high BP to greater decline were reported in each of the other studies. Schaie (1996) reported that hypertension predicted level and decline in Word Fluency for Seattle Longitudinal Study participants under age 60. In the Epidemiology of Vascular Aging Study, decline on the Mini-Mental State Exam (MMSE) over 4 years was associated with hypertension (Tzourio et al., 1999), and was greatest for hypertensive participants who were not being treated with antihypertensive medications. In the Cardiovascular Health Study, Haan et al. (1999) found that decline on both the modified MMSE and on the Digit Symbol Substitution Test over 5 to 7 years was associated with high systolic BP.

We now turn to the Maine-Syracuse studies involving three or more times of cognitive assessment. Findings for our first assessment of hypertensive vs. normotensive-related change for three assessments over 5 to 6-year intervals simply serves to illustrate why two times of assessment can mask trends that will be seen with a minimum of three assessment periods. Methodological details for this study (Schultz et al., 1989) are similar to those for the later study reported in the next section. This study involved a small number of hypertensive and normotensive individuals who participated in extensive hypertension diagnostic studies between 1976 and 1977 (baseline). For analyses that included subjects who developed hypertension-related complications after baseline, significant Hypertension by Time-of-Measurement interactions were observed for the Verbal scaled scores (Fig. 3) and the Performance scaled scores (Fig. 4). There were no hypertensive–normotensive differences at baseline for either WAIS score. For WAIS Verbal scaled scores, normotensive individuals improved and then declined over time whereas hypertensive subjects showed progressive but modest decline. For WAIS Performance scaled scores, the normotensive individuals improved in a non-significant manner and the hypertensive individuals showed significant decline. When subjects who developed hypertension-related complications during the longitudinal study were excluded from the analysis, the trends were exactly the same, although the interaction term was no longer significant. The latter phenomenon was most likely related to lack of adequate power to test the interaction. However, examination of change over time scores in a parallel study (Elias et al., 1989) using an index of cognitive impairment based on multiple

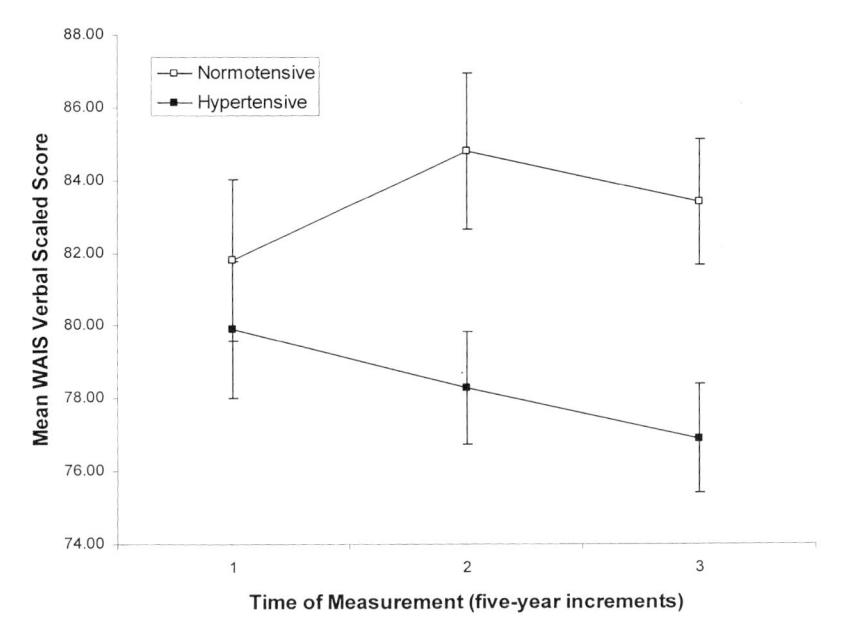

Fig. 3. Longitudinal WAIS Verbal Scale mean scores for Normotensive and Hypertensive Groups at each of three times of measurement ($n = 47$).

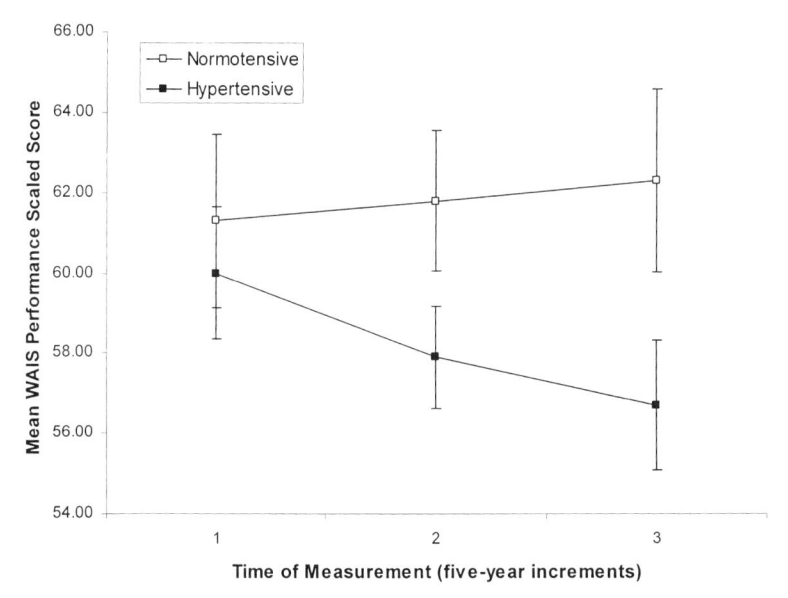

Fig. 4. Longitudinal WAIS Performance Scale mean scores for Normotensive and Hypertensive Groups at each of three times of measurement ($n = 47$).

neuropsychological tests, i.e. the Average Impairment Rating (AIR) (Russell et al., 1970) clearly indicated hypertension main effects and a parallel decline in cognitive functioning for hypertensive and normotensive individuals

Interestingly, for the longitudinal study with the WAIS (Figs. 3 and 4), hypertensive and normotensive individuals did not differ significantly at baseline for either the Verbal or Performance scaled scores. The same individuals were followed serially and thus the divergence of performance scores between hypertensive and normotensive individuals over time could not be attributed to selective volunteering or survival effects. Subsequent analyses indicated that failure to see baseline differences between hypertensive and normotensive groups were related to the fact that those who performed more poorly dropped out of the study, and the dropouts were characterized by a higher proportion of hypertensive individuals (McArdle et al., 1991).

These studies illustrate the importance of more than two waves of testing to detect other than linear trends, but they do not exemplify how one should proceed with a longitudinal study. We have learned much since then. Although significant effects were observed, sample sizes were small. More importantly, the analysis of variance techniques employed did not allow us to correct for disproportionate attrition by the poorest performing subjects, who were primarily hypertensive individuals (McArdle et al., 1991). Finally, all the subjects were carefully treated during the 10 to 12-year period of the study. All of these factors would lead to an underestimation of hypertension-related decline in cognitive function over time.

Our subsequent published longitudinal studies with the WAIS were designed to correct these deficiencies (McArdle et al., 1991; Elias et al., 1996, 1998a). We will focus on the less technical analysis represented by the Elias et al. (1998a) paper as it involved the longest period of longitudinal follow-up. Our objective was to explore mean *intra-individual* differences in hypertension-related change in cognitive functioning over time as opposed to examining mean differences at each examination. The sample was drawn from a subset of 246 community-dwelling individuals (aged 40–70 years) who were administered the WAIS in studies of endocrine function and hypertension conducted between 1975 and 1992 (Streeten et al., 1992).

To reduce the "background noise" from disease, all hypertensive and normotensive individuals who had diseases associated with medically complicated or secondary forms of hypertension, diagnosed dementia, treatment for alcoholism or drug abuse, or a psychiatric history were excluded. See Schultz et al. (1979) for a detailed list of exclusions via medical diagnosis. An additional requirement was that these participants either had no antihypertensive drug treatment history at baseline (Exam 1) or, if previously treated, were withdrawn from treatment (under their physician's supervision) 14–21 days prior to Exam 1 testing. Methodological detail with respect to BP assessments and measurement of cognitive functioning can be found in the original paper. Hypertension was defined as SBP ≥ 140 mmHg and/or DBP ≥ 90 mmHg based on the average of multiple sitting, standing, and reclining BP assessments. Individuals with both SBP and DBP levels less than defined hypertensive levels were classified as normotensive.

Of the 246 individuals who met these inclusion criteria at baseline, 36.2% were lost to attrition prior to Examination 2. Individuals lost to attrition (non-responders, $n=89$) exhibited lower occupation levels and Visualization-Performance composite scores ($p<0.05$) at baseline than those who participated in at least one additional examination (responders, $n=157$). For non-responders, increments in baseline diastolic BP were associated with lower levels of performance on the Visualization-Performance composite at baseline ($p<0.05$), but this was not true for responders.

Of the 157 longitudinal participants, 17 were excluded from the first-pass (primary) longitudinal analyses because they exhibited one or more of the following events or diseases during the longitudinal study: transient ischemic attack ($n=3$), cardiovascular disease ($n=13$), insulin-dependent diabetes ($n=2$), epilepsy ($n=1$) and stroke ($n=5$). These individuals were included in a secondary analysis. Of the remaining 140 longitudinal participants, 86 were tested twice, 26 were tested three times, and 28 were tested at a fourth and fifth time. The mean retest interval between successive examinations was 5.3 years (SD=0.62) and the mean interval between Exam 1 and Exam 5 was 18.8 years (SD=0.55). Of these 140 individuals, the attrition rate between baseline and Examination 5 was 25.1%. The major reasons for attrition were death and refusal.

Of the 77 participants who were diagnosed as hypertensive at Exam 1 or on at least one of the longitudinal examinations (Ever-Hypertensive), 40 were men and 37 were women. Sixty-three participants, 15 men and 48 women, were normotensive (Never-Hypertensive) throughout the longitudinal data collection. There were no statistically significant differences for education, age, or occupation between hypertensive and normotensive groups. The range of age at entry into the study was 40–70 years. The level of occupation ranged from unskilled to executive/professional, with mean level being clerical/skilled laborer. The average level of education was approximately 15 years. The ranges of BP values (relevant to regression analyses) averaged over all examinations were 96–178 mmHg for systolic BP and 54–113 mmHg for diastolic BP. For hypertensive participants, mean systolic BP was 146.5 (SD=14.7) mmHg and mean diastolic BP was 88.8 (SD=9.0). For normotensive participants, mean systolic BP was 118.4 (SD=12.4) mmHg and mean diastolic BP was 69.9 (SD=7.7). At Exam 1 the range for systolic BP was 83 to 210 mmHg and the range for diastolic BP was 53 to 124 mmHg.

In addition to age and the Ever vs. Never Hypertensive variable, two sets of DBP and SBP predictors were used: (1) averaged untreated BP at Exam 1 (Exam 1 BP); (2) averaged BP based on all examinations (All-Exam BP). A basic covariate set for all analyses was: Education (years), Occupation (level), Gender, and Ever-Treated vs. Never-Treated with antihypertensive drugs. Twenty-two percent of the Ever-Hypertensive individuals were not treated with antihypertensive drugs during the longitudinal study because many physicians did not aggressively treat mild isolated systolic hypertension during the early years of the study. Trait anxiety, depression, and alcohol consumption were included as statistical controls in preliminary models but were all unrelated to longitudinal change over time.

Table 4
Mean slope values for persons diagnosed as Ever-Hypertensive or Never-Hypertensive (Normotensive)

Variable	Normotensive ($n=63$)		Hypertensive ($n=77$)	
	Mean	SD	Mean	SD
Visualization/Performance	−0.007	1.16	−0.363*	1.15
Crystallized/Verbal	−0.003	1.50	−0.107	1.19
Memory-Span	−0.186	1.66	−0.175	1.16
Digit Symbol	−0.099	1.15	−0.294*	0.97

Note. Mean slope values are obtained by averaging the estimated slope values (scores) which constitute the basic longitudinal data for each individual.

A two-stage growth curve method was employed (Rogosa et al., 1982). Space does not permit a detailed presentation of this statistical method. Its important features are that it allows estimates of decline in performance for a given number of years, e.g. 10 or 20, even though not every subject has been in the study for that long. It does not require that all subjects complete every longitudinal examination as long as at least two examinations are completed at some point in the study, nor does it require equal time intervals between examinations. One significant advantage of this method of longitudinal analysis is that it adjusts for attrition because data for dropouts need not be discarded from the analysis as long as data are available at baseline and an additional time of measurement.

Stage 1 simply involves a calculation of slope and intercept values for each individual (intra-individual slopes and intercepts). These become the basic data, test score by test score, for each individual. In Stage 2 of the analysis, these intercept and slope values become the raw data for multiple regression analyses (or any other statistical method employed). Of course, one must have, for each subject, an intercept and a slope for each dependent variable.

Table 4 compares slope values (negative values indicate decrement in performance over time) for the Never-Hypertensive ($n=63$) and Ever-Hypertensive ($n=77$) individuals in the study. These are essentially mean slope values derived by adding the intra-individual slope values for each person in each group and dividing by the number of values. It is clear from the table that persons who were hypertensive on one or more examinations during the longitudinal study (Ever-Hypertensive) exhibited decline over time (significant negative slope values) for the Visualization-Performance composite score and for the Speed score (Digit Symbol Substitution). Figure 5 illustrates the estimated magnitude of differences between the hypertensive and normotensive cohorts over a 20-year period based on the data for change per year.

Table 5 describes these relationships in the context of the multiple regression analyses with statistical control for age, education, occupation, and treatment with antihypertensive drugs. The Visualization-Performance score was used as the outcome variable. No significant associations between the BP predictors and cognitive functioning were observed for intercepts (not shown). Now we consider the

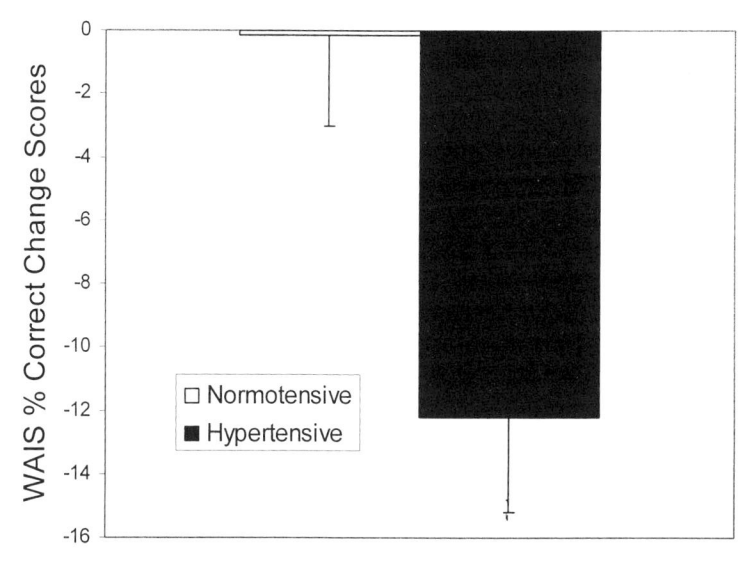

Fig. 5. Mean Visualization-Performance change scores over 20 years based upon slope values for Normotensive and Hypertensive groups ($n = 140$).

Table 5
Magnitude (b) and Strength (R^2) of association between the diagnosis of hypertension and BP level (10 mmHg) predictors and estimated intercept and slope values for the Visualization-Performance composite scores ($N = 140$)

	Slopes[a]			
Predictor	Age not controlled		Age controlled	
	b	R^2	b	R^2
Ever-Never Hypertensive	−0.733*	0.04	−0.603*	0.04
Exam 1 DBP	−0.223**	0.06	−0.159*	0.03
Exam 1 SBP	−0.132**	0.06	−0.084	0.02
All-Exam DBP	−0.413***	0.13	−0.340***	0.08
All-Exam SBP	−0.233***	0.11	−0.174**	0.05

Note. All regression coefficients (b) and R^2 values are adjusted for education, occupation, gender, and treatment with antihypertensive drugs. Values in the columns labeled age controlled are also adjusted for age.

[a]Slopes represent Hypertension-related or BP-related change in percent correct scores for each year of participation in the longitudinal study.

*$p < 0.05$, **$p < 0.01$, ***$p < 0.001$.

data for change over time (Table 5). It is important to note that the regression coefficients shown in the table express extent of change in the intra-individual slopes per unit increment (e.g. per 10 mmHg diastolic BP) in the predictor variable. In effect, the regression coefficients are slopes of slopes. That is, individual slope values for WAIS Visualization-Performance composite scores are regressed on the predictor variables and adjusted for the other variables in the multiple regression model. Obviously, with age in the regression model, effect sizes are smaller. With age controlled every BP measure is associated with negative change on the Visualization-Performance Composite over time (decline) except for Exam 1 Systolic BP. The Digit Symbol Substitution Test (Speed) is the only subtest which is included in the WAIS Performance Scale but excluded from the Visualization-Performance Composite. Only the Exam 1 DBP and All-Exam DBP variables were associated ($p<0.05$) with Digit Symbol slope values when age was excluded from the regression model ($b=-0.14$, $R^2=0.03$; $b=-0.21$, $R^2=0.04$). Only the association of All-Exam DBP with Digit Symbol slopes remained significant when age was included in the model ($b=-0.19$, $R^2=0.03$).

It is important not to lose track of an extremely important finding which relates back to the cross-sectional findings of increased vulnerability to hypertension in younger adults. For these analyses, age at entry into the study (40–70 years) did not interact with any of the BP variables in accounting for intercept values or slope (change over time) values. Although older persons at baseline declined more over time, the age-related decline was not more accelerated for persons with hypertensive status or higher BP values. This does not gainsay the fact that relations between BP and cognitive function were modestly attenuated by control for age at baseline and vice versa. Age and BP, particularly systolic BP are, of course, correlated ($r=0.23$).

Results obtained when we used the traditional Performance and Verbal Scale scores paralleled those obtained with the Visualization-Performance and the Crystallized-Verbal Composite scores. We added the 17 individuals who displayed one or more medical complications to the sample in a secondary analysis ($n=157$). Associations among the predictor variables and the dependent variables reported for the smaller sample ($n=140$) were not strengthened further with the addition of these subjects to the analysis. However, the higher the reported number of hypertension-related complications, the greater the decline over time on the Visualization-Performance composite ($b=-0.35$, $p<0.05$; $R^2=0.03$).

In summary, the WAIS composite scores showing more accelerated change over time in relation to the BP variables were Visualization-Performance (comprising the Picture Completion, Block Design, Picture Arrangement, and Object Assembly subtests) and Psychomotor Speed (measured by a single subtest, Digit Symbol Substitution). The Visualization-Performance composite taps executive functioning and fluid abilities in addition to visualization skills.

4.4.3. Wider age range and a larger sample

One may raise a question as to whether these findings are a product of the relatively small sample or the restricted age range studied. Subjects, regardless of hypertension-related complications or age were admitted to the study ($n=529$; age range = 18 to 83 years) and the analyses were repeated. Results were essentially the same (Elias et al., 1998b; Robbins et al., 2002).

4.4.4. Continuing work

This work is continuing as we are presently in a new wave of data collection. We did not adjust for attrition from baseline to the second exam, although poorer performers who were disproportionately hypertensive individuals were more likely to drop out. This would lead to an under-reporting, not an over-reporting, of effect sizes. However, there are longitudinal methods that will allow for an estimation and correction of attrition from baseline, including methods employed by McArdle and colleagues (e.g. McArdle and Hamagami, 1991). Many techniques, considerably more sophisticated than the two-stage growth curve analyses, have been described in two outstanding books on the topic (Collins and Horn, 1991; Collins and Sayer, 2001). A chapter by Elias and Robbins (1991b) deals with shrinking sample sizes associated with exclusion of subjects with hypertension-related co-morbidity ("reducing the noise"). The next two sections of this chapter deal with methodological issues affecting progress and the significance of these findings.

4.4.5. Decline in Blood Pressure over time

In the Maine-Syracuse study we routinely perform analyses designed to determine if *decline* in BP level over all or part (e.g. early examinations) of a specified surveillance period, is related to lower cognitive functioning at the end of that surveillance period. We also have related change in BP over time to change in cognitive functioning over time. Thus far we have found no evidence to support the hypothesis that falling BP is related to lower cognitive function. We have not yet reported these negative findings as they may be a function of the length of time employed in our surveillance period and the relative good health of our sample. This relationship has been reported in other laboratories.

Swan et al. (1998) compared persons who exhibited a decline in BP over an 18 to 24-year follow-up to persons who exhibited sustained hypertension or normal BPs over this same time period. Persons who showed BP decline over time performed at a significantly lower level on a psychomotor speed factor score. This "fall in BP–cognitive test decline" relationship was not observed for any other measure in the Swan et al. battery, and was tentatively explained in terms of the higher presence of hypertension-related morbidity in those who showed a fall in BP. In the Maine-Syracuse study, fall in BP from earlier higher levels is primarily attributable to successful treatment, not a higher prevalence of hypertension-related morbidity. Individuals who show a fall in BP do not exhibit lowered cognitive test performance. However, our subjects are younger, in better health, and have not as yet been followed as long as those studied by Swan et al. (1998). The data reported by Swan et al. (1998) illustrate the importance of tracking trajectories of BP change for significant periods of time. We will continue to explore the possibility that decline in BP level over time is associated with lower cognitive function at some later period of time.

5. Unresolved issues in hypertension and cognitive function research

Despite advances in the study of hypertension, particularly within a life span context, there are several issues that, surprisingly, still remain after 30 or more years of work.

5.1. Identifying abilities related to hypertension

Waldstein (1995) has done an excellent job of identifying cognitive abilities that exhibit strong and consistent associations with blood pressure and has attempted to classify these by the age range employed in the study samples. She correctly points out that information contributing to the success of this undertaking is limited for elderly individuals. It is clear from Tables 2 and 3 that many large epidemiological studies use only one or two cognitive measures or simply employ the MMSE, a test more properly defined as a measure of mental status than a global measure of intellectual functioning. This phenomenon is most likely related to the fact that investigators are using established archival data sets rather than a failure to recognize the importance of comprehensive test batteries.

Considering the body of literature available, it appears that almost all cognitive abilities, with the possible exception of Crystallized-Verbal abilities, have been related to hypertension or blood pressure. There are three possible explanations for this finding: (1) the effects of hypertension on brain are more diffuse than specific; (2) the literature is dominated by studies which use clinical measures of cognitive function, more specifically sub tests, that lack specificity; and (3) some of the important cognitive constructs, e.g. executive functioning, are so broadly conceptualized that it is difficult to identify tests that index them. In the next section we consider all three possibilities.

5.1.1. Predictions from the biology of hypertension

As discussed in previous sections, the biology of hypertension suggests that blood pressure effects on cognitive functioning should be seen across a broad array of cognitive functions, with perhaps cognitive abilities associated with frontal and subcortical areas being more affected, e.g. executive functioning and memory. Thus far the literature indicates that, for some age groups, crystallized-verbal abilities are resistant to hypertension effects.

In order to go beyond this generalization, if indeed there are more specific effects of hypertension within a framework of diffuse effects, we need to improve our measurement methods in three ways: (1) by use of sophisticated factor analysis methods designed to achieve variable reduction and the assignment of highly correlated tests to composite scores that have been constructed in a theoretically meaningful way; (2) by use of information processing tasks from the experimental psychology laboratory; and (3) by improving the specificity of theoretical constructs defining various cognitive abilities, particularly the construct labeled "executive functioning" or the "executor functions." We will briefly discuss these three issues.

5.1.2. Factor analysis studies

Factor analysis has been underutilized, although there are examples of principal components analyses used in the hypertension research literature (Blumenthal et al., 1993; Waldstein et al., 1996). The general absence of application of factor analytic methods to the study of risk factors and cognitive function is most likely related to the fact that sample sizes have been too small and that a range of cognitive abilities necessary to the success of this approach has not been included in the test batteries employed. Large samples and a mix of variables likely to separate into factors with non-overlap are requirements for a proper application of factor analysis. Alternatively, one may, as we have done with the WAIS in our studies, make use of available information on factors carefully developed by other researchers.

5.1.3. Information processing studies

The advantages and disadvantages of information processing paradigms as they apply to this literature have been discussed by Elias and Elias (1993) and good examples of the approach may be found in published papers (Madden and Blumenthal, 1989; Blumenthal et al., 1993). Briefly, this approach is limited by the fact that information processing tasks are often complex, time consuming, and high in task difficulty and thus cannot be utilized with poorly educated and clinical populations or in clinical trials where the focus is other than cognitive function. Until these problems are solved, and it is possible, the major advantage of information processing tasks seems to be in the context of functional imaging or cerebral blood flow studies where clinical tests are most always not useful or usable. Work by Jennings and colleagues (Jennings et al., 1998) on relations among cerebral blood flow, hypertension, treatment, and cognitive functioning provides a good example of how one can use information processing paradigms to understand biological mechanisms intervening between blood pressure and cognitive functioning for specific cognitive domains. These methods promise to be very useful in understanding which specific cognitive abilities are affected by hypertension and in investigations designed to identify biological, or other, mechanisms linking blood pressure and cognition.

5.1.4. Theoretical issues

The use of a template such as the construct labeled Vascular Cognitive Impairment (VCI) (Bowler and Hachinski, 1995; Inzitari et al., 2002) may be particularly useful with respect to predictions of which cognitive abilities are affected by hypertension. Hypertension is a cardiovascular disease. The syndrome of VCI may involve a form of memory deficit, but memory deficit is not the overriding and predominant cognitive deficit (Bowler and Hachinski, 1995). In addition to selective aspects of memory, executive ability and speed of performance are primary targets (Inzitari et al., 2002) associated with VCI. Executive ability has been singled out as an aspect of cognition which may be particularly vulnerable to vascular disease, whether diagnosed or silent. Unfortunately, there is a significant lack of agreement as to which tests actually measure executive functioning (Lyon, 1996; Paolo et al., 1996), and the list grows as time passes (Lamar et al., 2002).

The executor, by definition (Lezak, 1983; Lyon, 1996), "presides" over more specific brain functions and involves planning, organizing, integration, coordinating, and purposeful goal-directed behavior. The critical reader will realize that these functions are involved in almost every cognitive task except those requiring the most rudimentary abilities. In a recent objective and critical review of the executive functioning literature, Lyon (1996) remarks that it is presently impossible to separate attention, memory, and executive functioning in terms of current ways in which they are operationally defined. Even where there is good agreement that executive functioning has been affected by hypertension, on the basis of the pattern of cognitive deficit observed, one is reduced to speculation that this phenomenon relates to frontal lobe damage.

Lamar et al. (2002) point out that the tendency to equate executive functioning with frontal lobe function has introduced an unfortunate circularity into the literature. Executive function can be affected by brain injury in other brain areas; further, executive function can be impaired in the absence of any diagnosed frontal lobe injury (Lamar et al., 2002).

5.1.5. Is antihypertensive treatment an effective intervention and if so, for whom?

It is logical to assume that aggressive lowering of blood pressure via treatment will have a positive effect on the preservation of cognitive function at the population level and for individuals for whom controlled blood pressures are achieved. This is based on the logical assumption that if high BP is bad for cognitive functioning, prevention, or control of high BP will prevent hypertension related cognitive deficits. But, surprisingly, direct evidence in support of this assumption is not as strong as we expect it to be. Despite advances in our understanding of associations between BP levels and cognitive function, it is still not clear that treatment with antihypertensive medications slows the progression of cognitive decline within the normal range of functioning. Clinical trials have offered the promise of improvement in cognitive function after treatment with contemporary antihypertensive agents, but the benefit has been modest (Croog et al., 1986) and negative effects of treatment have been reported (Jonas et al., 2001). Where modest improvement has been seen, it is not clear whether improvements are due to the lowering of blood pressure. Thus far we have not found that treatment for hypertension is associated with cognitive deficit or decrement over time, nor has it been associated with improvement in cognitive functioning.

Consequently, a number of important questions remain to be conclusively answered by our studies and others: (1) is improvement in cognitive functioning dependent on age at treatment, how early in the progression of the disease treatment is initiated, or the level of cognitive impairment when treatment is initiated; (2) is there an optimal BP range for slowing progression of cognitive decline rather than the previously arbitrary definitions of normal BP and hypertension; (3) are there subtypes of hypertensive individuals for whom treatment results in better cognitive performance and subtypes for whom treatment is ineffective as a cognitive intervention; and (4) do particular classes of antihypertensive agents have particular advantages given their other pharmacological properties aside from BP lowering? The inclusion of cognitive batteries in current clinical trials of antihypertensive agents is aimed at answering these questions. However, the time limitations imposed by multiple outcome measurement often limit the number of cognitive tests that can be administered, and despite our urging and the urging of other investigators, there has not been much progress with respect to establishing a core battery of tests to be used in clinical trials of antihypertensive agents.

5.1.6. Summary

Unless we address some fundamental issues related to theory and measurement of cognitive abilities it is unlikely that we will advance much further in understanding which specific abilities are affected by hypertension. That said, we remain optimistic that ongoing and future studies will involve more ingenious psychometric strategies and thus shed more light on the adverse cognitive effects of hypertensive disease, especially among older individuals.

6. What are the clinical and population implications of high blood pressure?

One of the obvious conclusions we can reach from an overwhelming body of data is that hypertension is associated with lower levels of cognitive functioning and that individuals who remain free from it and otherwise in good health are likely to perform at normal cognitive levels for substantial periods of time. This is nicely illustrated by the previously presented bar graph (Fig. 5) based on Maine-Syracuse data (Elias et al., 1998a). This leads to three important questions. What are the implications for the individual, for the population, and for treatment? These questions need to be addressed separately because the answers are not the same in each case.

6.1. Individuals vs. groups

The implications of labeling hypertensive individuals as suffering cognitive deficit or impairment are serious and may affect employment, for example the performance of jobs that involve military defense and public safety, as well as the cost of health insurance. It seems apparent that no individual should be labeled as cognitively impaired or suffering from cognitive deficit unless this state has been clearly defined and diagnosed clinically. Reviews of the literature (Waldstein and Katzel, 2001) and our own studies (Elias et al., 1987b, 1993) indicate that *stroke-free and dementia-free hypertensive individuals* do not perform at a level indicative of clinical cognitive deficit. Most certainly it is not appropriate to characterize community-dwelling persons with well-controlled, medically uncomplicated, essential hypertension as cognitively impaired (Elias et al., 1987b). Differences between cohorts with diagnosed hypertension and cohorts with normal BP of as much as 1.0 SD have been reported, but effect sizes vary as a function of the design and recruitment procedures (Waldstein et al., 1991a; Waldstein and Katzel, 2001). Obviously, one must consider individual differences when applying group differences to the issue of clinical deficit in the individual. Light (1978) makes this point most effectively by showing a plot of her data as well as summary statistics. In Light's (1978) plot, "noise" (variability around the regression line) increased as a function of diastolic BP. Plotting one's data can be a sobering experience. Obviously, a host of individual difference variables, including education, training, and occupational experience, contribute to variability in cognitive test scores. Fortunately, we are blessed with the fact that many variables that are highly related to cognitive functioning protect against, or aid in compensation for, disease-related deficit (P.K. Elias et al., 1999; Christensen, 2001). Education is a good example (Elias et al., 1987b).

We are not arguing that statistically significant differences between hypertensive and normotensive cohorts are of no consequence, nor are we promoting the idea that cognitive decline associated with hypertension is of no practical or clinical importance. Our argument is that the importance of hypertension-cognitive performance data for people who are functioning normally lies with its significance at the population level. In order to assess this type of significance one must turn to statistics that help us to assess population risk.

6.2. The population and risk estimates

As an illustration of this point, we performed binary logistic regression analyses for the WAIS Performance Scale, the Visualization-Performance Composite score, and Speed of Performance score employed in our previously described cross-sectional analysis. These analyses yield, as descriptive statistics, odds ratios. Odds ratios are normally employed to describe the relative likelihood of a discrete event such as stroke or myocardial infarction (MI). Odds of 1.00 do not reflect no risk, but rather reflect a baseline risk ratio in the absence of the risk factor in question, e.g. stroke or MI. For purposes of our illustration we employed good vs. poor performance as our outcome variable and defined poor performance as a score in the lowest quartile of the distribution of scores for the 760 scores entering into this calculation.

These three measures showed the most consistent linear relationship to blood pressure variables in our studies with the Maine-Syracuse sample, and there was no evidence of a curvilinear relationship between BP and cognitive function for our data. Consequently, we summed over age for these analyses in order to benefit from large sample sizes ($N = 760$). The age range was 18 to 83 years, but odds ratios were adjusted for age, as well as education, gender, treatment, and other covariates.

Table 6 shows odds ratios (estimated risk of poor performance) in relation to each of the predictor variables. Hypertension was defined as systolic BP ≥ 140 mmHg or diastolic BP ≥ 90 mmHg compared to normotensive status (systolic BP < 140 mmHg and diastolic BP < 90 mmHg). The odds ratios provide an estimate of the risk of poorer performance for hypertensive individuals. So for example, hypertension was associated with a 74% increase in risk for poor cognitive performance for the WAIS Performance Scale. Each 10 mmHg increment in diastolic BP was associated with 20, 17, and 17% increments in risk of poor performance for the Performance Scale, Visualization-Performance Composite, and Speed score, respectively. Similar estimates of risk were associated with 20 mmHg increments in systolic BP.

Table 6
Estimated risk of performance in the lowest quartile of the distribution of score based on Odds Ratios[a,b]

Predictor variable	WAIS performance	Visualization-Performance	Speed
Systolic BP (20 mmHg)	1.18*,[c]	1.11	1.22*
Diastolic BP (10 mmHg)	1.20*	1.17*	1.17[†]
JNC 1997 Category	1.21*	1.18*	1.23*
Hypertension (> 140 or 90 mmHg)	1.74*	1.63*	1.67[†]
Ten years Age	1.58***	1.46***	1.85***
MAP (10 mmHg)	1.16*	1.13[†]	1.16*
Pulse pressure (10 mmHg)	1.04	1.00	1.10

[a]$N = 760$.
[b]The regression model consisted of one of the blood pressure variables, age, education level, occupation, gender, anti-hypertensive medication status, and trait anxiety and depression scores.
[c]1.18 = 18% increment in risk per 20 mmHg systolic BP.
[†]$p < 0.10$; *$p < 0.05$; ***$p < 0.001$.

By contrast each 10-year increment in age was associated with an estimated increase in risk of 58, 46, and 85%, respectively for the WAIS measures displayed in the table. Admittedly, the comparison between 10-year increments in chronological age and 10 mmHg increments in BP (Table 6) is an "apples and oranges comparison." It does, however, provide a sense of the relative cognitive deficit associated with increments in age and BP.

The odds ratios (risk estimates) obtained for the WAIS scores were remarkably similar to those obtained in a similar set of analyses using a sample of 1695 individuals, age 55 to 88 years, participating in the Framingham Heart Study sample (P.K. Elias et al., 1995, 1997). For instance, 10 mmHg increments in diastolic BP were associated with 20, 29, and 17% increments in risk of poor performance for Logical Memory-Immediate Recall, Logical Memory-Delayed Recall, and Visual Reproductions scores, respectively. In no case are the hypertension variables associated with double the risk of lowered cognitive function, but risk at the levels reported is of significant concern when considered in relationship to the population. It is of even greater concern if we consider the fact that hypertension is often present with one or more additional risk factors. The effect of multiple risk factors on cognitive function appears to be cumulative (Elias et al., 2001, 2003). The effects of diabetes and the effects of obesity on cognitive functioning are potentiated by the presence of hypertension (P.K. Elias et al., 1997; Elias et al., 2003). It is quite clear from our work with the Framingham Heart Study population that the risk of lowered cognitive functioning increased as a function of the total number of risk factors (hypertension, smoking, diabetes, obesity) present (Elias et al., 2001). For instance, the additional risk for poorer performance associated with each one-unit increment in the number of risk factors per examination was 15, 29, and 32%, respectively for the Logical Memory-Immediate Recall, Logical Memory-Delayed Recall, and Visual Reproductions scores. In terms of linear regression analyses, cognitive performance level was inversely related to the number of risk factors present. A more comprehensive explanation and summary of these data relevant to the issue of cardiovascular risk factors, cognition, and population risk are presented in the following publications: P.K. Elias et al. (1995), Elias et al. (2001) and Siegler et al. (2002).

6.3. Treatment

Assuming the correctness of our argument that associations between BP variables and cognitive performance are of population significance, i.e. of epidemiological concern, we must ask what this implies for treatment of hypertension to reduce blood pressure levels or prevent further rise in BP levels over time. It is obvious that reductions of even 10 mmHg diastolic BP should make a significant difference with regard to cognitive functioning in the population. And since we routinely treat hypertension for physical health reasons, we may see a beneficial side effect of treatment for the maintenance of cognitive health in the population as a whole, and, for a significant number of individuals. Thus, just as the potentially adverse physical effects of hypertension are a focus of concern within the physician-patient dialogue, so too should be the potentially adverse cognitive effects.

While it may seem contradictory to minimize the effects of hypertension with regard to cognitive deficits for the individual and then suggest that individual patients may benefit cognitively from treatment, it really is not. Ever since the early data from the Framingham Heart Study were presented, American medicine has been characterized by treatment of the individual based on population statistics. Moreover, prevention of cognitive deficit and other undesirable outcomes of hypertension in the population begins with treatment of the individual.

7. Where do we go from here?

Probably the most important question demanding of an immediate answer is as follows: why do some individuals with hypertension (and other cardiovascular risk factors) progress to dementia while others do not? One answer is that some individuals do not live long enough. Another is that treatment for hypertension, and co-risk factors, may actually help prevent this progression (Forette et al., 2002). Other answers will come with a better understanding of factors that precipitate, and those that protect against, this progression. Indeed, the true holy grail would be the ability to optimize each individual's state of cardiovascular adaptation with aging such that it promoted the maintenance of brain function whilst protecting against the evolution of progressive neuro-degenerative change. What may prove to be clinically accessible markers of this state (e.g. simple measures of brachial BP, cumulative indices of carotid atherosclerotic plaque load (Spence et al., 2002), or neuro-imaging derived indices of cerebral perfusion) will depend on our ingenuity in unraveling the multi-faceted causal evolution of the hypertensive cardiovascular syndrome.

The binding thesis in this chapter is that life span research on associations among blood pressure, related risk factors and cardiovascular disease, is necessary to understand the role of cardiovascular risk factors in cognitive aging, including the catastrophic cognitive deficits associated with dementia. As with all life span developmental issues, and as in life, one must understand what happens at the beginning to understand what happens at the end.

Acknowledgments

The preparation of this paper, and the Maine-Syracuse Studies reported in this paper, were supported by the National Institute on Aging (Project # R01-AG00868 and Project # 5R37-AG03055) and the National Heart, Lung, and Blood Institute (Project # 5R01-HL67358).

We authors gratefully acknowledge the following associates who are not listed as authors but have contributed in a significant manner to the Maine-Syracuse studies: Ms. Suzanne Brennan, Thomas W. Pierce, Ph.D., Judith Deking, Julie Hartsell, and Amy Wilson-Gudrun, Ph.D.

We also wish to recognize with great appreciation two colleagues and dear friends, David H. P. Streeten, MD and Norman R. Schultz, Jr., Ph.D. (deceased), without whom these studies would never have been done.

References

Alves de Moraes, S., Szklo, M., Knopman, D., Sato, R., 2002. The relationship between temporal changes in blood pressure and changes in cognitive function: Atherosclerosis Risk in Communities (ARIC) Study. Prev. Med. 35, 258–263.

American Heart Association, 1998. Heart and Stroke Statistical Update. American Heart Association, Dallas, TX.

Applegate, W.B., Pressel, S., Wittes, J., Luhr, J., Shekelle, R.B., Camel, G.H., Greenlick, M.R., Hadley, E., Moye, L., Perry, H.M., Schron, E., Wegener, V., 1994. Impact of the treatment of isolated systolic hypertension on behavioural variables. Results from the systolic hypertension in the elderly trial. Archives of Internal Medicine 154, 2154–2160.

Baumbach, G.L., Heistad, D.D., 1997. Mechanisms involved in the genesis of cerebral vascular damage in hypertension. In: Hanson, L., Birkenhäger, W.H. (Eds.), Handbook of Hypertension Volume 18: Assessment of Hypertensive Organ Damage. Elsevier Science B.V., Amsterdam, The Netherlands, pp. 249–268.

Blumenthal, J.A., Madden, D.J., Pierce, T.W., Siegel, W.C., Applebaum, M., 1993. Hypertension affects neurobehavioral functioning. Psychosomatic Medicine, 55, 44–50.

Bohannon, A.D., Fillenbaum, G.C., Pieper, C.F., Hanlon, J.T., Blazer, D.G., 2002. Relationship of race/ethnicity and blood pressure to change in cognitive function. Journal of the American Geriatric Society 50, 424–429.

Bowler, J.V. Hachinski, V., 1995. Vascular cognitive impairment: A new approach to vascular dementia. Bailliere's Clinical Neurology 4, 357–376.

Carmelli, D., Swan, G.E., Reed, T., Miller, B., Wolf, P.A., Jarvik, G.P., Schellenberg, G.D., 1998. Midlife cardiovascular risk factors, ApoE, and cognitive decline in elderly male twins. Neurology 50, 1580–1585.

Cervilla, J.A., Prince, M., Joels, S., Lovestone, S., Mann, A., 2000. Long-term predictors of cognitive outcome in a cohort of older people with hypertension. British Journal of Psychiatry 177, 66–71.

Christensen, H., 2001. What cognitive changes can be expected with normal ageing? Australian and New Zealand Journal of Psychiatry 35, 768–775.

Collins, L.M., Horn, J.L. (eds.), 1991. Best methods for the analysis of change: Recent advances, unanswered questions, future directions. American Psychological Association, Washington, DC.

Collins, L.M., Sayer, A.G. (eds.), 2001. New methods for the analysis of change. American Psychological Association, Washington, DC.

Croog, S.H., Elias, M.F., Colton, T., Baume, R.M., Lieblum, S.R., Jenkins, C.D., Perry, H.M., Hall, W.D., 1994. Effects of antihypertensive medications on quality of life in elderly hypertensive women. American Journal of Hypertension 7, 329–339.

Croog, S.H., Levine, S., Testa, M.A., Brown, B., Bulpitt, C.J., Jenkins, C.D., Klerman, G.L., William, G.H., 1986. The effects of antihypertensive therapy on the quality of life. New England Journal of Medicine 314, 1657–1664.

D'Agostino, R.B., Wolf, P.A., Belanger, A.J., Kannel, W.B., 1994. Stroke risk profile: Adjustment for antihypertensive medication. The Framingham Study. Stroke 25, 40–43.

Deary, I.J., Starr, J.M., MacLennan, W.J., 1998. Fluid intelligence, memory and blood pressure in cognitive aging. Personality and Individual Differences 25, 605–619.

De Carli, C., Murphy, D.G.M., Tranh, M., Grady, C.L., Haxby, J.V., Gillette, J.A., Salerno, J.A., Gonzales-Aviles, A., Horwitz, B., Rapoport, S.I., Schapiro, M.B., 1995. The effect of white matter hyperintensity volume on brain structure, cognitive performance, and cerebral metabolism of glucose in 51 healthy adults. Neurology 45, 2077–2084.

Dimsdale, J.E., Newton, R.P., 1992. Cognitive effects of beta blockers. Journal of Psychomatic Research 36, 229–236.

Dwyer, J., Feinleib, M., 1991. Introduction to statistical models for longitudinal observation. In: Dwyer, J.H., Feinleib, M., Lippert, P., Hoffmeister, H. (Eds), Statistical models for longitudinal studies of health. Oxford University Press, New York, pp. 3–48.

Elias, M.F., 1998. Effects of chronic hypertension on cognitive functioning. Geriatrics 53, Suppl. 1, S49–S52.

Elias, M.F., D'Agostino, R.B., Elias, P.K., Wolf, P.A., 1995a. Neuropsychological test performance, cognitive functioning, blood pressure and age: The Framingham Study. Experimental Aging Research 21, 369–391.

Elias, M.F., Elias, J.W., Elias, P.K., 1990b. Biological and health influences on behavior. In: Birren, J.E., Schaie, K.W. (Eds.), Handbook of the Psychology of Aging, 3rd ed. Academic Press, San Diego, pp. 79–102.

Elias, M.F., Elias, P.K., 1993. Hypertension effects neurobehavioral functioning: So what's new? Psychosomatic Medicine 55, 51–54.

Elias, M.F., Elias, P.K., Cobb, J., D'Agostino, R., White, L.R., Wolf, P.A., 1995b. Blood pressure affects cognitive functioning: The Framingham studies revisited. In: Dimsdale, J.E., Baum, A. (Eds.), Quality of Life in Behavioral Medicine Research. Lawrence-Erlbaum, Hillsdale, NJ, pp. 121–143.

Elias, M.F., Elias, P.K., D'Agostino, Wolf, P.A., 2000. Comparative effects of age and blood pressure on neuropsychological test performance: The Framingham Study. In: Manuck, S.B., Jennings, R., Rabin, B.S., Rabin, B.S., Baum, A. (Eds.), Behavior, health and aging. Lawrence Erlbaum Associates, Mahwah, NJ, pp. 199–223.

Elias, M.F., Elias, P.K., D'Agostino, R.B., Silbershatz, H., Wolf, P. A., 1997. The role of age, education, and gender on cognitive performance in the Framingham Heart Study: Community-based norms. Experimental Aging Research 23, 201–235.

Elias, M.F., Elias, P.K., Robbins, M.A., Wolf, P.A., D'Agostino, R.B., 2001. Cardiovascular risk factors and cognitive functioning: An epidemiological perspective. In: Waldstein, S.R., Elias, M.F. (Eds.), Neuropsychology of Cardiovascular Disease. Lawrence Erlbaum, Mahwah, NJ, pp. 83–104.

Elias, M.F., Elias, P.K., Sullivan, L.M., Wolf, P.A., D'Agostino, R.B., 2003. Lower cognitive function in the presence of obesity and hypertension: The Framingham Heart Study. International Journal of Obesity and Related Metabolic Disorders 27, 260–268.

Elias, M.F., Robbins, M.A., 1991a. Cardiovascular disease, hypertension, and cognitive function. In: Shapiro, A.P., Baum, A. (Eds.), Behavioral Aspects of Cardiovascular Disease. Lawrence Erlbaum Associates, Hillsdale, NJ, pp. 249–285.

Elias, M.F., Robbins, M.A., 1991b. Where have all the subjects gone? Longitudinal studies of disease and cognitive function. In: Collins, L.M., Horn, J.L. (Eds.), Best Methods for the Analysis of Change: Recent Advances, Unanswered Questions, Future Directions. American Psychological Association, Washington, DC, pp. 264–275.

Elias, M.F., Robbins, M.A., Elias, P.K., 1996. A 15-year longitudinal study of Halstead-Reitan Neuropsychological test performance. Journals of Gerontology Series B: Psychological Sciences and Social Sciences 51, P331–P334.

Elias, M.F., Robbins, M.A., Elias, P.K., Streeten, D.H.P., 1998a. A longitudinal study of blood pressure in relation to performance on the Wechsler Adult Intelligence Scale. Health Psychology 17, 486–493.

Elias, M.F., Robbins, M.A., Elias, P.K., Streeten, D.H.P., 1998b. Cognitive ability declines as a function of blood pressure level. Abstract 4512, Circulation 98 (Suppl.) I-860.

Elias, M.F., Robbins, M.A., Schultz, N.R., Jr., 1987a. The influence of essential hypertension on intellectual performance: Causation or speculation? In: Elias, J.W., Marshall, P.H. (Eds.), Cardiovascular disease and behavior. Hemisphere Publishing Corp., Washington, pp. 107–149.

Elias, M.F., Robbins, M.A., Schultz, N.R., Jr., Pierce, T.W., 1990a. Is blood pressure an important variable in research on aging and neuropsychological test performance? Journals of Gerontology Series B: Psychological Sciences and Social Sciences 45, P128–P135.

Elias, M.F., Robbins, M.A., Schultz, N.R., Jr., Streeten, D.H.P., 1986. A longitudinal study of neuropsychological test performance in hypertensives and normotensives: initial findings. Journal of Gerontology 41, 503–505.

Elias, M.F., Robbins, M.A., Schultz, N.R., Jr., Streeten, D.H.P., Elias, P.K., 1987b. Clinical significance of cognitive performance by hypertensive patients. Hypertension 9, 192–197.

Elias, M.F., Schultz, N.R., Jr., Robbins, M.A., Elias, P.K., 1989. A longitudinal study of neuropsychological performance by hypertensives and normotensives: A third measurement point. Journal of Gerontology 44, P25–P28.

Elias, M.F., Wolf, P.A., D'Agostino, R.B., Cobb, J., White, L.R., 1993. Untreated blood pressure level is inversely related to cognitive functioning: the Framingham Study. American Journal of Epidemiology 138, 353–364.

Elias, P.K., D'Agostino, R.B., Elias, M.F., Wolf, P.A., 1995. Blood pressure, hypertension and age as risk factors for poor cognitive performance. Experimental Aging Research 21, 393–417.

Elias, P.K., Elias, M.F., D'Agostino, R.B., Silbershatz, H., Wolf, P.A., 1999. Alcohol consumption and cognitive performance in the Framingham Heart Study. American Journal of Epidemiology 150, 580–589.

Elias, P.K., Elias, M.F., D'Agostino, R.B., Cupples, L.A., Wilson, P.W., Silbershatz, H., Wolf, P.A., 1997. NIDDM and blood pressure as risk factors for poor cognitive performance: The Framingham Study. Diabetes Care 20, 1388–1395.

Farmer, M.E., Kittner, S.J., Abbott, R.D., Wolz, M.M., Wolf, P.A., White, L.R., 1990. Longitudinally measured blood pressure, antihypertensive medication use, and cognitive performance: The Framingham Study. Journal of Clinical Epidemiology 43, 475–480.

Farmer, M.E., White, L.R., Abbott, R.D., Kittner, S.J., Kaplan, E., Wolz, M., Brody, J.A., Wolf, P.A., 1987. Blood pressure and cognitive performance: The Framingham Study. American Journal of Epidemiology 126, 1103–1114.

Fazekus, F., Niederkorn, K., Schmidt, R., Offenbacher, H., Horner, S., Bertha, G., Lechner, H., 1998. White matter signal abnormalities in normal individuals: correlation with carotid ultrasonography, cerebral blood flow measurements, and cerebrovascular risk factors. Stroke 19, 1285–1288.

Forette, F., Seux, M.L., Staessen, J.A., Thijs, L., Babarskiene, M.R., Babeanu, S., Bossini, A., Fagard, R., Gil-Extremera, B., Laks, T., Kobalava, Z., Sarti, C., Tuomilehto, J., Vanhanen, H., Webster, J., Yodfat, Y., Birkenhäger, W.H., 2002. The prevention of dementia with antihypertensive treatment: New evidence from the Systolic Hypertension in Europe (Syst-Eur) study. Archives of Internal Medicine 162, 2046–2052.

Gavras, H., Gavras, I., 1983. Hypertension in the elderly. John Wright, Boston, pp. 1–7.
Gifford, R.W., 1989. Core organ effects: Part II (Cerebral). In: Punzl, H.A., Flamenbaum, W. (Eds.), Clinical cardiovascular therapeutics. Vol. 1. Hypertension. Future, Mt. Kisco, NY, pp. 65–81.
Glynn, R.J., Beckett, L.A., Hebert, L.E., Morris, M.C., Scherr, P.A., Evans, D.A., 1999. Current and remote blood pressure and cognitive decline. Journal of the American Medical Association 281, 438–445.
Guo, Z., Fratiglioni, L., Winblad, B., Viitanen, M., 1997. Blood pressure and performance on the Mini-Mental State Examination in the very old. American Journal of Epidemiology 145,1106–1113.
Haan, M.N., Shemanski, L., Jagust, W.J., Manolio, T.A., Kuller, L., 1999. The role of APOE _4 in modulating effects of other risk factors for cognitive decline in elderly persons. Journal of the American Medical Association 282, 40–46.
Hansson, L., Himmelmann, A., Hedner, T., 1999. Hypertension and dementia: Can antihypertensive treatment preserve cognitive function? Blood Pressure 8, 196–197.
Horn, J.L., 1985. Remodeling old models of intelligence. In: Wolman, B. (Ed.), Handbook of intelligence: theories, measurements, and applications. Wiley, New York, pp. 267–300.
Horn, J.L., McArdle, J.J., 1980. Perspectives on mathematical/statistical model building (MASMOB) in research on aging. In: Poon, L.W. (Ed.), Aging in the 1980's: Psychological issues. American Psychological Association, Washington, DC, pp. 503–541.
Inzitari, D., Ballie, A.M., Carlucci, G., 2002. Vascular cognitive impairment and disability. In: Erkinjuntti, T., Gauthier, S. (Eds.), Vascular cognitive impairment. Martin Dunitz, London, pp. 227–237.
Izzo, J.L., Black, H.R., 1993. Hypertension Primer: the Essentials of High Blood Pressure. American Heart Association, Dallas.
Jennings, J.R., Muldoon, M.F., Ryan, C.M., Mintun, M.A., Meltzer, C.C., Townsend, D.W., Sutton-Tyrrell, K., Shapiro, A.P., Manuck, S.B., 1998. Cerebral blood flow in hypertensive patients: An initial report of reduced and compensatory blood flow responses during performance of two cognitive tasks. Hypertension 31, 1216–1222.
Jonas, D.L., Blumenthal, J.A., Madden, D.J., Serra, M., 2001. Cognitive consequences of antihypertensive medications. In: Waldstein, S.R., Elias, M.F. (Eds.). Neuropsychology of cardiovascular disease, Lawrence Erlbaum, Mahwah, NJ, pp. 167–188.
Kannel, W.B., Dawber, T.R., Sorlie, P., Wolf, P.A., McNamara, P.M., 1976. Components of blood pressure and risk for atheroembolic brain infarction. The Framingham Study. Stroke 7, 327–331.
Kannel, W.B., Wolf, P.A., Verter, J., McNamara, P.M., 1970. Epidemiologic assessment of the role of blood pressure in stroke. The Framingham Study. Journal of the American Medical Association 214, 301–310.
Kilander, L., Nyman, H., Boberg, M., Hansson, L., Lithell, H., 1998. Hypertension is related to cognitive impairment: a 20-year follow-up of 999 men. Hypertension 31, 780–786.
Knopman, D., Boland, L.L., Mosley, T., Howard, G., Liao, D., Szklo, M., McGovern, P., Folsom, A.R., 2001. Cardiovascular risk factors and cognitive decline in middle-aged adults. Neurology 56, 42–48.
Kuller, L.H., Shemanski, L., Manolio, T., Haan, M., Fried, L., Bryan, N., Burke, G.L., Tracy, R., Bhadelia, R., 1998. Relationship between ApoE, MRI findings, and cognitive function in the Cardiovascular Health Study. Stroke 29, 388–398.
LaCroix, A.L., 1993. Gender effects and hypertension in women. In: Izzo, J.L., Black, H.R. (Eds.). Hypertension primer. The essentials of high blood pressure. Council on High Blood Pressure Research: American Heart Association, Dallas, TX, pp. 150–153.
Lamar, M., Zonderman, A.B., Resnick, S., 2002. Contribution of specific cognitive processes to executive functioning in an aging population. Neuropsychology 16, 156–162.
Launer, L.J., Masaki, K., Petrovitch, H., Foley, D., Havlik, R.J., 1995. The association between midlife blood pressure levels and late-life cognitive function. The Honolulu-Asia Aging Study. Journal of the American Medical Association 274, 1846–1851.
Lezak, M.D., 1983. Neuropsychological assessment. Oxford University Press, New York, pp. 145–463.
Lezak, M.D., 1995. Neuropsychological assessment (3rd ed.). Oxford University Press, New York.
Liao, D., Cooper, L., Cai, J., et al., 1996, abstract. Population correlates of cerebral white matter lesions: The ARIC study. Circulation 93, 629.

Light, K.C., 1978. Effects of mild cardiovascular and cerebrovascular disorders on serial reaction time performance. Experimental Aging Research 4, 3–22.

Longstreth, W.T., Jr., Manolio, T.A., Arnold, A., Burke, G.L., Bryan, N., Jungreis, C.A., Enright, P.L., O'Leary, D., Fried, L., 1996. Clinical correlates of white matter findings on cranial magnetic resonance imaging of 3301 elderly people: The Cardiovascular Health Study. Stroke 27, 1274–1282.

Lyon, G.R., 1996. The need for conceptual and theoretical clarity in the study of attention, memory, and executive function. In: Lyon, G.R., Krasnegor, N.A. (Eds.), Attention, memory, and executive function. Paul H. Brooks, Baltimore, pp. 3–9.

Madden, D.J., Blumenthal, J.A., 1989. Slowing of memory-search performance in men with mild hypertension. Health Psychology 8, 131–142.

Madden, D.J., Blumenthal, J.A., 1998. Interaction of hypertension and age in visual selective performance. Health Psychol. 17, 76–83.

Manolio, T.A., Kronmal, R.A., Burke, G.L., Poirier, V., O'Leary, D.H., Gardin, J.M., Fried, L.P., Steinberg, E.P., Bryan, R. N., 1994. Magnetic resonance abnormalities and cardiovascular disease in older adults: The Cardiovascular Health Study. Stroke 25, 318–327.

McArdle, J.J., Hamagami, F., 1991. Modeling incomplete longitudinal and cross-sectional data using latent growth structural equation models. In: Collins, L.M., Horn, J.L. (Eds.). Best methods for the analysis of change: Recent advances, unanswered questions, future directions. American Psychological Association, Washington, DC, pp. 276–304.

McArdle, J.J., Hamagami, F., Elias, M.F., Robbins, M.A., 1991. Structural modeling of mixed longitudinal and cross-sectional data. Experimental Aging Research 17, 29–52.

Meissner, I., Whisnant, J.P., Sheps, S.G., Schwartz, G.L., O=Fallon, W.M., Covalt, J.L., Sicks, J.D., Bailey, K.R., Wiebers, D.O., 1999. Detection and control of high blood pressure in the community: do we need a wake-up call? Hypertension 34, 466–471.

Muldoon, M.F., Waldstein, S.R., Jennings, J.R., 1995. Neuropsychological consequences of antihypertensive medication use. Experimental Aging Research 21, 353–368.

O'Rourke, M.F., 2000. Editorial: Basis and implications of change in arterial pressure with age. Vascular Medicine 5, 209–211.

Paolo, A.M., Cluff, R.B., Ryan, J.J., 1996. Influence of perceptual organization and naming abilities on the Hooper Visual Organization Test: A replication and extension. Neuropsychiatry, Neuropsychology, and Behavioral Neurology 9, 254–257.

Patoni, L., Garcia, J.H., 1995. The significance of cerebral white matter abnormalities 100 years after Binswanger's report. A review. Stroke 26, 1293–1301.

Peila, R., White, L.R., Petrovich, H., Masaki, K., Ross, G.W., Havlik, R.J., Launer, L.J., 2001. Joint effect of the APOE gene and midlife systolic blood pressure on late-life cognitive impairment: The Honolulu-Asia aging study. Stroke 32, 2882–2889.

Pessina, A.C., Pauletto, P., 1997. Hypertension and atherosclerosis. In: Zanchetti, A., Mancia, G. (Eds.). Handbook of hypertension Vol. 17: Pathophysiology of hypertension. Elsevier Science B.V., Amsterdam, pp. 438–481.

Phillips, S.J., Whisnant, J.P., 1992. Hypertension and the brain. The National High Blood Pressure Education Program. Archives of Internal Medicine 157, 938–945.

Posner, H.B., Tang, M.X., Luchsinger, J., Lantigua, R., Stern, Y., Mayeux, R., 2002. The relationship of hypertension in the elderly to AD, vascular dementia, and cognitive function. Neurology 58, 1175–1181.

Prince, M., Lewis, G., Bird, A., Blizard, R., Mann, A., 1996. A longitudinal study of factors predicting change in cognitive test scores over time, in an older hypertensive population. Psychological Medicine 26, 555–568.

Prisant, L.M., Moser, M., 2000. Hypertension in the elderly: Can we improve results of therapy? Archives of Internal Medicine 160, 283–289.

Reitan, R.M., Wolfson, D., 1993. The Halstead-Reitan Neuropsychological Test Battery: Theory and clinical interpretation (2nd Edition). Neuropsychology Press, Tucson, AZ.

Robbins, M.A., Elias, M.F., Budge, M.M., Elias, P.K., 2002. Blood pressure related decline in cognitive performance over two decades. Gerontologist 42, 216.

Robbins, M.A., Elias, M.F., Croog, S.H., Colton, T., 1994. Unmedicated blood pressure levels and quality of life in elderly hypertensive women. Psychosomatic Medicine 56, 251–259.

Rogosa, D., Brandt, D., Zimowski, M., 1982. A growth curve approach to the measurement of change. Psychological Bulletin 92, 726–748.

Russell, E.W., Neuringer, C., Goldstein, G., 1970. Assessment of brain damage: A neuropsychological key approach. Wiley-Interscience, New York.

Salerno, J.A., Murphy, D.G., Horwitz, B., DeCarli, C., Haxby, J.V., Rapoport, S.I., Shapiro, M.B., 1992. Brain atrophy in hypertension: A volumetric magnetic resonance imaging study. Hypertension 20, 340–348.

Salthouse, T.A., 1992. What do adult age differences in the Digit Symbol Substitution test reflect? Journal of Gerontology 47, P121–P128.

Sands, L.P., Meredith, W., 1992. Blood pressure and intellectual functioning in late midlife. Journals of Gerontology Series B: Psychological Sciences and Social Sciences 47, P81–84.

Schaie, K.W., 1996. Intellectual development in adulthood. The Seattle longitudinal study. Cambridge University Press, New York.

Schmidt, R., Fazekas, F., Offenbacher, H., Lytwyn, H., Blematl, B., Niederkorn, K., Horner, S., Payer, F., Freidl, W., 1991. Magnetic resonance imaging, white matter lesions, and cognitive impairment in hypertensive individuals. Archives of Neurology 48, 417–420.

Schultz, N.R., Jr., Dineen, J.T., Elias, M.F., Pentz, C.A., III, Wood, W.G., 1979. WAIS performance for different age groups of hypertensive and control subjects during the administration of a diuretic. Journal of Gerontology 34, 246–253.

Schultz, N.R., Jr., Elias, M.F., Robbins, M.A., Streeten, D.H.P., Blakeman, N., 1989. A longitudinal study of the performance of hypertensive and normotensive subjects on the Wechsler Adult Intelligence Scale. Psychology and Aging 4, 496–499.

Siegler, I.C., 1975. The terminal drop hypothesis: Fact or artifact? Experimental Aging Research 1, 169–185.

Siegler, I.C., Botwinick, J., 1979. A long-term longitudinal study of intellectual ability of older adults: The matter of selective subject attrition. Journal of Gerontology 34, 242–245.

Siegler, I.S., Bosworth, H.B., Elias, M.F., 2002. Adult development and aging in health psychology. In: Nezu, A.M., Nezu, C.M., Geller, P.A. (Eds.). Comprehensive handbook of psychology, Vol. 9. Health Psychology. Wiley, New York, pp. 487–510.

Sixth Report of the Joint National Committee on Prevention, Detection, Evaluation, and Treatment of High Blood Pressure. NIH Publication, No. 98-4080, November 1997. Archives of Internal Medicine 157, 2413–2446.

Skoog, I., Lernfelt, B., Landahl, S., Palmertz, B., Andreasson, L.A., Nilsson, L., Persson, G., Oden, A., Svanborg, A., 1996. 15-year longitudinal study of blood pressure and dementia. Lancet 347, 1141–1145.

Spence, J.D., Eliasziw, M., DiCicco, M., Hackam, D.G., Galil, R., Lohmann, T., 2002. Carotid plaque area: A tool for targeting and evaluating vascular preventive therapy. Stroke 33, 2916–2922.

Starr, J.M., Whalley, L.J., 1992. Senile hypertension and cognitive impairment: An overview. Journal of Hypertension 10 (Suppl. 2), S31–S42.

Starr, J.M., Deary, I.J., Inch, S., Cross, S., MacLennan, W.J., 1997. Blood pressure and cognitive decline in healthy old people. J. Hum. Hypertens. 11, 777–781.

Stewart, R., Richards, M., Brayne, C., Mann, A., 2001. Vascular risk and cognitive impairment in an older, British, African-Caribbean population. Journal of the American Geriatrics Society 49, 263–269.

Streeten, D.H.P., Anderson, G.H., Jr., Elias, M.F., 1992. Special features of hypertension in the elderly. Geriatric Nephrology and Urology 2, 91–98.

Suzuki, H., Sweifach, B.W., Schmid-Schunbein, 1997. The multifaceted contribution of microvascular abnormalities to the pathophysiology of the hypertensive syndrome. In: Zanchetti, A., Mancia, G. (Eds.). Handbook of hypertension Vol. 17: Pathophysiology of hypertension. Elsevier Science B.V., Amsterdam, pp. 482–523.

Swan, G.E., Carmelli, D., LaRue, A., 1996. The relationship between blood pressure during middle age and cognitive impairment in old age: The Western Collaborative Group Study. Aging, Neuropsychology, and Cognition 3, 241–250.

Swan, G.E., Carmelli, D., LaRue, A., 1998. Systolic blood pressure tracking over 25 to 30 years and cognitive performance in older adults. Stroke 29, 2334–2340.

Tzourio, C., Dufouil, C., Ducimetière, P., Alpérovitch, A., 1999. Cognitive decline in individuals with high blood pressure: A longitudinal study in the elderly. Neurology 53, 1948–1952.

Waldstein, S.R., 1995. Hypertension and neuropsychological function: a lifespan perspective. Experimental Aging Research 21, 321–352.

Waldstein, S.R., 2000. Health effects on cognitive aging. In: Stern, P.C., Carstensen, L.L. (Eds.). The aging mind: Opportunities in cognitive research. National Academy Press, Washington, DC, pp. 189–217.

Waldstein, S.R., Elias, M.F. (eds.) 2001. Neuropsychology of cardiovascular disease. Lawrence Erlbaum, Mahwah, NJ.

Waldstein, S.R., Jennings, J.R., Ryan, C.M., Muldoon, M.F., Shapiro, A.P., Polefrone, J.M., Fazzari, T.V., Manuck, S.B., 1996. Hypertension and neuropsychological performance in men: Interactive effects of age. Health Psychology 15, 102–109.

Waldstein, S.R., Katzel, L.I., 2001. Hypertension and cognitive function. In: Waldstein, S.R., Elias, M.F. (Eds.), Neuropsychology of cardiovascular disease. Lawrence Erlbaum, Mahwah, NJ. pp. 15–36.

Waldstein, S.R., Manuck, S.B., Ryan, C.M., Muldoon, M.F., 1991a. Neuropsychological correlates of hypertension: Review and methodologic considerations. Psychological Bulletin 110, 451–468.

Waldstein, S.R., Ryan, C.M., Manuck, S.B., Parkinson, D.K., Bromet, E.J., 1991b. Learning and memory function in men with untreated blood pressure elevation. Journal of Consulting and Clinical Psychology 59, 513–517.

Wilkie, F., Eisdorfer, C., 1971. Intelligence and blood pressure in the aged. Science 172, 959–962.

Willett, J., 1988. Questions and answers in the measurement of change. In: Rothkopf, E.Z. (Ed.), Review of research in education, Vol. 15. American Educational Research Association, Washington, DC, pp. 345–422.

Wilson, P.W.F., 1993. Total cardiovascular risk. In: Izzo, J.L., Jr., Black, H.R. (Eds.), Hypertension primer: the essentials of high blood pressure. American Heart Association, Dallas, pp. 190–191.

Wolf, P.A., 1993. Cerebrovascular disease risks. In: Izzo, J.L., Jr., Black, H.R. (Eds.), Hypertension primer: the essentials of high blood pressure. American Heart Association, Dallas, pp. 180–182.

Wolf, P.A., D'Agostino, R.B., Belanger, A.J., Kannel, W.B., 1991. Probability of stroke: A risk profile from the Framingham Study. Stroke 22, 312–318.

Zelinski, E.M., Crimmins, E., Reynolds, S., Seeman, T., 1998. Do medical conditions affect cognition in older adults? Health Psychology 17, 504–512.

Zhu, L., Viitanen, M., Guo, Z., Winblad, B., Fratiglioni, L., 1998. Blood pressure reduction, cardiovascular diseases, and cognitive decline in the Mini-Mental State Examination in a community population of normal very old people: a three-year follow-up. Journal of Clinical Epidemiology 51, 385–391.

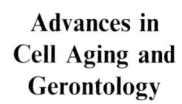

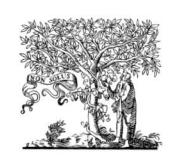

A life span view of emotional functioning in adulthood and old age

Susan T. Charles[1],* and Laura L. Carstensen[2]

[1]*Department of Psychology and Social Behavior, University of California, Irvine CA 924697, USA*
[2]*Department of Psychology, Stanford University, Bldg 420, Jordan Hall, Stanford, CA 94305, USA*

Contents

1. Introduction — 134
   1.1. The biological foundation of emotion — 134
   1.2. Affective processes across the adult life span — 136
   1.3. Psychological disorders — 138
2. Biological changes — 139
   2.1. Physiology — 139
   2.2. Biological changes: brain functioning — 140
   2.3. Emotional expression — 141
3. Potential mechanisms behind stable if not enhanced emotion regulation with age — 142
   3.1. Social processes — 142
   3.2. Social perceptions — 144
   3.3. Cognitive processes — 145
   3.4. General coping strategies — 146
   3.5. Memory — 147
4. Why are older adults doing so well? Theoretical explanations — 149
   4.1. Socioemotional selectivity theory — 150
   4.2. The cognitive-emotional integration model — 152
   4.3. Biological models — 153
   4.4. Declining inhibition — 154
   4.5. Summary and conclusion — 154
   References — 156

---

*Corresponding author. Department of Psychology and Social Behavior, University of California Irvine, 3340 Social Ecology II, Irvine, CA 92697-7085, USA. Tel: 949-824-1450. Fax: 949-824-3002. E-mail address: scharles@uci.edu (Susan T. Charles).

1. Introduction

Early theorists viewed emotions largely as the product of biological reactivity. Charles Darwin devoted an entire book to the subject of emotion and evolution (Darwin, 1872), and William James argued that physiological activation was the basis of emotional experience (James, 1884). Thus, when researchers began to consider emotional experience in later life, they reasoned that, in all likelihood, the emotion system would follow the same downward trajectory observed in other biological functions (Buhler, 1935; Banham, 1951; Frenkel-Brunswik, 1968). Indeed, initial theories of emotion were predicated on widespread evidence – most notably from studies of cognition, perception, and biology – for reduced efficiency, increased slowing and decreased elasticity in basic mental and physical processes with age. Developmental trajectories of social processes known to influence emotional experience failed to offer a more optimistic picture; research showed that social networks decreased in size, retirement lessened social power and prestige, and economic resources also grew more limited. Given this array of findings, the need for the empirical study of emotion was not terribly compelling. With answers presumably known, emotional functioning was rarely the focus of scientific inquiry prior to the 1990s (see review by Schulz, 1985). When emotional processes were examined directly, however, findings challenged initial assumptions. In contrast to other domains, the emotion system functioned well. Research pointed improved emotion regulation and stable, if not greater, subjective well-being in older adults.

In this chapter, we argue that changes in the emotion domain challenge pervasive loss models and represent an area that is better characterized by continued growth in the second half of life. In the first section, we propose that emotional processes represent biologically based affective tendencies apparent at birth that quickly come under cognitive and social control. We then review studies suggesting that emotion regulation improves with age, and argue that declines in emotion regulation occur only at the very end of life, when the cognitive and physical disabilities that often precede death in very old age overshadow previously vital areas of functioning (Baltes, 1998). In the second section, we discuss age-related biological changes to the peripheral nervous system, brain circuitry, and facial musculature that result in age differences in emotional circuitry, but not decrements in subjective experience. After describing these age-related patterns of emotional functioning, we then review in the third section studies examining developmental trends in social and cognitive processes that we believe are largely responsible for age-related improvements in emotion regulation. Finally, we describe several models often used to describe how these social and cognitive strategies follow predictable developmental patterns that preserve, and even increase, emotional functioning across the adult life span.

1.1. The biological foundation of emotion

From the moment of birth, infants display characteristics that highlight their individuality. Some children are very active, and others are more sedate. A noise that makes one child startle and cry serves as a mere point of interest for another. Researchers examining temperamental characteristics find that tendencies to behave and react in predictable patterns are present from birth and relatively consistent throughout childhood. Researchers have noted stability on measures of emotionality in studies of children ranging from 6 months to 2 years of age (Cyphers et al., 1990; Matheny et al., 1995). In studies of preadolescent children ranging from a little under two to a little over nine years old, relatively stable, shared heritability coefficients were present over time on measures of emotionality, fearfulness, and emotion regulation (Buss and Plomin, 1975; Plomin, 1976; Plomin and Rowe, 1977; Goldsmith and Gottesman, 1981; Goldsmith et al., 1997). Although children increase in their understanding and ability to control emotions as they grow older, the temperamental basis of their affective style reveals similarities across time.

Richard Davidson and his colleagues have conducted a series of studies examining individual differences in neurological activity in infancy. In their research on individual differences, one focus has been on hemispheric asymmetry. Individual differences in baseline activation of left and right hemispheres are associated with dispositional moods and affective reactivity (Davidson, 1992). Put simply, they find that hemispheric differentiation contributes to individual differences in affective style, where left hemispheric activation is involved with positive affect and approach behavior, and left hemispheric activation is involved in negative affect and withdrawal behavior (Davidson, 1995). Davidson and his colleagues have found that babies who smile quickly and are more social have greater baseline activation of their left hemisphere than other infants who do not show this asymmetry (Davidson and Fox, 1989). In contrast, those who are easily upset already exhibit greater baseline activation of their right prefrontal cortex. These patterns are similar to those of adults, where individual differences in approach (i.e. positive) and avoidance (i.e. negative) behavior, when operationalized by dispositional states and reactivity, are related to stable measure of baseline activation of left and right hemispheric activation (Davidson, 1992; see review by Davidson, 1995).

These preprogrammed, temperament characteristics documented among infants and continuing in childhood form the basis of relatively stable personality traits present throughout the life span (McCrae et al., 2000). Personality traits are linked to affective style (Carstensen et al., in press), specifically to the two primary dimensions of subjective emotional experience: positive and negative affect. The personality constructs most relevant to the study of emotion include neuroticism, correlating with negative affect, and extraversion, which correlates with positive affect. Neuroticism scores strongly relate to state levels of negative mood (Watson and Pennebaker, 1989), are correlated with stronger and more negative reactions to unpleasant stimuli (Gross et al., 1998), and in conjunction with extraversion, predict levels of happiness across periods as long as ten years (Costa and McCrae, 1980).

The above findings describe the temperamental basis for affective experience. This foundation serves as a source of affective continuity across the life span, but it is by no means immutable. Affective processes are shaped throughout life by external influences as well as internal motivational strivings that result in characteristic styles of self-regulation (see reviews by Bandura, 1997; McCrae and Costa, 1999). These external and internal influences interact with predispositions that allow for intra-individual change. For example, a considerable number of shy toddlers – roughly 40% – are no longer so by the time they enter preschool (Kagan et al., 1988). In addition to these intra-individual changes, group changes across people of different ages are also apparent. For example, levels of trait negative emotionality, as indexed by neuroticism, is systematically lower in older adults in samples representing differing cultures and ethnicities (McCrae et al., 2000). In addition, a number of studies have examined positive and negative affect across time and among people of different ages, revealing a consistent developmental pattern of increased emotional regulation (Carstensen et al., 2000; Charles et al., 2001b).

1.2. Affective processes across the adult life span

Earlier (Neugarten et al., 1961) and more recent studies (Malatesta and Kalnok, 1984; Diener and Diener, 1996; Lucas and Gohm, 2000) have found negligible age differences in life satisfaction and measures of overall well-being using cross-sectional data (For a complete review, refer to Diener and Suh, 1998). In slight contrast, studies that examine negative and positive affect separately reveal, for the most part, greater well-being among older adults, in that older adults report less anxiety and greater contentment (e.g. Lawton et al., 1993), and have a higher balance of positive to negative affect compared to their younger counterparts (Ryff, 1989).

Positive and negative affect are only moderately correlated with one another. In addition to different patterns of brain activity and different neuroanatomical pathways (see review by Davidson, 1999), they also distinguish themselves from each other in their associations with different types of life events. Whereas positive affect correlates with positive upturns and positive life events, negative affect is most aligned with negative stressors and negative life events (Stallings et al., 1997). Perhaps not surprising, then, is that these two valences also follow different trajectories throughout the life span.

For negative affect, frequency decreases among successively older age groups (Diener et al., 1985; Barrick et al., 1989; Gross et al., 1997) and over time (Charles et al., 2001b). Similarly, older adult couples express less negative affect when discussing areas of conflict with each other (Carstensen et al., 1996). This decrease in frequency does not suggest that the intensity of emotional experience diminishes with age. Based on subjective reports, Malatesta and Kalnok (1984) reported no age differences in emotional experience. And, in a study including over one thousand subjects, Lawton and colleagues (1992) found that the overall pattern of self-reported emotional experience was quite similar across adult age groups.

The exception to a general decrease in negative affect across adulthood occurs in the later years. A large study including participants from 43 nations found that self-reported negative affect decreased until about age 60, when it increased slightly with age up to the oldest group, comprised of people in their 80s (Diener and Suh, 1998). A closer examination, however, revealed that this slight rise after age 60 was only present among men (women ranging from those in their 60s to those in their 80s did not differ in frequency of negative affect), and never reached the levels of the youngest age group, comprised of people in their 20s (Diener and Suh, 1998). Another study that found a decrease in negative affect from age 18 until about age 60 but did not change from ages 60 to 94 for either men or women (Carstensen et al., 2000). Large, population-based cross-sectional studies have found that negative affect, defined by depressive symptoms, declines in the middle years but increases in very old age, with rates highest among the youngest and oldest age groups (Kessler et al., 1992; Gatz et al., 1993). This upturn in depressive symptoms, most notable among people in their 80s, has been documented in a sample with participants ranging from 70 to over 100 years old, where negative affect was higher for the old–old compared to the young–old adults (Smith and Baltes, 1993).

In contrast to negative affect, the pattern for positive affect is less clear, but for the most part is one of relative stability. In longitudinal analyzes, positive affect was stable across a 10-year span (Costa et al., 1987). Another study found that across 23 years, positive affect was relatively stable from early to middle-aged, and from middle-age to early older adulthood, but declined slightly among people followed from their early 60s to mid 80s (Charles et al., 2001b). Several cross-sectional studies have found no significant age differences in positive affect between younger and older adults (Vaux and Meddin, 1987; Barrick et al., 1989) and when comparing the old with the oldest–old (Smith and Baltes, 1993). However, other cross-sectional studies offer contradictory findings, where positive emotions are reported more often (e.g. Gross et al., 1997; Mroczek and Kolarz, 1998) or less often (Diener and Suh, 1998) among increasingly older adults. In sum, the findings are conflicting, but stability for the frequency of positive affect, with small decreases in later life, predominates in the existing literature. For the intensity of positive affect, age groups do not vary significantly from one another (Lawton et al., 1992; Carstensen et al., 2000).

Although negative and positive affect follow different trajectories throughout the life span, they are similar in two respects. First, age is not related to intensity of positive or negative affect in studies where people are asked to relive past experiences in a laboratory (Levenson et al., 1991), report on-line emotions throughout daily life (Carstensen et al., 2000) or answer questions about emotional experience on questionnaires (Malatesta and Kalnok, 1984; Lawton et al., 1992). Second, both valences reveal age-associated patterns for emotions of high arousal. Older adults, compared to younger adults, report reductions in the frequency of high intensity emotions regardless of affective valence, such as feeling positive, e.g. excitement, or negative, e.g. upset, high intensity emotions (Lawton et al., 1992).

The combination of lower negative affect and stable – if not greater – positive affect results in overall stability if not enhanced well-being across the adult life span. Perhaps this is one reason why, when asked about the ability to control emotions, older adults report better regulation than younger adults (Lawton et al., 1992; Gross et al., 1997). According to Gross et al. (1997), control is distinguished from the experience of emotion because, rather than referring to the intensity of the "feeling" of the emotion, control, instead refers to people trying to influence what emotions they experience and how the experience unfolds. Self-reports about emotional control are often assessed with questionnaire items such as "I try to stay neutral." Lawton et al. (1992) analyzed questionnaire data about emotional experiences that included questions regarding emotional control from a large sample of young, middle-aged, and old adults. Compared to younger adults, older adults reported that they had better control and were more likely than younger adults to remain "calm and cool." Gross et al. (1997) found converging evidence across five highly diverse samples. In each, older adults responded more positively than younger adults to a question concerning how well they are able to control their emotions overall (Gross et al., 1997).

Findings from an experience sampling study suggest that older adults are correct in their subjective accounts of control over their affective worlds. Using an experience-sampling paradigm, people ranging in age from 18 to 94 years old answered questions about their emotional experiences on randomly sampled occasions five times a day for one week (Carstensen et al., 2000). Once a negative or positive emotion was recorded, its duration was examined as a function of age. The duration of positive states was comparable across the age range; however the duration of negative states was shorter in older adults. The decreased length of time that negative affect is experienced, even in the absence of increases in positive affect, is impressive evidence for increased emotional control with age, especially in the light of shifts towards more losses relative to gains with age (Heckhausen et al., 1989).

1.3. Psychological disorders

At the extremes of emotional experience, older adults also fare better than their younger counterparts. With the exception of the dementias and other organically based brain syndromes, older adults experience lower levels of psychiatric disorders than younger adults (Regier et al., 1988; Fisher et al., 1993). Affective disorders, including major depression and the anxiety disorders, occur at lower rates in older than in younger cohorts. Researchers examining age differences in psychological disorders were particularly surprised by the relatively low rate of major affective disorders, long suspected to increase in prevalence linearly across the life span (e.g. Gurland, 1976). However, the life-time prevalence of depression in current cohorts of *adolescents* already matches the prevalence observed in the elderly (Klerman and Weissman, 1989), and more recently born cohorts are experiencing their first major depressive episodes at earlier ages than older cohorts (Wittchen et al., 1994). In addition, older adults also evince less severe forms of dysthmia, a disorder characterized by anhedonia and longstanding, low levels of depression (Oxman et al., 2000). Although cohort (as opposed to age) differences in psychopathology is certainly a plausible explanation for these findings, one longitudinal study suggests that this is not the case. Clinical ratings indicated improved emotion regulation, or psychological health, across time from adolescence into old age (Jones and Meredith, 2000). This robust finding of intact emotion regulation in old age is even present in people with severe physically degenerating diseases; emotional responsiveness, even in later stages of dementia, is relatively well-preserved (Magai et al., 1996).

2. Biological changes

2.1. Physiology

The overall improvement in subjective well-being at first seems at odds with a trajectory of biological decline with age. Emotional experience is linked to autonomic reactivity, and reductions in almost all areas of autonomic activity are reliably associated with age. For example, changes related to cardiovascular functioning, including reduced cardiac output, reduced muscle mass, reduced maximum capacity, increased resistance to blood flow and increased resting heart rate have been well documented (see review by Cacioppo et al., 1998). For this reason, emotional experience may become poorly regulated at a physiological level with age, particularly in the peripheral nervous system. In a test that addressed questions of emotional experience and aging, Levenson et al. (1991) examined subjective experience and physiological reactivity concomitantly under controlled laboratory conditions. Older participants came to the laboratory, identified events that had elicited a range of strong emotional reactions in the past, and were instructed through imagery to re-experience these emotions, one at a time, while they were videotaped. Measures of heart rate, somatic activity, blood pressure and respiration were simultaneously gathered. In addition, ratings of subjective intensity obtained after each emotional induction were computed. Findings suggest great similarity in subjective experience among older and younger adults. In addition, the psychophysiological profile associated with specific emotions in younger adults was also observed in this sample of elderly adults, suggesting maintenance of emotion-specific differentiation in psychophysiological patterning. One important age difference, however, was that the magnitude of the autonomic response was relatively subdued in older subjects. In other words, although emotion-specific patterns (e.g. heart rate increases more with anger than with disgust; somatic activity decreases more with fear than anger or surprise, etc.) are consistent for younger and older adults, the level of arousal is somewhat reduced in older adults, particularly in the cardiovascular response. This pattern of findings is consistent with reduction in general autonomic activity documented previously in studies of general functioning.

The findings of preserved emotional profiles, but overall reduced arousal, has now been replicated in older adults discussing marital conflicts with their spouses (Levenson et al., 1994) and older European- and Chinese-Americans viewing emotion-eliciting films (Tsai et al., 2000). Whether the reduction in arousal reflects general age-related depression of the autonomic nervous system, a circumscribed dampening of emotional arousal, or a combination of the two factors, remains unclear.

2.2. Biological changes: brain functioning

In addition to changes in the peripheral nervous system, changes in the central nervous system – particularly in the brain – inform discussions of emotion and aging. Although emotions are complex experiences dependent on many areas of brain functioning, certain regions – specifically the limbic system and the prefrontal cortex – have been the focus of studies concerning emotional functioning and are arguably the central areas involved in emotional processes (Davidson et al., 1998; Davidson, 2002; see reviews by Le Doux, 1992; Davidson et al., 2000). Within the limbic system, the hippocampus and amygdala have been regions of particular interest. The hippocampus plays a role in complex emotional experiences, such as conditioned fear (LaBar and LeDoux, 1997), and is linked to the amygdala, which is involved in emotional stimulus evaluation as well as long term emotional memory (LaBar and LeDoux, 1997; Le Doux, 1992).

Despite the robust findings that age is associated with decreases in total brain volume and loss of neurons (Dickson et al., 1992), both the hippocampus and the amygdala are relatively unscathed by the aging process compared to other brain regions (Benes et al., 1994; Good et al., 2001; see review by Mather, in press). Scheibel (1996) describes evidence pointing both to hippocampal atrophy as well as to hippocampal cell volume stability with aging. Other researchers, however, show that myelination of certain regions of the hippocampus appear to continue well into middle age, with a substantial increase in myelination occurring between the fourth and sixth decades (Benes et al., 1994). In addition, the amygdala is relatively spared from the predictable decrease in afferent fibers with age, despite experiencing some possible age-related neuronal loss (Scheibel, 1996).

In contrast to the findings for the relative sparing of the hippocampus and amygdala with age, research on changes to the prefrontal cortex overwhelmingly point to decline (see review by Raz, 2000). The prefrontal cortex is critical for emotion regulation, social functioning, and memory; damage to this area is associated with emotional dysregulation including depression, hostility, poor emotional judgment, and memory (see review by Davidson and Irwin, 1999). Given the robust and often disproportionate age-related loss in prefrontal volume with age compared to many other regions in the brain, a plausible deduction is that emotional functioning, particularly in the areas of regulation and social functioning, would exhibit the greatest age-related deficits. Empirical analyses, however, again does not support this logic. Emotion regulation, as we reviewed above, does not decline relative to the decreases in prefrontal cortex volume, and often improves with age. In addition, social cognition and socioemotional functioning, as we will review below, does not diminish with advanced age. Currently, this fundamental discrepancy between enhanced observed behavior and subjective experience in the emotion domain on the one hand, and decreases in prefrontal lobe cortex volume on the other, presents an intriguing question that has yet to be completely understood.

2.3. Emotional expression

The ability to express emotions is fundamental to affective experience, serving to communicate emotions both to others and even to the self (e.g. Darwin, 1872). Although societal norms and expectations often govern the display of emotions (e.g. Matsumoto, 1993), the ties between facial expression and physiological reactivity (see review by Ekman, 1999), coupled with its evolutionary origins (e.g. Darwin, 1872) and cross-cultural similarities (Elfenbein and Ambady, 2002) embed facial expression in the biological domain. For these reasons, age-related physical changes provide plausible reasons to believe that this form of non-verbal communication may decline with age. Decreased elasticity of skin tissue and consequent increased sagging and wrinkling may jeopardize the ability of others to interpret facial expressions. In addition, reduced physiological arousal may lead to reductions in the production of facial expressions.

Existing research on emotional expression, however, again contradicts assumptions of age related decline (for a review of age differences in emotional behavior, refer to Magai and Passman, 1998). In self-reports of expressive behavior, older adults are more likely than younger adults to assert that people of their age group need to conceal their emotions, but they are not more likely to report that they actually do hide their emotions from others (Malatesta and Kalnok, 1984). Thus, older adults are just as likely as younger adults to endorse a statement saying that they openly express what they are feeling, which the researchers interpret as older adults being less interested in adhering to societal restrictions on behavior but equally invested in conveying their current feelings to others. Indeed, laboratory research suggests that older adults are successful in this goal. In studies where older and younger adults experience emotions in a laboratory, expert coding of facial expressions reveal that older adults spontaneously display equal levels (Levenson et al., 1991) if not more frequent (Malatesta-Magai et al., 1992) facial expressions compared to younger adults. Moreover, the facial expressions of older adults are more complex, revealing a greater mix of emotional expressions during a relived emotion paradigm (Malatesta-Magai et al., 1992). Further observational research examining age differences in emotional expression during social interactions suggests that older adults may be better than middle-aged adults at regulating their emotions as they interact socially, at least with intimate partners (Levenson et al., 1993; Carstensen et al., 1995). From the observations of nonverbal and verbal emotional expression among couples discussing an area of conflict, findings indicate that older spouses (even unhappily married ones) express less anger, belligerence, and disgust to one another during the session compared to middle-aged adults (Carstensen et al., 1995).

Only two findings qualify the overall picture of stability, if not enhancement, of emotional expression in older age. The first concerns a task where participants are given instructions to move muscles in their faces to form emotional expressions. Unlike the relived emotion task, where old and younger adults were similar in the quality of their spontaneous facial expressions, this directed facial action task revealed a lower mean quality of facial expression among older adults relative to the normative performance of younger adults (Levenson et al., 1991). The concurrent subjective experience of older adults, however, was also lower among older adults relative to younger adults in the relived emotion task, which suggests that subjective experience may be partially responsible for these age differences; and, of course, because voluntary posing of expressions is unrelated to the quality of naturally occurring expressions, the meaning of this finding is unclear. The second, more interesting, finding concerns the ability of others to perceive facial expressions of people representing different age groups. Although older adults are equally adept at correctly identifying emotional facial expressions of people across the life span, younger adults are less able to identify correctly emotional facial expressions of older adults compared to those of younger adults (Malatesta et al., 1987). Because expert raters do not show age differences in the quality of expressions for relived emotions (Malatesta-Magai et al., 1992), this finding speaks more to the abilities of younger adults in detecting emotional expression, rather than the ability of older adults to express them.

3. Potential mechanisms behind stable if not enhanced emotion regulation with age

The above findings paint a relatively optimistic portrayal of emotional functioning in old age. Subjective well-being is equal if not enhanced among older adults, with decreasing negative affect largely responsible for the findings. And, despite biological changes that often result in general decline, emotional processes that rely on these biological processes remain relatively spared. Researchers interested in the mechanisms behind emotion regulation have turned to age-related changes in social and cognitive processes that are highly related to emotional functioning. These research directions have led to findings suggesting that older adults may be regulating their emotions by engaging in social processes aimed at avoiding potentially negative events, a strategy of antecedent emotion control (Carstensen et al., 1996). In addition, cognitive appraisals used by older adults also suggest that they may be engaging in more response-focused strategies of emotion regulation than younger adults, whereby they effectively reduce negative affect.

3.1. Social processes

In general, the most intense emotional experiences are social experiences. The most basic social stimulus – the human face – is thought to have evolved for the functional purpose of communicating emotions (Ekman, 1973). The primary functions of emotions, to motivate and communicate, are embedded within social processes and serve social goals. In daily life social and emotional processes are intertwined: emotion regulation relies heavily on the ability to navigate social environments, and social environments influence emotional experience. Antecedent emotion control refers to the process of proactively avoiding negative emotions, and regulating social contacts is among the most effective antecedent coping strategies. Age-associated changes in social network composition, and the emotional experience derived from social interactions, reveal that with age, people are more likely to structure their social worlds to optimize emotionally meaningful, and therefore gratifying, experiences and to avoid potentially negative interchanges.

Age-related reductions in social contact have been widely documented in both longitudinal (Palmore, 1981; Lee and Markides, 1990) and cross-sectional studies (Cumming and Henry, 1961; Lawton et al., 1987). Older people interact less with others and appear to resist efforts by others to make new friends (Carstensen, 1986). On the one hand, social connectedness clearly predicts mental health in the elderly (Lowenthal and Haven, 1968; Antonucci and Jackson, 1987). On the other hand, overall rates of interactions fail to predict social satisfaction (Chapell and Badger, 1989; Lee and Markides, 1990).

Presumably, older adults are more interested in maximizing emotionally meaningful experience (a point to which we return below), and for this reason their social preferences are biased towards well-known social partners compared to partner preferences of younger adults. Indeed, smaller social networks comprised of a greater proportion of meaningful social partners characterizes age differences in German, European-American, and African-American samples (Lang and Carstensen, 1994; Lang et al., 1998; Fung et al., 2001a). Moreover, these age-related patterns are not accounted for by personality (Lang et al., 1998) or selective mortality (Lang and Carstensen, 1994; Fung et al., 2001a). When peripheral partners disappear from the social networks of older adults, most often the loss represents an active move on the part of the older adult (Lang, 2000).

A series of studies including participants from the United States (Fredrickson and Carstensen, 1990), Hong Kong (Fung et al., 1999, Studies 2 and 4), Taiwan, and Beijing (Fung et al., 2001b) examine age differences in social partner preferences. In each of these studies, participants were asked to imagine that they had half an hour free with no pressing commitments and to choose one from among three potential social partners. Options were: (1) a member of your immediate family, (2) the author of a book you have read, and (3) an acquaintance with whom you seem to have much in common. These three prospective social partners were selected because they service different goals related, respectively, to deriving emotional meaning, gaining information, and expanding social horizons. In every one of these studies, when simply asked about their preferences, older adults but not their younger counterparts show a strong preference for spending time with emotionally close social partners.

Studies suggest that this age-associated reduction in peripheral social partners is beneficial to affective well-being. A longitudinal analysis assessing participants' frequency of contact and satisfaction with various types of social partners at ages 18, 30, 40, and 50 years revealed that both rates of interaction with acquaintances and the satisfaction derived from them declined from early to middle adulthood (Carstensen, 1992). Across the same period, however, interaction rates among emotionally close social partners – spouses, parents, and siblings – maintained or increased, as did the satisfaction they engendered. Average emotional closeness of social networks is positively related to social embeddedness, operationalized in our work by a composite index of social satisfaction, tenderness, and the absence of loneliness (Lang and Carstensen, 1994; Lang et al., 1998).

One recent study suggests that socioemotional processes during social interactions may be qualitatively different in younger and older adults. Pasupathi et al. (in press) compared the interactions of older and younger adults telling a story to a child. Younger and older women were given a picture book without text, asked to review it and then tell the story to a child (who was actually an experimental confederate in order to control for qualities of the child listener). Older women were more likely to tell the story around emotional themes and to emphasize positive emotions even when the scene also involved negative emotions.

In summary, age is related to social network composition. Older people do have smaller social networks, but the decrease in size is due to a reduction in acquaintances, as opposed to close social partners. Consequently, networks of older people are comprised primarily of well-known and emotionally close social partners. Research also suggests that social interactions are managed somewhat differently as well, with emphasis placed on emotional importance of topics. By constructing and managing social networks in this manner, older adults proactively avoid potentially negative interactions.

3.2. Social perceptions

Age differences are also found in the cognitive strategies people use to evaluate both strangers and well-known social partners. For example, in an impression formation task where participants read two short descriptions about a person and then were asked their opinions, older adults weigh negative information more heavily in evaluating others compared to younger adults, even when this information is later counterbalanced by positive information about the same person (Hess and Pullen, 1994). This age effect is most apparent when the information concerns characteristics regarding the morality of the person, e.g. their honesty, compared to information about their abilities, e.g. intelligence (Hess et al., 1999). A recent study of source memory also finds that honesty is particularly important to older adults (Rahhal et al., 2002). When the source is an honest or dishonest person, older adults are just as likely as younger adults to remember it, in contrast to situations where the source is a sensory or perceptual cue (see also Hashtroudi et al., 1990). A greater negative bias for strangers, particularly in a domain that would influence how one is treated by this stranger, may be a method employed by older adults more often to avoid potentially negative interactions. In another study, Fredrickson and Carstensen (1990) examined the use of emotional reasoning when people ranging from adolescents to octogenarians categorized prospective social partners.

Research participants sorted social partner descriptions according to how similarly they would feel interacting with them. Three general dimensions were revealed by the card sorts: an emotional or "like/dislike" dimension, an informational dimension, and a dimension characterized by future possibilities. Older people weighted the emotional dimension most heavily, followed by middle-aged and younger people.

3.3. Cognitive processes

Affective well-being influences, and is influenced by, the decisions people make, the problem-solving strategies they select, and the appraisal and memories of their prior events. Although emotions are integral to cognitive processing regardless of age (Zajonc, 1997), the salience of emotional material, relative to non-emotional material, appears to increase with age, as does the ability to integrate emotional material into logical reasoning. Labouvie-Vief and her colleagues have examined age differences in the processing of emotional material and have found that adults are more successful at understanding the emotional states of others than adolescents (Labouvie-Vief et al., 1989). When asked to focus on their own emotional experiences, younger adults reported control strategies when regulating emotions that focused on distraction, such as redirecting one's thoughts or ignoring the situation. Older adults more often mentioned that they acknowledge and focus on their emotional reactions to the emotion-eliciting event or experience (Diehl et al., 1996).

Older adults process information with a greater focus on subjective states and symbolic themes compared to younger adults (Labouvie-Vief, 1998). Several studies that have examined how people process short stories have found that older adults focus more on psychological themes and use metaphors when recalling and interpreting text (Labouvie-Vief and Hakim-Larson, 1989; Adams, 1991; Adams et al., 1997; see also Pasupathi et al., in press). In a further examination of problem-solving for highly emotional events, younger, middle-aged and older adults were asked to make attributions, either situational or dispositional, concerning the cause of interpersonal events (Blanchard-Fields and Norris, 1994). Results indicate that older adults use more interactive attributions, concluding that the event was caused by both the situation and the disposition of the primary character, compared to younger adults. This interactional attribution style is considered to reflect more sophisticated understanding of social situations, allowing the adoption of multiple perspectives (Labouvie-Vief, 1998). In addition, when faced with conflict, older adults show greater impulse control and are more likely to appraise conflict situations positively, whereas adults and adolescents express lower levels of impulse control and are more likely to display signs of aggression (Diehl et al., 1996).

This increased focus on emotions may result in greater emotional complexity among older adults relative to younger adults. Although younger adults do report experiencing a mix of both positive and negative emotions when faced with situations that are highly complex in the emotions they invoke, i.e. moving out of one's dorm and watching a movie that depicts a great victory at great cost (Larson et al., 2001), older adults report more co-occurring positive and negative emotions in their daily lives than younger adults (Carstensen et al., 2000). This greater frequency of mixed emotions may also be why, in a relived emotion task, the spontaneous facial expression of older adults reveal greater mixes of emotional displays compared to those of younger adults (Malatesta-Magai et al., 1992).

3.4. General coping strategies

Age differences in social cognition aid in the process of coping with problems in daily life. For example, social comparison is often used when people face both challenges and threats. Older people, compared to younger adults, engage in relatively more downward and less upward social comparison (Heckhausen and Kreuger, 1993). Whereas upward social comparison motivates future goal strivings, downward social comparison better serves emotion regulation. The emotion regulatory benefits of downward comparison for older adults are apparent in ratings of self-perceived health; ratings of health generally are more positive when older adults rate their health compared to others their age, than when they rate their health in general (Roberts, 1999).

Other studies examining coping strategies have found that older adults use both problem-focused and emotion-focused strategies and are more flexible in their problem-solving strategies than younger adults (Blanchard-Fields et al., 1997). When these problems focus on emotionally charged interpersonal issues with family and friends, however, older adults choose emotion-focused strategies. Research suggests that they do so to preserve harmony in their surroundings (Blanchard-Fields et al., 1997) and to regulate their own emotional experience (Heckhausen and Kreuger, 1993). In addition, when faced with highly emotional hypothetical situations that often include other people, older adults adopt emotion-focused strategies such as, "learn to live with infrequent visits," more often than younger adults (Blanchard-Fields et al., 1995). Older adults not only report engaging in these strategies more often than younger adults, but they also recommend these strategies to others as the best alternative to these difficult social situations (Charles et al., 2001a).

Older adults are more likely to choose problem-solving techniques that emphasize emotion regulation beyond the social domain, as well. Lazarus (1996) emphasizes the importance of choosing appropriate coping strategies based on the type of problem faced, and that old age is often a time when chronic, as opposed to acute, situations are more common. For problems with no simple solution or end in sight, emotion regulation is often highly prioritized for all people. For older adults, however, the coping strategies they employ in many situations suggest that emotion regulation may be even more valued than for younger adults. Flexible goal adjustment measured by items like, "I usually find something positive even after giving up something I cherish" increases from young to old age (Brandtstädter and Renner, 1990; Heckhausen and Schulz, 1995). Older people also endorse statements that suggest not engaging in negative emotional experiences (Lawton et al., 1992). Across a variety of stressful contexts experienced by people of all ages, older people report less confrontative coping and greater distancing and positive reappraisal than younger people (Folkman et al., 1987), a strategy which may help to "short circuit the stress process, so that incidents that might otherwise have been hassles [are] neutralized" (Folkman et al., 1987, p. 182). Indeed, research examining people of different ages faced with a similar stressful event suggest that these coping strategies are successful for older adults. Age was negatively related to distress among older adults who sustained property loss after a flood (Phifer, 1990). In another study, age was related to lower levels of hostility for adults ranging from middle to old age who were coping with chronic illness (Felton and Revenson, 1987).

3.5. Memory

Although rarely conceptualized as a self-regulatory process, the events, people, and places that individuals retrieve from memory clearly influence well-being. And, of course, memory itself is not simply a process of retrieval, but an elaborative process by which current goals influence constructions of the past (Johnson and Sherman, 1990). These goals have the potential of influencing the memorial processes at multiple levels, from the attention people place on specific stimuli, to the encoding, storage and retrieval processes. Although the mechanisms are not well-established at this point, a growing number of studies have found that age interacts with emotional material to create different patterns of performance. Specifically, age is associated with a relative increase in performance for emotional information relative to neutral material.

This phenomenon has been found on a number of memory tasks performed in the laboratory. One study using an incidental memory paradigm included people aged 20–83 years who first read a narrative drawn from a popular novel and were later asked to recall as much as they could from the passage. Of what people remembered, the proportion of emotional information, as opposed to neutral information, increased with each successively older age group (Carstensen and Turk-Charles, 1994). In another study, younger and older adults were asked to examine advertisements that varied in emotionality. Older people were more likely to remember advertisements with emotional slogans, like "Capture those special moments" more than information-related slogans, like "Capture the unexplored world." They also preferred the emotional framings more so than younger adults (Fung and Carstensen, in press). Similarly, in a source memory paradigm, younger people recalled more sensory and perceptual details about imagined and real experiences, but older adults recalled a greater number of feelings and evaluative statements (Hashtroudi et al., 1990). This greater emphasis on emotion is also documented in studies where people were asked to recall experiences from their past. In a collaborative story-telling study, younger and older couples were asked to describe a recent past vacation (Gould and Dixon, 1993). Most of the couples described fairly recent trips, and the experiences themselves seem similar enough to warrant age comparisons. In their descriptions, older couples provided more information on the subjective aspects, such as descriptions of people, and less information on the factual aspects, such as itineraries, than did younger couples. In another study showing similar increases in emotional salience for past experiences, older adults, compared to younger adults, rated songs from their youth as more emotional, and remembered more emotional songs better than less emotional songs (Schulkind et al., 1999).

These studies point to a general, age-related increase in memory for emotional material relative to neutral material. Other studies, however, suggest that findings are driven largely by the emphasis younger adults place for *negatively* valenced material. Older adults are more likely to show choice-supportive memory, i.e. attribute more positive and fewer negative features to a chosen option relative to a non-chosen option, than are younger adults (Mather and Johnson, 2000). Such memory is likely to optimize emotional experience by reducing regret and increasing satisfaction with past decisions. When recalling previously presented positive, negative, and neutral images, the proportion of correctly recognized and recalled negative, images declines linearly with age across younger, middle aged, and older adults (Charles et al., 2002b). Although older adults recalled fewer images of all valences, age differences were the greatest among the negative images. Age differences remained after controlling for current mood and depressive symptoms, indicating that this phenomenon cannot be accounted for by the effect of mood congruency.

This age difference, with memory becoming proportionally more positive with age, extends to autobiographical memory as well. When asked to recall the single most important experience in their moral development, older adults are more likely to cite a positive episode than adolescents and young adults (Quackenbush and Barnett, 2001). In longitudinal analyzes, autobiographical reports of the same event becomes more positive over time (Field, 1981; Kennedy et al., 2002), suggesting that the age-related increase in positive reports represents a developmental trend as opposed to a cohort effect. This reduction of negative events and resulting increased emphasis on positive events may be one reason why reminiscence – the process of recalling personal memories to connect people's past to their present – serves different therapeutic functions for younger and older adults. For younger adults, reminiscence serves to solidify identity and solve problems. Middle-aged adults too reminisce for the purpose of problem-solving to accomplish developmental tasks. Older adults also use reminisce as a life review strategy to accomplish a developmental task, but this task focuses on predominantly emotional goals of providing a sense of meaning, fulfillment, and integration to one's life journey (Lewis and Butler, 1974). Successful life review, then, is associated with increased life satisfaction for older adults (Webster, 1995).

This decrease in negative, as opposed to positive, material recalled appears in both laboratory tasks and autobiographical memory. The mechanism responsible for this age-related change, however, remains unclear. The few studies that have examined this question yield findings suggesting that more than one mechanism may be driving age-related changes. Findings from one study point to attentional processes in the age-related decrease in emphasis of negative information. In this study, participants saw a pair of faces, one emotional (happy, sad, or angry) and one neutral quickly flashed on the screen. Afterwards, a dot probe appeared on the screen, and participants were asked to report the emotion of the face that had appeared in the same location as the dot appearing before them. Attentional processes were calculated by the response time of the participant to specify the emotion of the face they had seen, with greater response time indicating more difficultly, hence less attention, to the original stimulus. Participants were also given a memory task, asking them to identify previously seen faces from a group that included novel as well as the familiar faces. Results indicate an age interaction, such that older adults attended to negative faces the least and remembered positive images better than negative images compared to the younger adults (Mather and Carstensen, in press).

Others find age-related decreases in memory for negative events, but these findings indicate mechanisms other than attention responsible for the phenomenon. In one study, adults who were endorsing a presidential candidate were asked about their emotions upon hearing that this person had withdrawn from the political race (Levine and Bluck, 1997). Soon after hearing about the withdrawal, young, middle, and older adults expressed similar levels of sadness, anger, and hopelessness, with sadness being the strongest emotion experienced by all age groups. In addition, older adults were less likely to redirect their energy towards a new candidate than younger and middle-aged adults. Four months later, however, of the people who still preferred the original candidate, older adults were more likely to underestimate the intensity of sadness they had originally experienced compared to their younger counterparts (Levine and Bluck, 1997). The researchers interpret these findings as older adults using strategies whereby their reappraise their past emotional reactions to enhance emotional well-being, a strategy that occurs after the attentional level and during the later stages – elaboration or retrieval – of the memory process. Moreover, findings suggest that these age differences occur routinely when recounting affective experiences of daily life. When people are asked about their immediate, on-line emotional reactions, or their reactions to the day's events, age effects are minimal (Almeida, 1998; Carstensen et al., 2000). Longer time frames, however, reveal greater age differences. When people are asked to recall the emotions of the week, age is associated with more positive reports (Almeida, 1998).

4. Why are older adults doing so well? Theoretical explanations

The research reviewed above provides converging evidence for improved emotion regulation with age. These findings are documented in studies of age differences in self-reported emotional well-being and evidenced in laboratory-based research as well as more naturalistic settings. Older adults use both antecedent emotion control strategies – as seen in their successful navigation of social partners to optimize meaningful experiences – as well as response-focused emotional control strategies, as evident by their increased emphasis on cognitive methods focused at minimizing negative affect. In response to the growing empirical evidence documenting affective experience in later life, researchers have formed models to explain these developmental trends. Below, we discuss three of these models – socioemotional selectivity theory, the cognitive-emotional integration model, and a model of biological change, that have been used to describe life span changes in emotional experience.

4.1. Socioemotional selectivity theory

The awareness of time, not just clock time or calendar time, but lifetime, is a fundamental human characteristic (Carstensen et al., 1999). This universal ability – considered by many to have been central in the evolution of human consciousness – plays an essential role in motivation. Socioemotional selectivity theory maintains that perceived limitations on time lead to motivational shifts that direct attention to emotional goals (Carstensen, 1993, 1995). This shift results in greater complexity of emotional experience and better regulation of emotions experienced in everyday life. Essentially, when people are relieved of concerns for the future, attention to current feeling-states heightens. Appreciation for the fragility and value of human life increases and long-term relationships with family and friends assume unmatched importance. The theory suggests that time perspective, not age per se, influences goal selection. Research has shown that younger people, as young as adolescents, who perceive time as limited also emphasize emotionally meaningful goals over informational goals (Carstensen and Fredrickson, 1998; Fung et al., 1999) and that older people who view time as expansive emphasize informational goals (Fung, et al., 1999). Time perspective is malleable. However, because mortality places constraints on time, there are reliable age differences in time perspective (Fung et al., 2001b; Lang and Carstensen, 2002) Because of the inextricable association between age and time left in life, chronological age – on average – is associated with increased preferences for and investment in emotionally meaningful goals. This age-related motivational shift leads to alterations in the dynamic interplay between individuals and their environments such that optimization of emotional experience is prioritized in later life.

According to the theory, goals are always set within temporal contexts, and goal selection depends fundamentally on the perception of time. When time is perceived as open-ended, goals related to the long-term future are prioritized. When time is perceived as limited, more immediate goals are pursued. Thus, although a reasonable stable set of goals – ranging from physical safety and sustenance to more psychological goals such as feeling comfortable and gaining information – motivates behavior throughout life, the perception of time influences which goal of these goals is adopted.

Socioemotional selectivity theory focuses on two main classes of psychological goals: one comprises expansive goals, such as acquiring knowledge or making new social contacts; the second comprises goals related to feelings, such as balancing emotional states or sensing that one is needed by others. Of course, approach and avoidance always involve the affective system (Zajonc, 1984), and therefore, classifying some social motives as "emotionally meaningful" and others as "knowledge-related" is, in some ways, artificial, but the distinction is intended heuristically to distinguish between goals that are pursued because of the accompanying feelings that ensue, and goals that are pursued to obtain novel information or experience.

Temporal appraisal allows people to balance long- and short-term needs in order to adapt effectively to their particular niche in the life cycle (Charles and Carstensen, 1999). Throughout life, goals vie with one another. Pursuing expansive goals (e.g. striking up a conversation with an attractive stranger) can, at times, entail negative emotions such as anxiety or shame. In contrast, goals related to feeling states (e.g. phoning a close friend who makes you feel good) usually offer less in the way of novel information but potentially more in realizing emotionally meaningful goals. Theoretically, in situations where goals compete with one another, a principle mechanism involved in goal selection is time perspective. When time is perceived as open-ended (as it typically is in youth), expansive goals are pursued. When boundaries on time are perceived, emotionally meaningful goals are pursued presumably because the pay-off is in the contact itself, not promised at some nebulous time in the future.

Early in life, time is typically perceived as expansive and people are motivated to prepare for a long and unknown future. With this future-orientation, developing organisms allocate considerable resources to obtaining knowledge and developing new skills and are motivated to do so particularly when knowledge is limited. Because knowledge striving is so important from late adolescence to middle adulthood, it is pursued relentlessly even at the cost of emotional satisfaction. In contrast, older people see fewer opportunities awaiting them and less time available to obtain and benefit from purely knowledge-related goals. Developmentally, the knowledge trajectory starts high during the early years of life and declines gradually over the life course as knowledge accrues and the future for which it is banked grows ever shorter.

Unlike knowledge-related goals, emotional goals follow a curvilinear trajectory. Socioemotional selectivity theory acknowledges that emotional needs are important throughout life, but posits that their relative salience among the constellation of social motives changes with age. The emotion trajectory is highest during infancy and early childhood when emotional trust and relatedness are initially established and rises again in old age when future-oriented strivings are less relevant. As people age, they realize that time, in a sense, is "running out" and begin to focus on the present as opposed to the future. Goals that are satisfied by the resulting feeling state are more likely to be pursued because they are experienced immediately, a valuable commodity in the face of limited time. Subsequently, as people realize they are gradually approaching the end of life, they care more about experiencing meaningful social ties and less about expanding their horizons. Older adults also reliably report the sense that time passes more and more quickly as they age; they foresee a relatively limited future, whereas younger adults envision a relatively expansive one (Lang and Carstensen, 2002). This motivational shift leads to a greater investment in the quality of important social relationships and a generally enhanced appreciation of life.

Resulting emotions are not purely positive; characterizing old age as "happy" does not do justice to the complex emotional states entailed in deriving meaning and satisfaction from life. What characterizes old age is not hedonism, but a desire to derive meaning and satisfaction from life. On balance, however, emotional states are more positive than negative. There is a quality of savoring the time left as opposed to fearing the end. This greater priority on emotional experience creates an age-related shift towards activities that serve to regulate emotions, decreasing negative affect and increasing positive affect. Older adults, recognizing that time is running out, choose emotional interactions that are meaningful and emotionally fulfilling. These goals also shift attentional processes, leading to greater emphasis on positive stimuli and greater importance placed on emotional information.

4.2. The cognitive-emotional integration model

Labouvie-Vief and her colleagues propose a cognitive-emotional integration theory to describe the development of emotion and cognition throughout adult development (see review by Labouvie-Vief et al., 1989; Labouvie-Vief and DeVoe, 1991; Labouvie-Vief, 1998). The cognitive-emotional integration model combines neo-Piagetian and psychodynamic constructs to explain how cognitions, specifically cognitions regarding interpersonal processes, are transformed throughout the life span from thinking characterized as concrete and ego-centered to a process described as increasingly complex and comprised of relativistic thinking. This model contends that cognitive abilities, as defined by ego level and intelligence, are responsible for age-related differences.

In this model, children first formulate their ideas about themselves and others using an ego-centered approach. They define themselves in conjunction with dyadic relationships, and interpret others based on their own beliefs and opinions. As they grow older and their ego level increases, they embed their impressions of themselves and others into social norms and absolute thinking. People are not seen as individuals, but as people who fulfill specific roles and engage in role-defined behavior. At this time, others are described as static and predictable based on their social roles. People are either "good" or "bad" and, once placed in these categories, rarely are reconsidered. Emotions, like people, are also viewed discretely.

As ego-level continues to develop, often across middle-age, others are viewed within increasingly broader social roles that extend beyond group membership. From a state where individuals do not distinguish self from others clearly and where they place people into specific categories with static dispositional traits, cognitive development allows people to incorporate a view where both self and other are seen abstractly, as products of history and culture, and with distinct internal conflicts and contradictions. This advanced understanding of emotions and more complex perception of self and others allows for greater insight into problem-solving and perspective taking. Finally, the self and others are viewed as individuals who experience complex, internal psychological processes that constantly interact with equally complex social partners. Emotional reasoning and emotional experience likewise increases in complexity. With this advanced reasoning, stories are viewed beyond simple structure to incorporate metaphors and relativistic thinking as well as more affectively laden content (Adams et al., 1990). In addition, people are able to experience several emotions simultaneously, recognizing and accepting contrasts in their evaluations of themselves and others (Labouvie-Vief et al., 1995).

Ego level is related to age, and middle-aged adults display this cognitive maturity to a greater degree than younger or older adults (Labouvie-Vief and Blanchard-Fields, 1982). Age, however, remains a unique predictor of this cognitive-emotional integration separate from either ego level or measures of intelligence. For example, more mature strategies of coping are linearly related to higher ego levels and older age (Diehl et al., 1996). Specifically, younger adults are more likely than older adults to use aggressive and defensive styles, whereas older adults are more likely to reinterpret the problems and delay making absolute judgments. Labouvie-Vief (1998) maintains that in addition to advanced ego level, age may bring a greater sense of mortality and a subsequent increased acceptance of emotions. She further contends that even if older adults do not perform as well on tasks of cognitive complexity and problem-solving in the laboratory (e.g. Labouvie-Vief et al., 1995), it may be because these tasks place more emphasis on goals relevant to middle-age, such as personal growth and defining oneself in a future oriented schema, and less on emotion-focused goals. In this way, cognitive-emotional integration may, like the coping styles related to them, continue to evidence gains with age, once the emphasis is placed on emotional goals. Indeed, although cognitive complexity appears to peak in middle-aged and then decline slightly thereafter when evaluated using laboratory measures, this curvilinear finding does not reflect a pattern fitting emotion regulation with age. In studies of emotion regulation, feelings of aggression are reduced, and positive reappraisals are more common among successively older age groups (Diehl et al., 1996).

4.3. Biological models

As stated in the introduction, biological decline was once thought to cause emotional dysregulation (e.g. Buhler, 1935; Banham, 1951). Now, ironically, some researchers view biological decline as potentially helpful to emotion regulation (see review by Levenson, 2000). In other words, particular age differences do not necessarily oppose, and may even contribute to, self-perceived maintained or improved emotional functioning and control with age. Using this argument, decreases in physiological arousal may well facilitate the ability to control strong emotional reactions. Put simply, older adults control their emotions better because there is less physiological reactivity to control. Of course, the entire physical system decreases, so reductions in arousal in the emotional system may not be as pronounced in an organism where homeostasis is harder to maintain. Nevertheless, the findings that several physiological indicators necessary for emotional reactivity, such as cardiovascular functioning, show a greater decrease in arousal with age relative to other systems (see review by Cacioppo et al., 1998), coupled with the findings that certain regions of the brain necessary for emotional experience, i.e. the limbic system, may be less sensitive to age-related decline (see review by Mather, in press), make this a viable model.

4.4. Declining inhibition

Other researchers focus directly on changes in cognition that are posited to have the unintended consequence of increasing the salience of emotional material. Specifically, failures of executive functioning, specifically the inhibitory mechanisms, may lead to age-related increases in reports of emotional detail at the expense of other information (Hasher and Zacks, 1988; Zacks and Hasher, 1997). In this model, inhibitory mechanisms are hypothesized to become less effective as people get older. Because inhibitory mechanisms determine what enters working memory in the first place by excluding irrelevant stimuli, they promote efficient (and presumably faster) cognitive processing of target stimuli. Inhibition failures thus permit task-irrelevant material to receive more sustained activation than it would otherwise, resulting in heightened distractibility, increased forgetfulness, and longer response latencies (Hasher and Zacks, 1988; Stoltzfus et al., 1993). Hashtroudi et al. (1990) raised the interesting possibility that older adults' relatively good recall for thoughts and feelings may, in fact, represent failures of inhibitory mechanisms to ignore this less important material relative to factual, neutral information. If so, emotional disinhibition could account for the apparent age-related increased salience of emotion in cognitive processing previously described.

Cognitive failures associated with inefficient inhibitory mechanisms, however, are now thought to be fairly domain specific and not to generalize widely across stimuli (Connelly and Hasher, 1993; Kane et al., 1994). Thus, evidence for *emotional* disinhibition per se would be needed in order to make a compelling case that disinhibition accounts for heightened attention to emotion in older adults. In addition, a general emotional disinhibition would presumably lead to a global increase in all emotional material, regardless of valence. Findings that older adults are more likely to focus on positive information than negative information, compared to younger adults (Mather and Johnson, 2000), cast doubt on an overarching cognitive decrement responsible for decrements that have differential effects on positive and negative emotions.

5. Summary and conclusion

In the study of aging, quite legitimately, research often focuses on physical deterioration and disease. Prevalence rates of physical disease and impairment increase with age and are central issues in societies where an increasing average life expectancy is leading to unprecedented growth in the proportion of older adults in the population. Still, these decrements are not ubiquitous to all processes, and emotional experience is one area that offers a welcome reprieve from the majority of studies showing age-related decline.

Given that emotions are largely determined by biological substrates and influenced by social factors, the stable, and often improved, emotional experience with age often surprises both laymen and scientists alike. Upon hearing the news about age differences in emotions, many people are reluctant to dismiss the stereotype that older adults become more depressed, anxious, and lonely with age. The evidence, however, cannot be ignored. A growing number of studies based in Europe and the United States have found improved levels of affective well-being, and lower rates of affective disorders, across the adult life span. Both cohort differences and developmental processes have been documented: more recent cohorts are experiencing clinical levels of depression at early ages and in greater percentages than older adults (Wittchen et al., 1994), and rates of negative affect decline over time. Only at the very end of life, when presumably the physical and cognitive changes signaling terminal decline appear, does negative affect appear to increase and even at this point, it occurs at lower levels than observed in younger adults. Rates of depression, for example, even in advanced old age do not reach those observed in early adulthood; and in studies of normal populations, frequencies of negative emotions slightly increase in very old age, but do not approach frequencies of younger adults. Importantly, the subjective intensity of emotion, positive and negative, does not differ by age, despite reductions in physiological arousal and decreases in brain volume in processes implicated in the emotional system. In other words, the emotion system works. The complexity of experienced emotions seems to increase, emotional poignancy is more frequent, and more complex combinations of emotions appear on peoples' faces.

We highlighted several strategies that older adults use to regulate their emotions. Older adults engage in more proactive strategies to avoid negative emotional experience, specifically in the area of social interactions. In addition, they respond to negative emotional experience with less hostility and aggression. Their cognitions regarding emotional problems are complex and indicate greater insight into analyzing problems from multiple perspectives. Three models were then described that offer unifying explanations for these findings. Socioemotional selectivity theory emphasizes time perspective as the motivating force behind the central goals that direct human behavior. When time is limited, emotions become increasingly important, and emotional goals focused on regulation assume primacy. The cognition-emotional integration model discusses a developmental trajectory where ego level drives greater complexity of emotional experience with age. This model describes a cognitive developmental processes that begins with simple, insular concepts of discrete emotions and ego-centered world views, and grows into a more individualistic broader view where inconsistencies and multiple perspective taking is achieved. Lastly, models of biological decline discuss how greater importance on emotional processes may be the result of reduced physiological arousal – and therefore more easily controlled emotions – as well as cognitive decline that leads to increases in the saliency of emotional material as an unintended consequence. Together, these models offer structure from which to continue the study of the complex nature of emotions and aging. The study of how emotions unfold across the adult life span provides a rich interdisciplinary study incorporating physical, social, and cognitive processes, and one which constantly provides new findings that force scientists to rethink the nature of aging.

References

Adams, C., 1991. Qualitative age differences in memory for text: A life-span developmental perspective. Psychol. Aging 6, 323–336.
Adams, C., Labouvie-Vief, G., Hobart, C.J., Dorosz, M., 1990. Adult age group differences in story recall style. J. Gerontol. Psychol. Sci. 45, 17–27.
Adams, C., Smith, M.C., Nyquist, L., Perlmutter, M., 1997. Adult age-group differences in recall for the literal and interpretive meanings of narrative text. J. Gerontol. Psychol. Sci. 52, 187–195.
Almeida, D.M., 1998. Age differences in daily weekly and monthly estimates of psychological distress. In: Fleeson, A., Mroczek, D. (Chairs), Intraindividual Variability and Change Processes: New Directions in Understanding Personality. Symposium presented at the meetings of the American Psychological Association Meetings, San Francisco, CA.
Antonucci, T.C., Jackson, J.S., 1987. Social support, interpersonal efficacy, and health. In: Carstensen, L.L., Edelstein, B. (Eds.), Handbook of Clinical Gerontology Pergamon Press. New York, pp. 291–311.
Baltes, M.M., 1998. The psychology of the oldest old: The fourth age. Curr. Opin. Psychiatry 11, 411–415.
Bandura, A., 1997. Self-efficacy: The Exercise of Control. W.H. Freeman and Co., New York.
Banham, K.M., 1951. Senescence and the emotions: A genetic theory. J. Genet. Psychol. 78, 175–183.
Barrick, A.L., Hutchinson, R.L., Deckers, L.H., 1989. Age effects on positive and negative emotions. J. Social Behav. Pers. 4, 421–429.
Benes, F.M., Turtle, M., Khan, Y., Farol, P., 1994. Myelination of a key relay zone in the hippocampal formation occurs in the human brain during childhood, adolescence, and adulthood. Arch. Gen. Psychiatry 51, 477–484.
Blanchard-Fields, F., Chen, Y., Norris, L., 1997. Everyday problem solving across the adult life span: Influence of domain specificity and cognitive appraisal. Psychol. Aging 12, 684–693.
Blanchard-Fields, F., Jahnke, H.C., Camp, C., 1995. Age differences in problem-solving style: The role of emotional salience. Psychol. Aging 10, 173–180.
Blanchard-Fields, F., Norris, L., 1994. Causal attributions from adolescence through adulthood: Age differences, ego level, and generalized response style. Aging Cognit. 1, 67–86.
Brandtstädter, J., Renner, G., 1990. Tenacious goal pursuit and flexible goal adjustment: Explication and age-related analysis of assimilative and accommodative strategies of coping. Psychol. Aging 5, 58–67.
Buhler, C., 1935. The curve of life as studied in biographies. J. Appl. Psychol. 1, 184–211.
Buss, A.H., Plomin, R., 1975. A Temperament Theory of Personality Development. Wiley-Interscience, New York.
Cacioppo, J.T., Berntsen, G.B., Klein, D.J., Poehlmann, K.M., 1998. Psychophysiology of emotion across the life span. In: Schaie, K.W., Lawton, M.P. (Eds.), Annual Review of Gerontology and Geriatrics: Focus on Emotion and Adult Development, Vol. 17. Springer, New York, pp. 27–74.
Carstensen, L.L., 1986. Social support among the elderly: Limitations of behavioral interventions. Behav. Ther. 6, 111–113.
Carstensen, L.L., 1992. Social and emotional patterns in adulthood: Support for socioemotional selectivity theory. Psychol. Aging 7, 331–338.
Carstensen, L.L., 1993. Motivation for social contact across the life span: A theory of socioemotional selectivity. In: Jacobs, J. (Ed.), Nebraska Symposium on Motivation: Vol. 40. Developmental Perspectives on Motivation. University of Nebraska Press, Lincoln, NE, pp. 209–254.

Carstensen, L.L., 1995. Evidence for a life-span theory of socioemotional selectivity. Curr. Dir. Psychol. Sci. 4, 151–156.
Carstensen, L.L, Charles, S.T., Isaacowitz, D.M., Kennedy, Q., 2003. Life-span personality development and emotion. In: Davidson, R.J., Goldsmith, H.H., Scherer, K. (Eds.), The Handbook of Affective Sciences. Oxford University Press, Oxford, England. pp. 726–744.
Carstensen, L.L., Fredrickson, B.F., 1998. Influence of HIV status and age on cognitive representations of others. Health Psychol. 17, 494–503.
Carstensen, L.L., Gottman, J.M., Levenson, R.W., 1995. Emotional behavior in long-term marriage. Psychol. Aging 10, 140–149.
Carstensen, L.L., Graff, J., Levenson, R.W., Gottman, J.M., 1996. Affect in intimate relationship: A developmental course of marriage. In: Magai, C., McFadden, S.H. (Eds.), Handbook of Emotion, Adult Development, and Aging . Academic Press, New York, pp. 227–247.
Carstensen, L.L., Isaacowitz, D.M., Charles, S.T., 1999. Taking time seriously: A theory of socioemotional selectivity. Am. Psychol. 54, 165–181.
Carstensen, L.L., Pasupathi, M., Mayr, U., Nesselroade, J., 2000. Emotion experience in the daily lives of older and younger adults. J. Pers. Social Psychol. 79, 1–12.
Carstensen, L.L., Turk-Charles, S., 1994. The salience of emotion across the adult life span. Psychol. Aging 9, 259–264.
Chapell, N.L., Badger, M., 1989. Social isolation and well-being. J. Gerontol. Social Sci. 44, 169–176.
Charles, S.T., Carstensen, L.L., 1999. The role of time in the setting of social goals across the life span. In: Blanchard-Fields, F., Hess, T. (Eds.), Social Cognition and Aging. Academic Press, New York, pp. 319–342.
Charles, S.T., Carstensen, L.L., McFall, R., 2001a. Age differences problem-solving in the nursing home environment: Age and experience differences in emotional reactions and responses. J. Clin. Geropsychol. 7, 319–330.
Charles, S.T., Mather, M., Carstensen, L.L., 2003. Aging and emotional memory: the forgettable nature of negative images for older adults. J. Experimental Psychol. 132, 310–324.
Charles, S.T., Reynolds, C.A., Gatz, M., 2001b. Age-related differences and change in positive and negative affect over 23 years. J. Pers. Social Psychol. 80, 136–151.
Connelly, S.L., Hasher, L., 1993. Aging and the inhibition of spatial location. J. Exp. Psychol. Human Percept. Perform. 19, 1238–1250.
Costa, P.T., Jr., , McCrae, R.R., 1980. Influence of extraversion and neuroticism on subjective well-being. J. Pers. Social Psychol. 38, 668–678.
Costa, P.T., Zonderman, A.B., McCrae, R.R., Cornoni-Huntley, J., Locke, B.Z., Barbano, H.E., 1987. Longitudinal analyses of psychological well-being in a national sample: Stability of mean levels. J. Gerontol. Psychol. Sci. 42, 50–55.
Cumming, E., Henry, W.E., 1961. Growing Old: The Process of Disengagement. Basic Books, New York.
Cyphers, L.H., Phillips, K., Fulker, D.W., Mrazek, D.A., 1990. Twin temperament during the transition from infancy to early childhood. J. Am. Acad. Child Adoles. Psychiatry 29, 392–397.
Darwin, C., 1872. The Expression of the Emotions in Man and Animals. Murray, London.
Davidson, R.J., 1992. Emotion and affective style: Hemispheric substrates. Psychol. Sci. 3, 39–43.
Davidson, R.J., 1995. Cerebral asymmetry, emotion, and affective style. In: Davidson, R.J., Hugdahl, K. (Eds.), Brain Asymmetry. The MIT Press, Cambridge, MA, pp. 361–387.
Davidson, R.J., 1999. Neuropsychological perspectives on affective styles and their cognitive consequences. In: Dalgleish, T., Power, M.J. (Eds.), Handbook of Cognition and Emotion. John Wiley and Sons, New York, pp. 103–123.
Davidson, R.J., 2002. Anxiety and affective style: Role of prefrontal cortex and amygdala. Biol. Psychiatry 51, 68–80.
Davidson, R.J., Fox, N., 1989. Frontal brain asymmetry predicts infants' response to maternal separation. J. Abnormal Psychol. 98, 127–131.
Davidson, R.J., Hugdahl, K. (Eds.), 1995. Brain Asymmetry. The MIT Press, Cambridge, MA.
Davidson, R.J., Irwin, W., 1999. The functional neuroanatomy of emotion and affective style. Trends Cogn. Sci. 3, 11–21.

Davidson, R.J., Irwin, W., Eisenberg, N., Fabes, R., Shepard, S., Murphy, B., Jones, S., Guthrie, I., 1998. Contemporaneous and longitudinal prediction of children's sympathy from dispositional regulation and emotionality. Dev. Psychol. 34, 910–924.

Davidson, R.J., Jackson, D.C., Kalin, N.H., 2000. Emotion, plasticity, context, and regulation: Perspectives from affective neuroscience. Psychol. Bull. Special Issue: Psychology in the 21st Century 126, 890–909.

Dickson, D.W., Crystal, H.A., Mattiace, L.A., Masur, D.M., Blau, A.D., Davies, P., Yen, S.H., Aronson, M.K., 1992. Identification of normal and pathological aging in prospectively studies nondemented elderly humans. Neurobiol. Aging 13, 179–189.

Diehl, M., Coyle, N., Labouvie-Vief, G., 1996. Age and sex differences in strategies of coping and defense across the life span. Psychol. Aging 11, 127-139.

Diener, E., Diener, C., 1996. Most people are happy. Psychol. Sci. 7, 181–185.

Diener, E., Sandvik, E., Larsen, R.J., 1985. Age and sex differences for emotional intensity. Dev. Psychol. 21, 542–546.

Diener, E., Suh, E., 1998. Measuring quality of life: Economic, social, and subjective indicators. Social Indicators Res. 40, 189–216.

Ekman, P., 1999. Facial expressions. In: Dalgleish, T., Power, M.J. (Eds.), Handbook of Cognition and Emotion. John Wiley and Sons, New York, pp. 301–320.

Ekman, P., 1973. Universal facial expressions in emotion. Studia Psychologica 15, 140–147.

Elfenbein, H.A., Ambady, N., 2002. On the universality and cultural specificity of emotion recognition: A meta-analysis. Psychol. Bull. 128, 203–235.

Felton, B.J., Revenson, T.A., 1987. Age differences in coping with chronic illness. Psychol. Aging 2, 164–170.

Field, D., 1981. Retrospective reports by healthy intelligent elderly people of personal events of their adult lives. Int. J. Behav. Dev. 4, 77–97.

Fisher, J.E., Zeiss, A.M., Carstensen, L.L., 1993. Psychopathology in the aged. In: Sutker, P.B., Adams, H.E. (Eds.), Comprehensive Handbook of Psychopathology, 2nd ed. Plenum Press, New York, pp. 815–842.

Folkman, S., Lazarus, R.S., Pimley, D., Novacek, J., 1987. Age differences in stress and coping processes. Psychol. Aging 2, 171–184.

Fredrickson, B.L., Carstensen, L.L., 1990. Choosing social partners: How age and anticipated endings make people more selective. Psychol. Aging 5, 335–347.

Frenkel-Brunswik, E, 1968. Adjustments and reorientation in the course of the life span. In: Neugarten, B.L. (Eds.), Middle Age and Aging. University of Chicago Press, Chicago, pp. 77–84.

Fung, H.H., Carstensen, L.L., 2003. Sending memorable messages to the old: Age differences in preferences and memory for advertisements. J. Pers. Social Psychol. 85, 163–178.

Fung, H.H., Carstensen, L.L., Lang, F.R., 2001a. Age-related patterns of social relationships among African-Americans and Caucasian-Americans: Implications for socioemotional selectivity across the life span. Int. J. Aging Human Dev. 52, 185–206.

Fung, H.H., Carstensen, L.L., Lutz, M.A., 1999. Influence of time on social preferences: Implications for life-span development. Psychol. Aging 14, 595–604.

Fung, H.H., Lai, P., Ng, R., 2001b. Age differences in social preferences among Taiwanese and Mainland Chinese: The role of perceived time. Psychol. Aging 16, 351–356.

Gatz, M., Johansson, B., Pedersen, N., Berg, S., Reynolds, C., 1993. A cross-national self-report measure of depressive symptomatology. Int. Psychogeriatr. 5, 14–156.

Goldsmith, H.H., Buss, K.A., Lemery, K.S., 1997. Toddler and childhood temperament: Expanded content, stronger genetic evidence, new evidence for the importance of environment. Dev. Psychol. 33, 891–905.

Goldsmith, H.H., Gottesman, I.I., 1981. Origins of variation in behavioral style: A longitudinal study of temperament in young twins. Child Dev. 52, 91–103.

Good, C.D., Johnsrude, I.S., Ashburner, J., Henson, R.N.A., Friston, K.J., Frackowiak, R.S.J., 2001. A voxel-based morphometric study of ageing in 465 normal adult human brains. NeuroImage 14, 21–36.

Gould, O.N., Dixon, R.A., 1993. How we spent our vacation: collaborative storytelling by young and older adults. Psychol. Aging 6, 93–99.

Gross, J.J., Carstensen, L.C., Pasupathi, M., Tsai, J., Götestam-Skorpen, K., Hsu, A.Y.C., 1997. Emotion and aging: Experience, expression, and control. Psychol. Aging 12, 590–599.

Gross, J.J., Sutton, S.K., Ketelaar, T., 1998. Relationship between affect and personality: Support for the affect-level and affective-reactivity view. Pers. Social Psychol. Bull. 24, 279–288.

Gurland, B., 1976. The comparative frequency of depression in various adult age groups. J. Gerontol. 31, 283–292.

Hasher, L., Zacks, R.T., 1988. Working memory, comprehension, and aging: A review and a new view. In: Bower, G.G. (Eds.), The Psychology of Learning and Motivation, Vol. 22. Academic Press, San Diego, CA, pp. 193–225.

Hashtroudi, S., Johnson, M.K., Chrosniak, L.D., 1990. Aging and qualitative characteristics of memories for perceived and imagined complex events. Psychol. Aging 5, 119–126.

Heckhausen, J., Dixon, R.A., Baltes, P.B., 1989. Gains and losses in development throughout adulthood as perceived by different adult age groups. Dev. Psychol. 25, 109–121.

Heckhausen, J., Kreuger, J., 1993. Developmental expectations for the self and most other people: Age grading in three functions of social comparison. Dev. Psychol. 29, 539–548.

Heckhausen, J., Schulz, R., 1995. A life-span theory of control. Psychol. Rev. 102, 284–304.

Hess, T.M., Bolstad, C.A., Woodburn, S.M., Auman, C., 1999. Trait diagnosticity versus behavior consistency as determinants of impression change in adulthood. Psychol. Aging 14, 77–89.

Hess, T.M., Pullen, S.M., 1994. Adult age difference in informational biases during impression formation. Psychol. Aging 9, 237–250.

James, W., 1884. What is an emotion? Mind 19, 188–205.

Johnson, M.K., Sherman, S.J., 1990. Constructing and reconstructing the past and the future in the present. In: Higgins, E.T., Sorrentino, R.M. (Eds.), Handbook of Motivation and Cognition: Foundations of Social Behavior. Guilford Press, New York, pp. 482–526.

Jones, C.J., Meredith, W., 2000. Developmental paths of psychological health from early adolescence to later adulthood. Psychol. Aging 15, 351–360.

Kagan, J., Reznick, J.S., Snidman, N., Gibbons, J., Johnson, M., 1988. Childhood derivatives of inhibition and lack of inhibition to the unfamiliar. Child Dev. 59, 1580–1589.

Kane, M.J., Hasher, L., Stoltzfus, E.R., Zacks, R.T., Connelly, S.L., 1994. Inhibitory attentional mechanisms and aging. Psychol. Aging 9, 103–112.

Kennedy, Q., Mather, M., Carstensen, L.L., 2002. The role of motivation in the age-related positive memory bias in long-term autobiographical memory. Psychol. Science. In press.

Kessler, R.C., Foster, C., Webster, P.S., House, J.S., 1992. The relationship between age and depressive symptoms in two national surveys. Psychol. Aging 7, 119–126.

Klerman, G.L., Weissman, M.M., 1989. Increasing rates of depression. JAMA 261, 2229–2235.

LaBar, K.S., LeDoux, J.E., 1997. Partial disruption of fear conditioning in rats with unilateral amygdala damage: Correspondence with unilateral temporal lobectomy in humans. Behav. Neurosci. 110, 991–997.

Labouvie-Vief, G., 1998. Cognitive-emotional integration in adulthood. In: Schaie, K.W., Lawton, M.P. (Eds.), Annual Review of Gerontology and Geriatrics: Focus on Emotion and Adult Development, Vol. 17. Springer, New York, pp. 206–237.

Labouvie-Vief, G., Blanchard-Fields, F., 1982. Cognitive aging and psychological growth. Aging Soc. 2, 183–209.

Labouvie-Vief, G., Chiodo, L.M., Goguen, L.A., Diehl, M., Orwoll, L., 1995. Representations of self across the life span. Psychol. Aging 10, 404–415.

Labouvie-Vief, G., DeVoe, M., 1991. Emotional regulation in adulthood and later life: A Developmental View. Annual Review of Gerontology and Geriatrics, Vol. 11. Springer, New York, pp. 172–194.

Labouvie-Vief, G., DeVoe, M., Bulka, D., 1989. Speaking about feelings: Conceptions of emotion across the lifespan. Psychol. Aging 4, 425–437.

Labouvie-Vief, G., Hakim-Larson, J., 1989. Developmental shifts in adult thought. In: Hunter, S., Sundel, M. (Eds.), Midlife Myths. Sage, Newbury Park, CA, pp. 69–96.

Lang, F.R., 2000. Endings and Continuity of Social Relationships: Maximizing Intrinsic Benefits Within Personal Networks When Feeling Near to Death? J. Social Pers. Relation. 17, 157–184.

Lang, F.R., Carstensen, L.L., 2002. Time counts: Future time perspective, goals, and social relationships. Psychol. Aging 17, 125–139.

Lang, F.R., Carstensen, L.L., 1994. Close emotional relationships in late life: Further support for proactive aging in the social domain. Psychol. Aging 9, 315–324.

Lang, F.R., Staudinger, U.M., Carstensen, L.L., 1998. Perspectives on socioemotional selectivity in late life: How personality and social context do (and do not) make a difference. J. Gerontol. Psychol. Sci. 53, 21–30.

Larson, J.T., McGraw, A.P., Cacioppo, J.T., 2001. Can people feel happy and sad at the same time? J. Pers. Social Psychol. 81, 684–696.

Lazarus, R.S., 1996. The role of coping in the emotions and how coping changes over the life course. In: Magai, C., McFadden, S.H. (Eds.), Handbook of Emotion, Adult Development, and Aging. Academic Press, San Diego, CA, pp. 289–306.

Lawton, M.P., Kleban, M.H., Dean, J., 1993. Affect and age: Cross-sectional comparisons of structure and prevalence. Psychol. Aging 8, 165–175.

Lawton, M.P., Kleban, M.H., Rajagopal, D., Dean, J., 1992. The dimensions of affective experience in three age groups. Psychol. Aging 7, 171–184.

Lawton, M.P., Moss, M., Fulcomer, M., 1987. Objective and subjective uses of time by older people. Int. J. Aging Hum. Dev. 24, 171–188.

Le Doux, J.E., 1992. Emotion and the amygdala. In: Aggleton, J.P. (Eds.), The Amygdala: Neurobiological aspects of emotion, memory, and mental dysfunction. Wiley-Liss, New York, pp. 339–351.

Lee, D.J., Markides, K.S., 1990. Activity and mortality among aged persons over an eight-year period. J. Gerontol. Social Sci. 45, 39–42.

Levenson, R.W., 2000. Expressive, physiological, and subjective changes in emotion across adulthood. In: Qualls, S.H., Abeles, N. (Eds.), Psychology and the aging revolution: How we adapt to longer life. American Psychological Association, Washington, D.C., pp. 123–140.

Levenson, R.W., Carstensen, L.L., Friesen, W.V., Ekman, P., 1991. Emotion, physiology, and expression in old age. Psychol. Aging 6, 28–35.

Levenson, R.W., Carstensen, L.L., Gottman, J.M., 1993. Long-term marriage: Age, gender, and satisfaction. Psychol. Aging 8, 301–313.

Levenson, R.W., Carstensen, L.L., Gottman, J.M., 1994. Influence of age and gender on affect, physiology, and their interrelations: A study of long-term marriages. J. Pers. Social Psychol. 67, 56–68.

Levine, L.J., Bluck, S., 1997. Experienced and remembered emotional intensity in older adults. Psychol. Aging 12, 514–523.

Lewis, M.I., Butler, R.N., 1974. Life review therapy: Putting memories to work in individual and group psychotherapy. Geriatrics, 165–173.

Lowenthal, M., Haven, C., 1968. Interaction and adaptation: Intimacy as a critical variable. In: Neugarten, B.L. (Eds.), Middle Age and Aging: A Reader in Social Psychology. University of Chicago Press, Chicago, pp. 390–400.

Lucas, R.E., Gohm, C., 2000. Age and sex differences in subjective well-being across cultures. In: Diener, E., Suh, E.M. (Eds.), Subjective Well-being Across Nations and Cultures. MIT Press, Cambridge, MA, pp. 291–317.

Magai, C., Cohen, C., Gomberg, D., Malatesta, C., Culver, C., 1996. Emotional expression during mid- to late-stage dementia. Int. Psychogeriatr. 8, 383–395.

Magai, C., Passman, V., 1998. The interpersonal basis of emotional behavior and emotion regulation in adulthood. In: Schaie, K.W., Lawton, M.P. (Eds.), Annual Review of Gerontology and Geriatrics, Vol. 17: Focus on Emotion and Adult Development. Springer, New York, pp. 104–137.

Malatesta, C.Z., Fiore, M.J., Messina, J.L., 1987. Affect, personality, and facial expressive characteristics of older people. Psychol. Aging 2, 64–69.

Malatesta, C.Z., Kalnok, M., 1984. Emotional experience in younger and older adults. J. Gerontol. Psychol. Sci. 39, 301–308.

Malatesta-Magai, C., Jonas, R., Shepard, B., Culver, L.C., 1992. Type A behavior pattern and emotion expression in younger and older adults. Psychol. Aging 7, 551–561.

Matheny, A.P., Wachs, T.D., Ludwig, J.L., Phillips, K., 1995. Bringing order out of chaos: Psychometric characteristics of the confusion, hubbub, and order scale. J. Appl. Dev. Psychol. 16, 429–444.

Mather, M. (in press). Aging and emotional memory. To appear in Reisberg, D, Hertel, P. (Eds.), Memory and Emotion. Oxford University Press, Oxford.

Matsumoto, D., 1993. Ethnic differences in affect intensity, emotion judgments, display rule attitudes, and self-reported emotional expression in an American sample. Motiv. Emotion 17, 107–123.

Mather, M., Carstensen, L.L., 2003. Aging and attentional biases for emotional faces. Psychol. Sci. 14, 409–415.

Mather, M., Johnson, M.K., 2000. Choice-supportive source monitoring: Do our decisions seem better to us as we age? Psychol. Aging 15, 596–606.

McCrae, R.R., Costa Jr., P.T., 1999. A five-factor theory of personality. In: Pervin, L., John, O.P. (Eds.), Handbook of Personality, 2nd ed. Guilford Press, New York, pp. 139–153.

McCrae, R.R., Costa Jr., P.T., Ostendorf, F., Angleitner, A., Hrebickova, M., Avia, M.D., Sanz, J., Sanchez-Bernardos, M.L., 2000. Nature over nurture: Temperament, personality, and life span development. J. Pers. Social Psychol. 1, 173–186.

Mroczek, D.K., Kolarz, C.M., 1998. The effect of age on positive and negative affect: A developmental perspective on happiness. J. Pers. Social Psychol. 75, 1333–1349.

Neugarten, B.L., Havighurst, R.J., Tobin, S.S., 1961. The measurement of life satisfaction. J. Gerontol. 16, 134–143.

Oxman, T.E., Barrett, J.E., Sengupta, A., Williams, J.W., 2000. The relationship of aging and dysthymia in primary care. Am. J. Geriatr. Psychiatry 8, 318–326.

Palmore, E., 1981. Social Patterns in Normal Aging: Findings from the Duke Longitudinal Study. Duke University Press, Durham, NC.

Pasupathi, M., Henry, R., Carstensen, L.L., 2002. Age and ethnicity differences in storytelling to young children: Emotionality, relationality and socialization. Psychol. Aging. 17(4), 610–621.

Phifer, J.F., 1990. Psychological distress and somatic symptoms after natural disaster: Differential vulnerability among older adults. Psychol. Aging 5, 412–420.

Plomin, R., 1976. A twin and family study of personality in young children. J. Psychol. 94, 233–235.

Plomin, R., Rowe, D.C., 1977. A twin study of temperament in young children. J. Psychol. 97, 107–113.

Quackenbush, S.W., Barnett, M.A., 2001. Recollection and evaluation of critical experiences in moral development: A cross-sectional examination. Basic Appl. Social Psychol. 23, 55–64.

Rahhal, T., May, C.P., Hasher, L., 2002. Truth and character: Sources that older adults can remember. Psychol. Sci. 13, 101–105.

Raz, N., 2000. Aging of the brain and its impact on cognitive performance: Integration of structural and functional findings. In: Craik, F.I.M., Salthouse, T.A. (Eds.), Handbook of Aging and Cognition, 2nd ed. Lawrence Erlbaum, Mahwah, NJ, pp. 1–90.

Regier, D.A., Boyd, H.J., Burke, J.D., Rae, D.S., Myers, J.K., Kramer, M., Robins, L.N., George, L.K., Karno, M., Locke, B.Z., 1988. One-month prevalence of mental disorders in the United States. Arch. Gen. Psychiatry 45, 977–986.

Roberts, G., 1999. Age effects and health appraisal: A meta-analysis. J. Gerontol. 54, S24–S30.

Ryff, C.D., 1989. Happiness is everything, or is it? Explorations on the meaning of psychological well-being. J. Pers. Social Psychol. 57, 1069–1081.

Scheibel, A.B., 1996. Structural and functional changes in the aging brain. In: Birren, J.E., Schaie, K.W. (Eds.), Handbook of the Psychology of Aging, Vol. 4. Academic Press, San Diego, pp. 105–128.

Schulkind, M.D., Hennis, L.K., Rubin, D.C., 1999. Music, emotion and autobiographical memory: They're playing your song. Mem. Cognit. 27, 948–955.

Schulz, R., 1985. Emotion and affect. In: Birren, J.E., Schaie, W.K. (Eds.), Handbook of the Psychology of Aging, 2nd ed. Van Nostrand Reinhold, New York, pp. 531–543.

Smith, J., Baltes, P.B., 1993. Differential psychological aging: Profiles of the old and very old. Ageing Soc. 13, 551–587.
Stallings, M.C., Dunham, C.C., Gatz, M., Baker, L.A., Bengtson, V.L., 1997. Relationships among life events and psychological well-being: More evidence for a two factor theory of well-being. J. Appl. Gerontol. 16, 104–119.
Stoltzfus, E.R., Hasher, L., Zacks, R.T., Ulivi, M.S., Goldstein, D., 1993. Investigations of inhibition and interference in younger and older adults. J. Gerontol. Psychol. Sci. 48, 179–188.
Tsai, J.L., Levenson, R.W., Carstensen, L.L., 2000. Autonomic, subjective, and expressive responses to emotional films in older and younger Chinese Americans and European Americans. Psychol. Aging 15, 684–693.
Vaux, A., Meddin, J., 1987. Positive and negative life change and positive and negative affect among the rural elderly. J. Community Psychol. 15, 447–458.
Watson, D., Pennebaker, J.W., 1989. Health complaints, stress, and distress: Exploring the central role of negative affectivity. Psychol. Rev. 96, 234–254.
Webster, J.D., 1995. Adult age differences in reminiscence functions. In: Haight., B.K., Webster, J.D. (Eds.), The Art and Science of Reminiscing: Theory, Research, Methods, and Applications. Taylor & Francis, Philadelphia, pp. 89–102.
Wittchen, H., Knauper, B., Kessler, R.C., 1994. Lifetime risk of depression. Br. J. Psychiatry 165, 16–22.
Zacks, R.T., Hasher, L., 1997. Cognitive gerontology and attentional inhibition: A reply to Burke and McDowd. J. Gerontol. Psychol. Sci. 52, 274–283.
Zajonc, R.B., 1984. On the primacy of affect. Am. Psychol. 39, 117–123.
Zajonc, R., 1997. Emotions. In: Gilbert, D., Fiske, S.T., Lindzey, G. (Eds.), Handbook of Social Psychology, 4th ed. McGraw-Hill, Cambridge, MA, pp. 591–631.

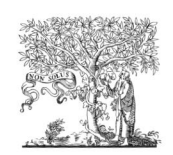

Personality and self-esteem development across the life span

Kali H. Trzesniewski[1]*, Richard W. Robins[1], Brent W. Roberts[2] and Avshalom Caspi[3]

[1]*Department of Psychology, University of California, One Shields Ave., Davis, CA 95616-8686, USA*
[2]*University of Illinois, Urbana-Champaign, USA*
[3]*Institute of Psychiatry, King's College London and University of Wisconsin, Madison, USA*

Contents

1. Rank-order stability of personality and self-esteem across the life span	164
1.1. Personality	165
1.2. Self-esteem	166
2. Mean-level changes in personality and self-esteem across the life course	168
2.1. Personality	169
2.2. Self-esteem	173
2.2.1. Childhood	173
2.2.2. Adolescence	174
2.2.3. Adulthood	174
2.2.4. Old age	175
3. Socio-contextual factors that influence personality and self-esteem change	176
3.1. Work experiences	176
3.2. Relationship experiences	177
4. Conclusion	180
References	181

Over the past few decades, there has been an explosion of longitudinal research on the consistency of personality and related constructs such as self-esteem. This plethora of studies has provided sufficient evidence to move researchers toward consensus about the degree to which personality characteristics change over the life course. The emerging story, based on an accumulating body of empirical research, is that personality and self-esteem show remarkable continuity given the vast array of experiences that impinge upon a lived life. At the same time, research also reveals

*Corresponding author. Tel.: 530-754-8287; fax: 530-752-2087;
E-mail address: kftrzesniewski@ucdavis.edu (K.H. Trzesniewski).

that personality and self-esteem show important and systematic changes that are meaningfully connected to particular life experiences and contexts.

In the first section of this chapter, we review longitudinal evidence that personality and self-esteem show moderate levels of rank-order stability across the life span. This moderate level of stability demonstrates continuity in the way that individuals behave, think, and feel as they age. However, this continuity does not imply that personality and self-esteem are immutable.

Indeed, most studies of personality and self-esteem development reveal interesting patterns of normative change. These systematic normative changes illustrate the role of personality and self as organizational constructs that influence how individuals orient their behavior to meet environmental demands and new developmental challenges (Funder, 1991). In turn, personality and self-esteem are developmental constructs in that they demonstrate changes across the life course (Roberts and Caspi, 2001; Robins, Trzesniewski, Tracy, Gosling, and Potter, 2002), often in response to the environments being mastered (Roberts, 1997). Thus, as individuals experience normative developmental transitions, normative changes in related areas of personality and the self will occur. In the second part of this chapter, we review cross-sectional and longitudinal research on the normative development of personality and self-esteem across the life span.

Normative patterns of change imply a dynamic relation between life events and personality. However, not everyone experiences the same life events at the same time, and consequently there are individual differences in personality and self-esteem change. In the last section of the chapter, we review findings from longitudinal studies that have investigated the impact of socio-contextual factors on personality and self-esteem change. In this section, we explore how different life experiences across generations and across individuals lead to varying patterns of personality and self-esteem change.

1. Rank-order stability of personality and self-esteem across the life span

We first consider the rank-order stability of personality and self-esteem from childhood through adulthood. Rank-order stability is typically assessed using test–retest correlations (i.e. the correlation between scores across two time points). Test–retest correlations reflect the degree to which the relative ordering of individuals is maintained over time; that is, individuals who are high (or low) relative to others at Time 1 remain high (or low) relative to others at Time 2.

High rank-order stability indicates that (a) individuals did not change much over time *or* (b) individuals changed over time, but in more or less the same way (i.e. everyone increased or decreased to the same extent). The latter situation ("b") can occur when a normative developmental event such as puberty impacts all individuals in the same way (e.g. if puberty causes everyone to decline in self-esteem by the same amount). Low rank-order stability indicates that individuals changed over time *and* there were individual differences in the direction of change (i.e. some individuals increased while others decreased). This situation can occur when non-normative developmental events impact the trait being studied (e.g. if some individuals experience parental divorce and decline in self-esteem whereas others do not experience parental divorce and maintain the same self-esteem level). Low rank-order stability can also occur when the factors that influence the trait are normative but individuals have unique reactions to these events (e.g. if puberty causes some individuals to increase in self-esteem but causes others to decrease in self-esteem). Finally, a low test–retest correlation could simply reflect measurement error; less reliable measures will show lower test–retest correlations.

Below we review the evidence for the rank-order stability of personality and self-esteem, drawing heavily on the findings of two recent meta-analyses (Roberts and DelVecchio, 2000; Trzesniewski et al., in press).

1.1. Personality

Over the past few decades, researchers have debated the degree to which individual differences in personality are stable across the life span. Two contradictory perspectives have been advanced. The *classical trait perspective* states that personality traits are highly heritable, biologically based "temperaments" that are relatively impervious to the influence of the environment during adulthood (McCrae et al., 2000). From this "essentialist" perspective, we would expect to find high rank-order stability, particularly after age 30, when personality is assumed to become "set like plaster" (Costa and McCrae, 1994). In contrast, the *contextual perspective* emphasizes the importance of life changes and role transitions in personality development and suggests that personality should be fluid, prone to change, and yield low test–retest correlation coefficients, particularly during adolescence and young adulthood (Lewis, 1999).

Existing longitudinal studies do not support either of these extreme positions. The findings of a recent meta-analysis of the rank-order stability of personality confirmed several general conclusions (Roberts and DelVecchio, 2000). First, rank-order stability is not as high as the classical trait perspective claims, nor as low as the contextual perspective suggests. Overall, test–retest correlations are moderate in magnitude; across all age groups, the median test–retest correlation (unadjusted for measurement error) was 0.50. Thus, the magnitude of rank-order stability, although far from perfect, is still remarkably high. The only psychological construct more consistent than personality is cognitive ability (Conley, 1984).

Second, rank-order stability generally increased across the life span. Test–retest correlations (unadjusted for measurement error) increased from 0.41 in childhood to 0.55 at age 30, and then reached a plateau around 0.70 between ages 50 and 70 (see Fig. 1). This developmental trend points to several interesting findings. Most notably, the level of continuity in childhood and adolescence is much higher than originally expected (cf. Lewis, 1999, 2001). Although childhood character is by no means fate, there are striking continuities that point to the importance of childhood temperament and the effects of cumulative continuity from childhood through adulthood (Caspi, 2000). Even more impressive is the fact that the level of

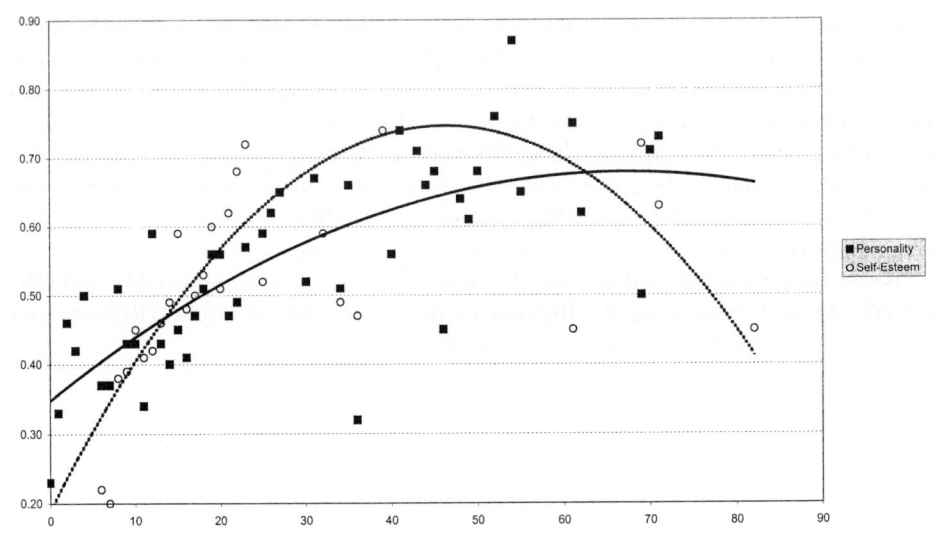

Fig. 1. Personality and self-esteem test-retest correlations by age.

consistency increases in a relatively linear fashion through adolescence and young adulthood. Young adulthood has been described as demographically dense, such that people make more life-changing decisions (to marry, one's career, children, etc.) during this period than at any other time in the life course (Rindfuss, 1991; Arnett, 2000). Yet, despite these dramatic demographic shifts, personality differences remain remarkably consistent. Finally, the developmental trend in stability suggests that personality continuity in adulthood peaks later than expected. Contrary to the claim that personality traits are essentially fixed and unchanging after age 30 (McCrae and Costa, 1994), the meta-analytic findings show that rank-order stability peaks some time after age 50, but at a level well below unity. Thus, personality traits continue to change throughout adulthood, but only modestly after age 50.

Third, rank-order stability did not vary markedly across the Big Five trait domains, across different assessment methods (i.e. self-reports, observer ratings, and projective tests), or by gender. Moreover, the levels of consistency found in this meta-analysis replicated smaller studies dating back to 1941 (Crook, 1943; Conley, 1984; Schuerger et al., 1989). Apparently, there have been few if any cohort shifts in the level of rank-order stability in personality traits over the past 60 years.

1.2. Self-esteem

Mirroring the debate that occurred in personality psychology, some researchers have argued that self-esteem is a trait-like construct that remains relatively stable over time (e.g. Coopersmith, 1967; Rosenberg, 1986), whereas others have argued that self-esteem should be conceptualized as a state-like process that continually fluctuates in response to environmental stimuli (e.g. Kernis et al., 1992;

Leary and Baumeister, 2000). If the long-term stability of self-esteem is much lower than other trait-like constructs (e.g. personality traits), then self-esteem should not be considered a stable individual-difference construct and should not be used to predict future behavior (Conley, 1984).

Again, a recent meta-analysis has helped to clarify the debate. Trzesniewski et al. (in press) examined the rank-order stability of self-esteem using data from 50 published articles ($N=29,839$). Overall, the findings support the view that self-esteem is a stable individual-difference construct. Test–retest correlations are moderate in magnitude and comparable to those found for personality traits; across all age groups, the median correlation (unadjusted for measurement error) was 0.47.

In contrast to personality, which showed an increasing linear trend, the rank-order stability of self-esteem showed a robust curvilinear trend (see Fig. 1): self-esteem stability (uncorrected for measurement error) was relatively low during early childhood (0.40), increased throughout adolescence (0.51) and early adulthood (0.55 during the college years and 0.65 during the 20s), and then declined during midlife (0.55) and old age (0.48). This curvilinear trend could not be explained by age differences in the reliability of self-esteem measures and generally replicated across different self-esteem scales, gender, ethnicity (Caucasian vs. African-American), nationality (U.S. vs. non-U.S.), and the year the study was conducted.

Several aspects of these findings are noteworthy. First, self-esteem was least stable during childhood. Although the analyses rule out low reliability (defined in terms of internal consistency) as an explanation for this effect, it is possible that the stabilities during childhood were attenuated by other measurement factors, such as poor validity of self-esteem scales for this age group.

Second, self-esteem stability decreased from adulthood to old age. This decline may reflect the dramatic life changes and shifting social circumstances that characterize later adulthood and old age. For example, normative life events such as children moving out of the home, retirement, and death of a loved one, may lead to changes in social roles and corresponding shifts in identity during old age. In addition, maturational changes again become common, such as health problems, which can result in greater dependency on others and reduced feelings of personal agency. These changes may challenge some individuals' view of themselves and thus produce idiosyncratic changes that reduce the stability of self-esteem. Another possibility is that as individuals age they may begin to review their lifelong accomplishments and experiences, leading in some cases to more critical self-appraisals and in other cases to greater acceptance of their faults and limitations. This process would be consistent with Erikson's (1985) notion of old age as a time when people reflect on their lived life. Some individuals may decide that their life has been a success (i.e. develop ego integrity) and thus maintain or increase their self-esteem whereas others may decide that they have failed (i.e. suffer despair) and experience a decline in self-esteem. Thus, a developmental shift toward greater self-reflection in old age may produce increases in self-esteem for some individuals but decreases for others, contributing to lower levels of stability.

Third, at no age did the stability of self-esteem reach unity, even after disattenuating the test-retest correlations for measurement error. Thus, self-esteem continues to change across the life span. The evidence suggests that self-esteem, much like personality traits, is never set like plaster and, in fact, shows even lower levels of stability in old age.

What are the implications of these findings for self-esteem's position in the hierarchy of consistency (e.g. Kelly, 1955; Conley, 1984)? Roberts and DelVecchio's (2000) meta-analysis of personality trait stability provides a useful comparison point. In general, self-esteem and personality traits show similar levels of stability (see Fig. 1). Roberts and DelVecchio (2000) reported uncorrected personality test-retest correlations (controlling for time interval) of 0.43 in childhood, 0.44 in adolescence, 0.54 during the college years, 0.60 for ages 22 to 29, and 0.64 during the 30s. Similarly, Trzesniewski et al. (in press) found uncorrected correlations (controlling for time interval) of 0.40 in childhood, 0.48 in adolescence, 0.55 during the college years, 0.65 for ages 22 to 29, and 0.62 during the 30s. However, Roberts and DelVecchio (2000) reported a test-retest correlation of 0.74 for adults between the ages of 50 and 70 whereas Trzesniewski et al. (2003) found a test-retest correlation of 0.49 for this same age range.

Considering the similarity in the stability of self-esteem and personality throughout most of the life span, this large divergence during late adulthood seems puzzling. It is possible that a developmental shift toward greater self-reflection during late adulthood and old age produces changes in self-esteem, but not in basic personality traits. Indeed, reflecting on the overall worthiness of your life may change your self-esteem but it is not likely to have a powerful impact on how sociable, conscientious, and creative you are.

In summary, for both personality and self-esteem neither extreme perspective was supported: both constructs showed moderate stability overall and increasing stability from childhood to adulthood. Interestingly, at no time did the stability of personality or self-esteem reach unity. The evidence suggests that personality and self-esteem never become set like plaster. Nonetheless, we did find substantial levels of continuity across decades of life, suggesting that personality and self-esteem are best characterized as showing both continuity and change across the life span.

2. Mean-level changes in personality and self-esteem across the life course

In the previous section we showed that personality and self-esteem show moderate levels of continuity across the life span when continuity is defined by rank-order stability. We next discuss research in which continuity is defined by mean-level changes. Mean-level change refers to changes in the average trait level of a population, and is typically assessed by mean-level differences in specific traits over time, which indicates whether the sample as a whole is increasing or decreasing on a trait. Mean-level change is conceptually and statistically distinct from rank-order stability (e.g. Caspi and Roberts, 1999; Robins et al., 2001). For example, individuals in a sample could increase substantially on a trait but the rank ordering of individuals would be maintained if everyone increased by the same amount. Similarly, the rank ordering of individuals in a sample could change substantially over time without producing any aggregate increases or decreases (e.g. if the number of people who decreased offset the number of people who increased). Mean-level changes result from maturational processes or social-contextual factors that influence a population.

2.1. Personality

In this section, we summarize and expand upon our previous extensive review of mean-level changes in personality traits across the life course using the Big Five taxonomy as an organizing framework (Roberts, Robins, Caspi, and Trzesniewski, in press). The Big Five taxonomy is one of the most significant developments in the field of personality psychology in the last few decades. Many personality researchers now believe that the majority of personality traits can be categorized into five broad superordinate categories: extraversion, agreeableness, conscientiousness, neuroticism (or its opposite emotional stability), and openness to experience. One of the primary advantages of the Big Five framework is its ability to organize previous research findings on the development of personality traits into a manageable number of conceptually coherent domains. So, rather than review the voluminous literature on mean-level change for all possible traits, we can examine the evidence within these five broad domains.

Extraversion refers to individual differences in the propensity to be sociable, active, assertive, and to experience positive affect (John and Srivastava, 1999). Roberts et al. (in press) report conflicting patterns of findings across cross-sectional and longitudinal studies that track changes in extraversion. Some cross-sectional and longitudinal studies show decreases with age (Field and Millsap, 1991; McCrae et al., 1999; Lamb et al., 2002), whereas others show no change in measures of extraversion in young adulthood (Robins et al., 2001), middle age (Pedersen and Reynolds, 1998), or old age (Nilsson and Persson, 1984). Some studies have even found increases in extraversion during college and early adulthood (e.g. Haan et al., 1986; Vaidya et al., in press). One possible explanation for the inconsistency could be a gender difference. Two studies that examined gender differences found that women decreased in extraversion and men increased from late adolescence to late adulthood (Goldberg et al., 1998; Srivastava et al., 2002).

A second possibility is that inconsistencies in the literature are due to the multifaceted nature of extraversion. Helson and Kwan (2000) have argued for dividing extraversion into two constituent elements: social dominance and social vitality. Social dominance reflects traits such as dominance, independence, and self-confidence, especially in social contexts. Social vitality corresponds more closely to traits like sociability, positive affect, gregariousness, and energy level. Roberts et al. (in press) report that studies measuring both facets have found divergent trajectories for social dominance and social vitality in cross-sectional (e.g. Goldberg et al., 1998) and longitudinal studies (Helson et al., 2002). A meta-analysis of the existing literature could provide a clearer picture of the overall extraversion trajectory and help determine whether the facets of extraversion show divergent developmental paths.

The second domain of the Big Five, Agreeableness, refers to traits that reflect individual differences in the propensity to be altruistic, trusting, modest, and warm (John and Srivastava, 1999). Roberts et al. (in press) report consistent evidence for increases in agreeableness. Several large cross-sectional studies have shown that agreeableness increases with age (e.g. Goldberg et al., 1998; McCrae et al., 1999). In addition, longitudinal studies have reported increases in agreeableness in young adulthood (Stein et al., 1986), middle age (Haan et al., 1986), and old age (Field and Millsap, 1991). The finding that agreeableness increases across the life course was substantiated by the largest cross-sectional study performed to date (Srivastava et al., 2002). Srivastava et al. (2002) found that agreeableness increased from age 21 to 60 with accelerated growth occurring between the late 20s and the 40s.

Conscientiousness, the third Big Five domain, refers to the propensity to be self-controlled, task-oriented, goal-directed, planful, and rule-following (John and Srivastava, 1999). Like agreeableness, conscientiousness seems to increase with age (Roberts et al., in press). Several cross-sectional studies have found a positive relationship between age and conscientiousness (e.g. Goldberg et al., 1998; McCrae et al., 1999). Closer examination of the age trajectory shows that although conscientiousness increases throughout the life course, most of the growth occurs in the 20s and then slows throughout the 30s, 40s and 50s (Srivastava et al., 2002).

Longitudinal research supports the inference that conscientiousness increases most in young adulthood and tapers off in middle and old age. For example, the evidence for increasing conscientiousness is most consistent in young adulthood across numerous longitudinal studies (e.g. Haan et al., 1986; Stein et al., 1986; Helson and Moane, 1987; McGue et al., 1993; Roberts et al., 2001; Robins et al., 2001; Vaidya et al., in press). In contrast, longitudinal studies tracking change in conscientiousness in middle age and beyond show somewhat contradictory patterns. Some studies show increases (Helson and Wink, 1992; Cartwright and Wink, 1994), whereas others find decreases (Costa et al., 2000). More recently, Helson et al. (2002) examined several facets of conscientiousness in a sample of 21- to 75-year-olds followed for up to 40 years, and found that four facets increased with age (self-control, good impression, achievement via conformance, and inflexibility) and two facets decreased (responsibility and socialization).

In summary, previous studies consistently show increases in conscientiousness during adolescence and early adulthood and a majority of studies show increases in conscientiousness during adulthood and old age. However, more research is needed throughout adulthood and later life before firm conclusions can be made about how conscientiousness changes beyond age 30. In particular, research is needed that tracks the developmental trajectory of specific facets of conscientiousness.

The fourth domain of the Big Five is Neuroticism or its converse, Emotional Stability. This domain contrasts even-temperedness with the experience of anxiety, worry, anger, and depression (John and Srivastava, 1999). Findings from several large cross-sectional studies suggest that neuroticism decreases with age from late adolescence to old age (Goldberg et al., 1998; McCrae et al., 1999). However, Carstensen et al. (2000) found a curvilinear developmental trajectory for negative emotions: decreasing neuroticism up to age 60 and then a slight increase after age 60.

Roberts et al. (in press) reported that the longitudinal evidence points to declines in neuroticism during late adolescence and early adulthood (Baltes and Nesselroade, 1972; McGue et al., 1993; Carmichael and McGue, 1994; Viken et al., 1994; Watson and Walker, 1996; Roberts et al., 2001; Robins et al., 2001) and midlife (Costa et al., 2000). However, the evidence for change in old age is equivocal with many studies showing no change (Field and Millsap, 1991) or increases (Leon et al., 1979).

In summary, neuroticism tends to decrease from adolescence to midlife and then remains stable or slightly increases during old age. However, some studies have found a gender difference in the neuroticism trajectory. Both Goldberg et al. (1998) and Srivastava et al. (2002) found a stronger decline in neuroticism for women than for men. Thus, it is possible that some of the inconsistencies found in previous research may be due to underlying gender differences. More research is needed to examine the role of gender before firm conclusions can be made about the trajectory of neuroticism across the life course.

The final domain of personality traits is Openness to experience, which refers to individual differences in the propensity to be original, complex, creative, and open to new ideas (John and Srivastava, 1999). Roberts et al. (in press) report that cross-sectional studies do not provide a clear picture of age differences in openness to experience. Costa and McCrae (1988) and McCrae et al. (1999, 2000) found a negative relation between openness to experience and age, in samples drawn from nine countries. Similarly, Srivastava et al. (2002) found that openness to experience decreased from age 21 to 60. However, Goldberg et al. (1998) and Helson and Kwan (2000) did not find any significant relation between measures of openness to experience and age in samples ranging in age from 18 to 75.

Unfortunately, longitudinal studies do little to clarify the nature of age-related changes in openness to experience. Studies of adolescents and young adults generally show increases in openness to experience (Baltes and Nesselroade, 1972; Robins et al., 2001; Vaidya et al., in press); however, the evidence for increases in openness during this age period is confounded by the fact that all of these studies tracked personality change in college students who are ostensibly being socialized to be more open to experience (Sanford, 1956). Beyond the college years, Roberts et al. (in press) report that the evidence is equivocal, with some studies demonstrating increases (Helson et al., 2002), some decreases (Field and Millsap, 1991), and others no change (Costa and McCrae, 1988).

Thus, a murky picture emerges with regard to mean-level changes in openness to experience. It is possible that the relation between age and openness is non-linear or that the same construct is not being measured across studies or age periods. Like other Big Five dimensions, future developmental research might benefit from differentiating among the facets of openness. For example, it may be that wisdom increases with age (Baltes and Staudinger, 2000), but traits like creativity, openness to feelings, and openness to ideas may decrease.

The previous sections focused on whether or not personality changes throughout the life course. Although the findings were not unequivocal, they do suggest that personality continues to show some changes throughout the life course. However, the research we have reviewed so far does not provide a direct test of the classical trait perspective. Recently, Srivastava et al. (2002) tested two hypotheses related to the classical trait perspective using data from a large cross-sectional sample of individuals ranging in age from 21 to 60: (1) there is no change in personality after age 30 (i.e. the slope after age 30 is not significantly different from zero), and (2) change after age 30 is smaller than change prior to age 30 (i.e. the slope for ages 31–60 is significantly smaller than the slope for ages 21–30). They found that change in each trait after age 30 was significantly different from zero, except for neuroticism for men. Thus, they did not find support for the hypothesis that traits stop changing after age 30. There was mixed support for their second hypothesis that the rate of change after age 30 is slower than the rate of change prior to age 30. For some traits, the rate of change after age 30 was slower (conscientiousness for men and women and extraversion for men), but other traits showed an increase in rate of change after age 30 (agreeableness for men and women and openness for men), and others showed an equal rate of change before and after age 30 (neuroticism for men and women and openness and extraversion for women).

In conclusion, our review of the literature on mean-level changes in personality leads us to conclude that personality continues to change throughout the life course, however the rate of change may slow after early adulthood. Although there were some contradictory findings for each trait, we can nonetheless reach some tentative conclusions about the general pattern of change. Overall, the research suggests that extraversion decreases and agreeableness and conscientiousness increase from early childhood to old age. Neuroticism increases in early childhood, decreases from adolescence to midlife, and appears to plateau or increase into old age. The results for openness to experience were too mixed to draw any conclusions about its normative trajectory.

Overall, age-related changes in personality generally replicate across gender, country, and study design. This consistency lends strength to the argument that the observed normative changes are maturational and not the result of social influences. For example, results based just on cross-sectional studies confound age and cohort and results based just on longitudinal studies confound age and time of measurement. The combination of both types of studies affords the most robust test of whether personality demonstrates coherent patterns of change with age (Schaie, 1965). That is, finding consistency across cross-sectional and longitudinal studies lends confidence to the interpretation that the change observed is attributable to age, not cohort or time of measurement effects.

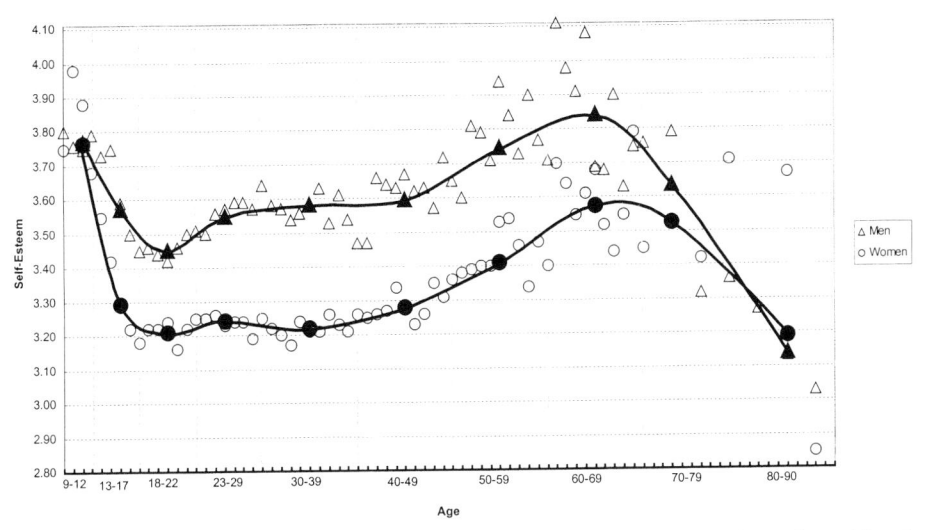

Fig. 2. Mean level of self-esteem as a function of developmental period, separately for males and females. Also plotted are year-by-year means, separately for males (open triangles) and females (open circles). From *self-esteem across the life span*, by R.W. Robins, K.M. Trzesniewski, J.L. Tracy, S.D. Gosling and J. Potter, 2002b. Psychology and Aging 17, 428. © 2002 by the American Psychological Association. Reprinted with permission.

2.2. Self-esteem

Researchers have long debated whether self-esteem shows normative age changes. Wylie (1979) initiated this debate with her influential review of the self-esteem literature. She concluded that there are no systematic age differences in self-esteem. Although this conclusion has been widely debated (e.g. McCarthy and Hoge, 1982; O'Malley and Bachman, 1983; Rosenberg, 1986; Demo, 1992; Twenge and Campbell, 2001), these debates have failed to lead to any consensus about the normative development of self-esteem.

To obtain a more comprehensive picture of normative age differences in self-esteem, we review the findings from two recent studies of self-esteem development, a meta-analysis of 86 published articles (Trzesniewski et al., 2001) and a large, cross-sectional study ($N = 326{,}641$) of individuals aged 9 to 90 (Robins et al., 2002a). The two studies generally converged in their findings, and together help clear up inconsistencies in the extant literature and suggest several conclusions about the way self-esteem develops from childhood to old age. Below we describe the findings within developmental periods (childhood, adolescence, adulthood, old age). Figure 2 shows the trajectory of self-esteem across the life course, separately for males and females, based on findings from the cross-sectional study.

2.2.1. Childhood

Both studies indicated that young children have relatively high self-esteem, which gradually declines over the course of childhood. The meta-analysis showed a moderate drop in self-esteem between ages 7 and 8 and ages 8 and 9 (1/3 and 1/4 standard deviation, respectively), followed by smaller yearly drops between the ages of 9 and 12. Beginning at age 9, the cross-sectional study showed that children (aged 9–12) rated themselves well above the scale midpoint and higher than during any subsequent period in the life span.

Some researchers have speculated that children have high self-esteem because it is artificially inflated, and that the subsequent decline reflects an increasing reliance on more realistic information about the self (Harter, 1998). For example, as children develop cognitively, they begin to base their evaluations of self-worth on external feedback and social comparisons, which may produce more accurate judgments of where they stand in relation to others (Ruble et al., 1980). It is also possible that as children transition from preschool to elementary school they experience more negative feedback from teachers, parents, and peers, and their self-evaluations correspondingly become more negative (Eccles et al., 1993).

2.2.2. Adolescence

The decline in self-esteem that began during childhood continues into adolescence, producing a substantial cumulative drop. For example, the meta-analysis revealed a one full standard deviation drop when 7- and 8-year-olds are compared to 13- and 14-year-olds. Similarly, the cross-sectional study showed a half standard deviation drop from its high point at age 10 to its low point at age 17.

The adolescent drop in self-esteem appears to be particularly robust. It replicates across gender, although it is much more pronounced for girls, across several ethnic groups (Blacks, Whites, Latinos, Asians), and across U.S. and non-U.S. citizens. Researchers have attributed the adolescent decline in self-esteem to maturational changes associated with puberty, cognitive changes associated with the emergence of formal operational thinking, and socio-contextual changes associated with the transition from grade school to junior high school (Simmons et al., 1979; Wigfield et al., 1991; Harter, 1998). Although our findings do not point to any particular explanation for why self-esteem declines during adolescence, they do raise questions about the validity of certain theoretical explanations. For example, the claim that the decline represents the transition from grade school to junior high school needs to be reconciled with the fact that the decline also occurs for non-U.S. participants whose educational systems may not involve such transitions.

2.2.3. Adulthood

The meta-analysis included few studies that examined self-esteem during adulthood. These studies showed slight increases from young adulthood to middle adulthood and slight decreases from middle adulthood to old age (up to age 87). The findings from the cross-sectional study replicated the gradual increase throughout adulthood. In addition, the cross-sectional study showed that adult self-esteem peaked during late adulthood. Thus, other than childhood, the mid-60s seem to represent the apex of self-esteem across the life course.

General theories of adult development provide some explanation for why self-esteem peaks during midlife. Erikson (1968), Jung (1958), Neugarten (1977),

Levinson (1978), and others have theorized that mid-life is characterized by a focus on activity, achievement, power, and control. For example, Erikson suggested that the maturity and superior functioning associated with mid-life is linked to the "generativity" stage, during which individuals tend to be increasingly productive and creative at work, while at the same time promoting and guiding the next generation. Similarly, Mitchell and Helson (1990) described the latter part of midlife as a period characterized by higher levels of psychological maturity and adjustment, and noted that during the post-parental period "the energy that went to children is redirected to the partner, work, the community, or self-development" (p. 453). Role theories of aging suggest that over the course of adulthood individuals increasingly occupy positions of power and status, which might convey a sense of self-worth (Sarbin, 1964; Dannefer, 1984; Helson et al., 1984; Hogan and Roberts, in press). As Gove et al. (1989) noted, "during the productive adult years, when persons are engaged in a full set of instrumental and social roles, their sense of self will reflect the fullness of this role repertoire... there will be high levels of instrumentality, competitiveness, and socioemotional support. Levels of life satisfaction and self-esteem will also be high" (p. 1122).

2.2.4. Old age
The meta-analysis did not turn up enough studies of self-esteem during old age to be informative. However, the cross-sectional study showed that self-esteem dropped substantially beginning around age 70. Interestingly, the majority of the decline occurred between the 70s and 80s (about one-third of a standard deviation), rather than between the 60s and 70s (about one-tenth of a standard deviation). By the 80s, self-esteem levels were as low as those found during adolescence. Nonetheless, self-esteem levels in the oldest age groups still averaged above the midpoint of the scale, and only 26% of the 70 to 90-year-olds reported low self-esteem (either a 1 or a 2).

Old age involves a number of changes that might contribute to declines in self-esteem, including spousal loss, decreased social support, declining physical health, cognitive impairments, an increase in elder abuse, and a downward shift in socioeconomic status. However, several theories of aging suggest an alternative view. Jung (1958), Erikson (1968), Neugarten (1977), Levinson (1978), Baltes and Mayer (1999), and others hold that persons in old age tend to be wiser and more comfortable with themselves. According to Erikson (1968), the final stage of life is a time of "post-narcissistic love of the human ego – not of the self – as an experience which conveys some world order and spiritual sense" (p. 81). Erikson thus provides an alternative interpretation of the self-esteem drop: it is not that deep-seated feelings of self-worth are declining in old age, but rather that older persons increasingly accept their faults and limitations and correspondingly have a diminished need for self-promotion and self-aggrandisement, which might artificially boost reports of self-esteem earlier in life. This suggests that during old age defense mechanisms such as denial might no longer inflate feelings of self-worth. Thus, the decline in self-esteem might not be part of a larger pattern of deteriorating emotional health in old age, but rather a specific shift in self-conceptions that contributes to a more modest, humble, and balanced view of the self.

Overall, our review of the literature on personality and self-esteem development suggests that these characteristics generally change in a positive direction, at least over the first 40 years of adulthood. Once people emerge from adolescence, they become warmer, more responsible, more emotionally stable, and more confident as they progress through young adulthood and enter middle age. However, it is important to note that this positive portrait may not hold into old age. As the findings for neuroticism and self-esteem suggest, the direction of change shifts after age 60 or 70. During this latter part of life, neuroticism increases and self-esteem decreases. However, these findings are based on a small set of studies and strong conclusions cannot be made. Thus, more research is needed beyond age 60 to better understand how we grow throughout our life span. Importantly, these findings show that personality characteristics, long thought to be immutable, not only change, but also continue to develop later in the life course than most theorists suggested. It appears that development does not end with the advent of adulthood.

3. Socio-contextual factors that influence personality and self-esteem change

Our review of the literature demonstrates that personality and self-esteem are stable individual-difference constructs that show systematic change across the life course. We found that as people move through adulthood, they become less sociable, more agreeable, more responsible, less anxious and neurotic, and more confident and secure.

These patterns reflect changes that occur at the group level. However, based on different life experiences, individuals may vary in the extent to which they experience these changes, producing individual differences in change. That is, factors in addition to chronological age, such as key social roles and events, define and shape one's position in the life course, and thereby determine the way personality and self develop (Caspi and Roberts, 2001). When these factors are non-age-dependent (e.g. divorce) or non-normative (e.g. early death of a spouse), they will differentially impact people's life trajectories and thus produce individual differences in intra-individual change.

From a sociogenic perspective, the social structure is, in part, responsible for personality and self-esteem development; that is, psychological change results from the way a person interfaces with society through their ongoing participation in social roles (Aldwin and Levenson, 1994; Caspi and Roberts, 1999). There is now a growing body of research demonstrating non-trivial relationships between changes in personality and self-esteem and sociogenic factors. The two main sociogenic factors associated with personality and self-esteem change are work and relationship experiences.

3.1. Work experiences

Individuals are assumed to change their personality and self-conceptions as they learn the norms associated with their work roles (Sarbin, 1964). In addition, many self-esteem theories suggest that mastery experiences in work and achievement domains contribute to feelings of self-worth, whereas failure experiences negatively impact self-esteem (Coopersmith, 1967; Rosenberg, 1979; Covington, 1992; Dweck, 1999; Harter, 1999). Thus, over time, positive experiences at work are likely to engender higher levels of conscientiousness and self-esteem. Previous longitudinal research generally supports this assumption. For example, having a high status job predicts increased dependability and responsibility (e.g. Elder, 1969; Roberts, 1997) and increased self-esteem (Bachman and O'Malley, 1977; Owens, 1994; Elliott, 1996). In addition, work satisfaction is associated with decreases in neuroticism (Roberts and Chapman, 2000) and increases in self-esteem (Mortimer et al., 1982).

3.2. Relationship experiences

Individuals may change their personality traits based on feedback they receive in their social roles from peers, which is one of the essential ideas of symbolic interactionism (Stryker and Statham, 1985). Moreover, self-esteem is generally believed to derive in part from feeling loved and accepted by others (Mead, 1934; Rogers, 1959; Coopersmith, 1967; Rosenberg, 1986; Felson, 1989; Leary and Downs, 1995; Harter, 1999). For example, according to Murray et al.'s (2000) dependency model, how you feel about yourself is regulated by how you think your close relationship partner feels about you. Thus, satisfying and supportive relationships should promote feelings of self-worth. Consistent with this, several longitudinal studies have shown that healthy social relationships prospectively predict increasing emotional stability and self-esteem. For example, positive relationship experiences (e.g. low martial tension, high martial satisfaction) are related to decreases in neuroticism and increases in self-esteem (Andrews and Brown, 1995; Roberts and Chapman, 2000). Similarly, positive relationships with family and peers is related to better adjustment during difficult transitions, such as the transition to junior high school and from college to the work force (e.g. Mortimer et al., 1982; Fenzel, 2000).

Consistent with these findings, Robins, Caspi, and Moffitt (in press) found that relationship experiences during young adulthood could serve as a catalyst for personality change. Young adults in dissatisfying and abusive relationships became more anxious, angry, and alienated over time. In contrast, young adults who remained in a stable relationship during their 20s became more cautious and restrained in their thoughts, feelings, and behaviors. This finding provides a plausible causal account for a particular intra-individual developmental pathway. Impulse control tends to increase in young adulthood, but the reason for this change is not fully understood (Roberts et al., 2001). Robins et al.'s findings suggest that settling down in an intimate relationship may be a contributory cause. It may be that the norms, expectations, and sex-role stereotypes associated with intimate relationships create an environmental press for a more controlled, cautious, and traditional approach to life. Likewise, the finding that individuals in unhappy relationships tend to become more hostile, anxious, and alienated over time dovetails with recent research on depression. Negative relationship experiences – including dissatisfaction (Whisman and Bruce, 1999) and dissolution (Monroe et al., 1999) – increase the risk of depression. However, the mediating mechanism remains to be understood. Repeated acts of aggression, recurrent negative emotional states, and other aversive experiences that chronically occur in maladaptive intimate relationships may increase an individual's disposition toward negative emotionality, which is a risk factor for depression (Krueger, 1999).

One additional sociogenic factor, historical context, has been long identified as a critical influence on personality development (Stewart and Healy, 1989). Different historical periods bring different opportunities, values, and social roles that are thought to influence the personalities of individuals living through those times (Baltes and Nesselroade, 1972; Twenge, 2001). Elder's (1979) study of the Great Depression is a classic example of how pervasive deprivation had differential developmental influences on the personality development of younger vs. older children. More recent research has demonstrated the influence of modern historical phenomena. For example, Agronick and Duncan (1998) investigated the personality changes associated with the perceived importance of the women's movement of the 1960s and 1970s. Women who felt that the women's movement was important showed increases in social poise and self-assurance and decreases in several measures of norm-adherence. Roberts and Helson (1997) explored the antecedents and consequences of changes in culture or climate that occurred in the United States between 1950 and 1985, described as the "culture of narcissism." They found that changes in cultural climate were associated with increases in narcissism and decreases in social responsibility (e.g. decreasing psychological maturity). Similarly, Twenge and Campbell (2001) found that college students' self-esteem rose between 1968 and 1994, a time during which a "culture of self-worth" presumably emerged.

These studies demonstrate that changes in personality and self-esteem are associated with experiences in careers, marriage, and the culture at large. Several aspects of these studies are worth highlighting. It seems apparent that certain life experiences are associated with increases in traits related to the functional definition of maturity. People who achieve more in work and remain in stable relationships become more conscientious (Roberts, 1997; Robins et al., 2002b). In addition, people who have satisfying jobs and marriages tend to increase in emotional stability and gain self-esteem (Roberts and Chapman, 2000; Robins et al., in press). It should also be noted that life experiences can counteract the developmental trends toward maturity. For example, the culture of narcissism in the United States during the 1960s, 1970s, and 1980s was associated with decreases in norm-adherence – a facet of conscientiousness (Roberts and Helson, 1997). Thus, although developmental changes oriented toward increasing maturity may be normative, countervailing societal or other socio-contextual forces may thwart these changes.

One problematic aspect of most research exploring the relationship between social structures and personality development is the assumption that environments only affect change in personality. We describe this perspective as the "exposure" model of personality development in which it is often assumed that mere exposure to the social structure, role, or context will facilitate change in personality. Exposure models ignore the fact that personality and social structure are often reciprocally related (Kohn and Schooler, 1978, 1982; Schooler et al., 1999). Roberts, Caspi, and Moffitt (2001) have proposed that the most likely effect of life experience on personality development is to deepen the characteristics that lead people to those experiences in the first place. Roberts, Caspi, and Moffitt (in press) characterized this pattern of development as "corresponsive." For example, individuals drawn to stimulating work because of their own intellectual complexity will become more intellectually complex because of their experiences. Similarly, individuals with low self-esteem will seek out information and interaction partners who confirm their negative self-views, just as individuals with high self-esteem will seek out contexts that confirm their positive self-views (Swann, 1996). Thus, people are not rudderless ships buffeted by the whims of the social context. Rather, the type of change they demonstrate will often grow out of their individuality and will therefore be somewhat predictable.

Exposure models also overlook the fact that social contexts may facilitate the more ubiquitous psychological phenomenon of adulthood: consistency. We believe that this more common effect of social context arises from people's attempts to build a personal niche that fits with their values, goals, and personality traits. At its broadest level the personal niche is built around primary social roles found in one's marriage, career, family, and community (e.g. religious, volunteer, and leisure time roles). To the extent that people can build a niche that fits with their psychological profile, then psychological adjustment should be facilitated, as should growth in the direction of the expectations of the social roles selected. In addition, because this niche should successfully reinforce a person's already existing dispositions, there should be less need for change and thus greater levels of consistency.

In our most recent research we tested these ideas by examining whether a person's fit with their school environment influenced the way their personality and values changed during college (Roberts and Robins, 2002). Consistent with our expectations, students who fit better with the school environment changed in the direction of the values of the school environment, becoming more competitive and more emotionally stable. Person–environment fit was also related to satisfaction with college, higher levels of self-esteem, and higher overall levels of personality consistency. This is one of the first studies to identify and test an environmental mechanism that is simultaneously associated with both change and continuity in personality over time.

Finally, the fact that personality change is associated with life experiences has important ramifications for how one conceptualizes the field of personality psychology and personality development in particular. From a theoretical perspective, we must ask why personality would remain an open system that is characterized by both consistency and change? What factors contribute to increasing consistency? What adaptive function, if any, does malleability serve in old age? Answering these questions entails a stark revision of our modal conceptualization of traits that is intrinsically more dynamic (e.g. Pervin, 1994). Rather than simply assuming that traits are consistent because they are traits, we need to understand the processes that account for continuity and change in personality (Whitbourne, 2001). From an applied perspective, we can speculate that developmental periods during which stability is relatively low may be ideal targets for intervention programs because it is during these times when personality and self-esteem may be particularly malleable.

4. Conclusion

In summary, although previous research provides some insight into the developmental course of personality and self-esteem, the field has not yet reached consensus on the overall trajectory of these constructs across the life span. As our review suggests, inconsistencies and gaps in the literature limit the conclusions that can be reached about personality and self-esteem development. For example, the meta-analyses revealed a lack of longitudinal studies of the rank-order stability of personality and self-esteem during childhood and old age. These age groups are marked by numerous maturational and interpersonal changes, and may be periods of rapid transformation and instability. Thus, more longitudinal studies are needed during these age groups before we fully understand the stability of personality and self-esteem across the entire life span.

Our qualitative review of mean-level personality change also revealed inconsistencies and gaps in the literature. Although we were able to discern some consistent developmental changes for the Big Five dimensions, the findings were often equivocal. Meta-analytic techniques are needed to more accurately quantify the findings from the existing research literature, and gain a more precise picture of the trajectory of personality across the life span. A meta-analysis would also help identify relevant moderators. For example, the few studies that examined change separately for males and females suggest that gender may be a significant moderator of the developmental trajectory (e.g. extraversion increases for males and decreases for females). Finally, a meta-analysis would reveal gaps in the literature. For example, our qualitative review turned up only a few studies of childhood and adolescent personality development. The results from a quantitative review would provide a foundation for future studies of personality development, and eventually contribute to a complete understanding of how personality changes from conception to death.

The research literature provides a somewhat clearer picture of the normative development of self-esteem. Self-esteem appears to be relatively high in childhood, drop during adolescence, rise gradually throughout adulthood, and then decline sharply in old age. However, the findings for old age were based on relatively few studies. Moreover, the bulk of the self-esteem literature relies on non-representative samples of particular age cohorts. An important direction for future research is to examine age differences in self-esteem across the entire life span, particularly into old age, using a cross-sequential design and more representative samples. By following multiple cohorts over time, we could tease apart aging and cohort effects and thus determine if the old age drop is (a) replicable and (b) due to maturational or cohort effects. Moreover, future studies could begin to ask what are the mechanisms of self-esteem change and identify the factors that promote or diminish self-esteem across the life span.

References

Agronick, G.S., Duncan, L.E., 1998. Personality and social change: Individual differences, life path, and importance attributed to the women's movement. J. Pers. Soc. Psychol. 74, 1545–1555.

Aldwin, C.M., Levenson, M.R., 1994. Aging and personality assessment. In: Lawton, M.P., Teresi, J.A. (Eds.), Annual Review of Gerontology and Geriatrics: Focus on Assessment. Springer Publishing, New York, pp. 182–209.

Andrews, B., Brown, G.W., 1995. Stability and change in low self-esteem: The role of psychosocial factors. Psychol. Med. 25, 23–31.

Arnett, J.J., 2000. Emerging adulthood: A theory of development from the late teens through the twenties. Am. Psychol. 55, 469–480.

Bachman, J.G., O'Malley, P.M., 1977. Self-esteem in young men: A longitudinal analysis of the impact of educational and occupational attainment. J. Pers. Soc. Psychol. 35, 365–380.

Baltes, P.B., Mayer, K.U. (Eds.) 1999. The Berlin Aging Study: Aging from 70 to 100. Cambridge University Press, Cambridge, England.

Baltes, P.B., Nesselroade, J.R., 1972. Cultural change and adolescent personality development: An application of longitudinal sequences. Dev. Psychol. 7, 244–256.

Baltes, P.B., Staudinger, U.M., 2000. Wisdom: A metaheuristic (pragmatic) to orchestrate mind and virtue toward excellence. Am. Psychol. 55, 122–136.

Carmichael, C.M., McGue, M., 1994. A longitudinal family study of personality change and stability. J. Pers. 62, 1–20.

Carstensen, L.L., Pasupathi, M., Mayr, U., Nesselroade, J.R., 2000. Emotional experience in everyday life across the adult life span. J. Pers. Soc. Psychol. 79, 644–655.

Cartwright, L.K., Wink, P., 1994. Personality change in women physicians from medical student years to mid-40s. Psychol. Women Q. 18, 291–308.

Caspi, A., 2000. The child is father of the man: Personality continuities from childhood to adulthood. J. Pers. Soc. Psychol. 78, 158–172.

Caspi, A., Roberts, B.W., 1999. Personality change and continuity across the life course. In: Pervin, L.A., John, O.P. (Eds.), Handbook of Personality Theory and Research. Guilford Press, New York, pp. 300–326.

Caspi, A., Roberts, B.W., 2001. Personality development across the life course: The argument for change and continuity. Psychol. Inq. 12, 49–66.

Conley, J.J., 1984. The hierarchy of consistency: A review and model of longitudinal findings on adult individual differences in intelligence, personality, and self-opinion. Pers. Individ. Diff. 5, 11–26.

Coopersmith, S., 1967. The Antecedents of Self-esteem. Freeman, San Francisco.

Costa Jr., P.T., Herbst, J.H., McCrae, R.R., Siegler, I.C., 2000. Personality at midlife: Stability, intrinsic maturation, and response to life events. Assessment 7, 365–378.

Costa, P.T., McCrae, R.R., 1994. Set like plaster: Evidence for the stability of adult personality. In: Heatherton, T.F., Weinberger, J.L. (Eds.), Can Personality Change? American Psychological Association, Washington, DC, pp. 21–40.

Costa, P.T., McCrae, R.R., 1988. Personality in adulthood: A six-year longitudinal study of self-reports and spouse ratings on the NEO Personality Inventory. J. Pers. Soc. Psychol. 54, 853–863.

Covington, M.V., 1992. Making the Grade: A Self-worth Perspective on Motivation and School Reform. Cambridge University Press, New York.

Crook, M.N., 1943. A retest with the Thurstone Personality Schedule after six and one-half years. J. Gen. Psychol. 28, 111–120.
Dannefer, D., 1984. Adult development and social theory: A paradigmatic reappraisal. Am. Sociol. Rev. 49, 100–116.
Demo, D.H., 1992. The self-concept over time: Research issues and directions. Annu. Rev. Sociol. 18, 303–326.
Dweck, C.S., 1999. Self-theories: Their role in motivation, personality and development. Psychology Press, Philadelphia.
Eccles, J., Wigfield, A., Harold, R.D., Blumenfeld, P., 1993. Age and gender differences in children's self- and task perceptions during elementary school. Child Dev. 64, 830–847.
Elder Jr., G.H., 1969. Occupational mobility, life patterns, and personality. J. Health Soc. Behav. 10, 308–323.
Elder Jr., G.H., 1979. Historical change in life patterns and personality. In: Baltes, P.B., Brim Jr.O.G. (Eds.), Life-span Development and Behavior, Vol. 2. Academic Press, New York, pp. 117–159.
Elliott, M., 1996. Impact of work, family, and welfare receipt on women's self-esteem in young adulthood. Soc. Psychol. Q. 59, 80–95.
Erikson, E.H., 1968. Identity, Youth, and Crisis, 1st ed. W.W. Norton, New York.
Erikson, E.H., 1985. The Life Cycle Completed: A Review. W.W. Norton, New York.
Felson, R.B., 1989. Parents and the reflected appraisal process: A longitudinal analysis. J. Pers. Soc. Psychol. 56, 965–971.
Fenzel, L.M., 2000. Prospective study of changes in global self-worth and strain during the transition to middle school. J. Early Adolesc. 20, 93–116.
Field, D., Millsap, R.E., 1991. Personality in advanced old age: Continuity or change? J. Gerontol. 46, 299–308.
Funder, D.C., 1991. Global traits: A neo-Allportian approach to personality. Psychol. Sci. 2, 31–39.
Goldberg, L.R., Sweeney, D., Merenda, P.F., Hughes Jr., J.E., 1998. Demographic variables and personality: The effects of gender, age, education, and ethnic/racial status on self-descriptions of personality attributes. Pers. Individ. Diff. 24, 393–403.
Gove, W.R., Ortega, S.T., Style, C.B., 1989. The maturational and role perspectives on aging and self through the adult years: An empirical evaluation. Am. J. Sociol. 94, 1117–1145.
Haan, N., Millsap, R., Hartka, E., 1986. As time goes by: Change and stability in personality over fifty years. Psychol. Aging 1, 220–232.
Harter, S., 1998. The development of self-representations. In: Damon, W., Eisenberg, N. (Eds.), Handbook of Child Psychology. Wiley, New York, pp. 553–617.
Harter, S., 1999. The Construction of the Self: A Developmental Perspective. Guilford, New York.
Helson, R., Jones, C., Kwan, V.S.Y., 2002. Personality change over 40 years of adulthood: HLM analyses of two longitudinal samples. J. Pers. Soc. Psychol. 83, 752–766.
Helson, R., Kwan, V.S.Y., 2000. Personality development in adulthood: The broad picture and processes in one longitudinal sample. In: Hampson, S. (Ed.), Advances in Personality Psychology, Vol. 1. Routledge, London, pp. 77–106.
Helson, R., Mitchell, V., Moane, G., 1984. Personality and patterns of adherence and nonadherence to the social clock. J. Pers. Soc. Psychol. 46, 1079–1096.
Helson, R., Moane, G., 1987. Personality change in women from college to midlife. J. Pers. Soc. Psychol. 53, 176–186.
Helson, R., Wink, P., 1992. Personality change in women from the early 40s to the early 50s. Psychol. Aging 7, 46–55.
Hogan, R., Roberts, B.W., In press. A socioanalytic model of maturity. J. Career Assess.
John, O.P., Srivastava, S., 1999. The Big Five trait taxonomy; History, measurement, and theoretical perspectives. In: Pervin, L.A., John, O.P. (Eds.), Handbook of Personality Theory and Research, Vol. 2. Guilford Press, New York, pp. 102–138.
Jung, C.G., 1958. The Undiscovered Self. Little Brown, Boston, MA.
Kelly, E.L., 1955. Consistency of adult personality. Am. Psychol. 10, 659–681.

Kernis, M.H., Grannemann, B.D., Barclay, L.C., 1992. Stability of self-esteem: Assessment, correlates, and excuse making. J. Pers. 60, 621–644.

Kohn, M.L., Schooler, C., 1978. The reciprocal effects of the substantive complexity of work and intellectual flexibility: A longitudinal assessment. Am. J. Sociol. 84, 24–52.

Kohn, M.L., Schooler, C., 1982. Job conditions and personality: A longitudinal assessment of their reciprocal effects. Am. J. Sociol. 87, 1257–1286.

Krueger, R.F., 1999. Personality traits in late adolescence predict mental disorders in early adulthood: A prospective-epidemiological study. J. Pers. 67, 39–65.

Lamb, M.E., Chuang, S.S., Wessels, H., Broberg, A.G., Hwang, C.P., 2002. Emergence and Construct Validation of the Big Five Factors in Early Childhood: A Longitudinal Analysis of Their Ontogeny in Sweden. Child Dev. 73, 1517–1524.

Leary, M.R., Baumeister, R.F., 2000. The nature and function of self-esteem: Sociometer theory. In: Zanna, M.P. (Ed.), Advances in Experimental Social Psychology. Academic Press, San Diego, CA, pp. 1–62.

Leary, M.R., Downs, D.L., 1995. Interpersonal functions of the self-esteem motive: The self-esteem system as a sociometer. In: Kernis, M. (Ed.), Efficacy, Agency, and Self-esteem. Plenum, New York, pp. 123–144.

Leon, G.R., Gillum, B., Gillum, R., Gouze, M., 1979. Personality stability and change over a 30 year period-Middle age to old age. J. Consult. Clin. Psychol. 47, 517–524.

Levinson, D. (in collaboration with Charlotte Darrow, Edward Klein, Maria Levinson, and Braxton McKee). (1978). Seasons of a Man's Life. Knopf, New York.

Lewis, M., 1999. On the development of personality. In: Pervin, L.A., John, O.P. (Eds.), Handbook of Personality Theory and Research. The Guilford Press, New York, pp. 327–346.

Lewis, M., 2001. Issues in the study of personality development. Psychol. Inq. 12, 67–83.

McCrae, R.R., Costa, P.T., 1994. The stability of personality: Observation and evaluations. Curr. Dir. Psychol. Sci. 3, 173–175.

McCrae, R.R., Costa, P.T., Jr., Pedroso de Lima, M., Simoes, A., Ostendorf, F., Angleitner, A., Marusic, I., Bratko, D., Caprara, G.V., Barbaranelli, C., Chae, J.-H., Piedmont, R.L., 1999. Age differences in personality across the adult life span: Parallels in five cultures. Dev. Psychol. 35, 466–477.

McCrae, R.R., Costa Jr., P.T., Ostendorf, F., Angleitner, A., Hrebrickova, M., Avia, M.D., Sanz, J., Sanchez-Bernardos, M.L., Kusdil, M.E., Woodfield, R., Saunders, P.R., Smith, P.B., 2000. Nature over nurture: Temperament, personality, and life span development. J. Pers. Soc. Psychol. 78, 173–186.

McCarthy, J.D., Hoge, D.R., 1982. Analysis of age effects in longitudinal studies of adolescent self-esteem. Dev. Psychol. 18, 372–379.

McGue, M., Bacon, S., Lykken, D.T., 1993. Personality stability and change in early adulthood: A behavioral genetic analysis. Dev. Psychol. 29, 96–109.

Mead, G.H., 1934. Mind, Self, and Society from the Standpoint of a Social Behaviorist. University of Chicago Press, Chicago.

Mitchell, V., Helson, R., 1990. Women's prime of life: Is it the 50's? Psychol. Women Q. 14, 451–470.

Mortimer, J.T., Finch, M.D., Kumka, D., 1982. Persistence and change in development: The multidimensional self-concept. Life-Span Dev. Behav. 4, 263–313.

Monroe, S.M., Rohde, P., Seeley, J.R., Lewinsohn, P.M., 1999. Life events and depression in adolescence: Relationship loss as a prospective risk factor for first onset of major depressive disorder. J. Abnorm. Psychol. 108, 606–614.

Murray, S.L., Holmes, J.G., Griffin, D.W., 2000. Self-esteem and the quest for felt security: How perceived regard regulates attachment processes. J. Pers. Soc. Psychol. 78, 478–498.

Neugarten, B.L., 1977. The awareness of middle age. In: Owen, R. (Ed.), Middle Age. BBC, London.

Nilsson, L.V., Persson, B., 1984. Personality changes in the aged. Acta Psychiatrica Scandanavica 69, 182–189.

O'Malley, P.M., Bachman, J.G., 1983. Self-esteem: Change and stability between ages 13 and 23. Dev. Psychol. 19, 257–268.

Owens, T.J., 1994. Two dimensions of self-esteem: Reciprocal effects of positive self-worth and self-deprecation on adolescent problems. Am. Soc. Rev. 59, 391–407.

Pedersen, N.L., Reynolds, C.A., 1998. Stability and change in adult personality: Genetic and environmental components. Eur. J. Pers. 12, 365–386.

Pervin, L.A., 1994. A critical analysis of current trait theory. Psychol. Inq. 5, 103–113.

Rindfuss, R.R., 1991. The young-adult years – Diversity, structural-change, and fertility. Demography 28, 493–512.

Roberts, B.W., 1997. Plaster or plasticity: Are work experiences associated with personality change in women? J. Pers. 65, 205–232.

Roberts, B.W., Caspi, A., 2001. Personality development and the person-situation debate: It's deja vu all over again. Psychol. Inq. 12, 104–109.

Roberts, B.W., Caspi, A., Moffitt, T., 2001. The kids are alright: Growth and stability in personality development from adolescence to adulthood. J. Pers. Soc. Psychol. 81, 670–683.

Roberts, B.W., Caspi, A., Moffitt, T. (in press). Work experiences and personality development in young adulthood. J. Pers. Soc. Psychol. 84, 582–593.

Roberts, B.W., Chapman, C., 2000. Change in dispositional well-being and its relation to role quality: A 30-year longitudinal study. J. Res. Pers. 34, 26–41.

Roberts, B.W., DelVecchio, W.F., 2000. The rank-order consistency of personality from childhood to old age: A quantitative review of longitudinal studies. Psychol. Bull. 126, 3–25.

Roberts, B.W., Helson, R., 1997. Changes in culture, changes in personality: The influence of individualism in a longitudinal study of women. J. Pers. Soc. Psychol. 72, 641–651.

Roberts, B.W., Robins, R.W. (2002). Person-environment fit and its implications for personality development: A longitudinal study. Unpublished manuscript, University of Illinois, Urbana-Champaign.

Roberts, B.W., Robins, R.W., Caspi, A., Trzesniewski, K.H. (in press). Personality trait development in adulthood. In: Mortimer, J.T., Shanahan, M. (Eds.), Handbook of the Life Course. Plenum, New York.

Robins, R.W., Caspi, A., Moffitt, T., 2002a. It's not just who you're with, it's who you are: Personality and relationship experiences across multiple relationships. J. Pers 70, 423–434.

Robins, R.W., Fraley, R.C., Roberts, B.W., Trzesniewski., K., 2001. A longitudinal study of personality change in young adulthood. J. Pers. 69, 617–640.

Robins, R.W., Trzesniewski, K.H., Tracy, J.L., Gosling, S.D., Potter, J., 2002b. Self-esteem across the life span. Psychol. Aging. 17, 423–434.

Rogers, C.R., 1959. A theory of therapy, personality, and interpersonal relations, developed in the client-centered framework. In: Koch, S. (Ed.), Psychology: A Study of a Science, Vol. 3. McGraw-Hill, New York, pp. 185–256.

Rosenberg, M., 1979. Conceiving the Self. Basic Books, New York.

Rosenberg, M., 1986. Self-concept from middle childhood through adolescence. In: Suls, J., Greenwald, A.G. (Eds.), Psychological Perspectives on the Self. Erlbaum, Hillsdale, NJ, pp. 107–136.

Ruble, D.N., Boggiano, A.K., Feldman, N.S., Loebl, J.H., 1980. Developmental analysis of the role of social comparison in self-evaluation. Dev. Psychol. 16, 105–115.

Sanford, N., 1956. Personality development during the college years. J. Social Issues 12, 3–70.

Sarbin, T.R., 1964. Role theoretical interpretation of psychological change. In: Worchel, P., Byrne, D. (Eds.), Personality Change. John Wiley, New York, pp. 176–219.

Schaie, K.W., 1965. A general model for the study of developmental problems. Psychol. Bull. 64, 92–107.

Schooler, C., Mulatu, M.S., Oates, G., 1999. The continuing effects of substantively complex work on the intellectual functioning of older workers. Psychol. Aging 14, 483–506.

Schuerger, J.M., Zarrella, K.L., Hotz, A.S., 1989. Factors that influence the temporal stability of personality by questionnaire. J. Pers. Soc. Psychol. 56, 777–783.

Simmons, R.G., Blyth, D.A., Van Cleave, E.F., Bush, D.M., 1979. Entry into early adolescence: The impact of school structure, puberty, and early dating on self-esteem. American Sociological Review 44, 948–967.

Srivastava, S., John, O.P., Gosling, S.D., Potter, J., 2002. Development of personality in early and middle adulthood: Set like plaster or persistent change? J. Pers. Soc. Psychol. 84, 1041–1053.

Stein, J.A., Newcomb, M.D., Bentler, P.M., 1986. Stability and change in personality: A longitudinal study from early adolescence to young adulthood. J. Res. Pers. 20, 276–291.

Stewart, A.J., Healy, J.M., 1989. Linking individual development and social changes. Am. Psychol. 44, 30–42.

Stryker, S., Statham, A., 1985. Symbolic interaction role theory. In: Lindzey, G., Aronson, E. (Eds.), Handbook of Social Psychology. Erlbaum, Hillsdale, NJ, pp. 311–378.

Swann, W.B., 1996. Self-traps: The Elusive Quest for Higher Self-esteem. Freeham, New York.

Trzesniewski, K.H., Donnellan, M.B., Robins, R.W. (2001, April). Self-esteem across the life span: A meta-analysis. Poster presented at the biannual meeting of the Society for Research on Child Development. Minneapolis, Minnesota.

Trzesniewski, K.H., Donnellan, M.B., Robins, R.W., 2003. Stability of self-esteem across the lifespan. J. Pers. Soc. Psychol. 84, 205–220.

Twenge, J.M., 2001. Changes in women's assertiveness in response to status and roles: A cross-temporal meta-analysis, 1931–1993. J. Pers. Soc. Psychol. 81, 133–145.

Twenge, J.M., Campbell, W.K., 2001. Age and birth cohort differences in self-esteem: A cross-temporal meta-analysis. Pers. Soc. Psychol. Rev. 5, 321–344.

Vaidya, J.G., Gray, E.K., Haig, J., Watson, D., 2003. On the temporal stability of personality: Evidence for differential stability and the role of life experiences. J. Pers. Soc. Psychol. 83, 1469–1484.

Viken, R.J., Rose, R.J., Kaprio, J., Koskenvuo, M., 1994. A developmental genetic analysis of adult personality: Extraversion and neuroticism from 18 to 59 years of age. J. Pers. Soc. Psychol. 66, 722–730.

Watson, D., Walker, L.M., 1996. The long-term stability and predictive validity of trait measures of affect. J. Pers. Soc. Psychol. 70, 567–577.

Whisman, M.A., Bruce, M.L., 1999. Marital dissatisfaction and incidence of major depressive episode in a community sample. J. Abnorm. Psychol. 108, 674–678.

Whitbourne, S.K., 2001. Stability and change in adult personality: Contributions of process-oriented perspectives. Psychol. Inq. 12, 101–103.

Wigfield, A., Eccles, J.S., Mac Iver, D., Reuman, D.A., Midgley, C., 1991. Transitions during early adolescence: Changes in children's domain-specific self-perceptions and general self-esteem across the transition to junior high school. Dev. Psychol. 27, 552–565.

Wylie, R.C., 1979. The Self-concept. University of Nebraska Press, Lincoln, Nebraska.

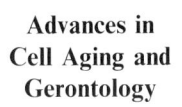

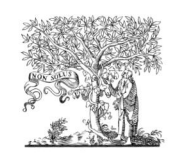

The evolving concept of subjective well-being: the multifaceted nature of happiness

Ed Diener[1]*, Christie Napa Scollon[1] and Richard E. Lucas[2]

[1]*Psychology Department, University of Illinois, 603 E. Daniel St. Champaign IL 61820, USA*
[2]*Psychology Department, Michigan State University, East Larsing, MI 48824, USA*

Contents

1. Evolving conceptions of subjective well-being: The multifaceted nature of happiness ... *188*
   - 1.1. Concern about happiness and the good life throughout history ... *188*
   - 1.2. Chapter overview ... *190*
2. Hierarchical structure: the components of SWB ... *191*
   - 2.1. Positive and negative affect ... *191*
     - 2.1.1. Frequency and intensity of positive and negative affect ... *194*
     - 2.1.2. Recommendations ... *195*
   - 2.2. Life satisfaction ... *196*
   - 2.3. Domain satisfactions ... *198*
   - 2.4. Convergent and discriminant validity of SWB components ... *198*
   - 2.5. Summary ... *199*
3. Temporal sequence and stages ... *199*
4. Stability and consistency of SWB ... *203*
5. Affect vs. cognition ... *204*
6. The functioning mood system ... *206*
7. Tradeoffs ... *207*
8. Implications for measurement ... *208*
9. Implications for research on aging ... *211*
10. Conclusions: the take-home message(s) and directions for future research ... *213*
    - References ... *214*

*Corresponding author. Alumni Professor of Psychology, Department of Psychology, University of Illinois, 603 E. Daniel Street, Champaign, IL 61820, USA. Tel.: 217-333-4804; fax: 217-244-5876.
  E-mail address: ediener@s.psych.uiuc.edu (E. Diener).

1. Evolving conceptions of subjective well-being: The multifaceted nature of happiness

Subjective well-being (SWB) is the field in the behavioral sciences in which people's evaluations of their lives are studied. SWB includes diverse concepts ranging from momentary moods to global judgments of life satisfaction, and from depression to euphoria. The field has grown rapidly in the last decade, so that there are now thousands of studies on topics such as life satisfaction and happiness. Scientists who study aging have shown particular interest in SWB, perhaps because of concern that declines in old age could be accompanied by deteriorating happiness. In this chapter we touch upon age trends in SWB, but our major goal is to alert researchers to the intriguing multi-faceted nature of this concept that has emerged in recent years.

1.1. Concern about happiness and the good life throughout history

A widely presumed component of the good life is happiness. Unfortunately, the nature of happiness has not been defined in a uniform way. Happiness can mean pleasure, life satisfaction, positive emotions, a meaningful life, or a feeling of contentment, among other concepts. In fact, for as long as philosophers have been discussing happiness, its definition has been debated. One of the earliest thinkers on the subject of happiness, the pre-Socratic philosopher Democritus, maintained that the happy life was enjoyable, not because of what the happy person possessed, but because of the way the happy person reacted to his/her life circumstances (Tatarkiewicz, 1976). Incorporated in Democritus's definition of happiness were ideas about disposition, pleasure, satisfaction, and subjectivity. However, this view was buried for centuries as Socrates, Plato, and Aristotle championed the eudemonia definition of happiness in which happiness consisted of possessing the greatest goods available (Tatarkiewicz, 1976).

Although there was little agreement among classical thinkers as to what the highest goods were, for Aristotle, they involved realizing one's fullest potential (Waterman, 1990). Most important, this view defined happiness according to objective standards, and pleasure was not considered central to this definition. In contrast, Aristippus advanced an extreme form of hedonism, the unrestrained pursuit of immediate pleasure and enjoyment (Tatarkiewicz, 1976). Happiness, for hedonists, was simply the sum of many pleasurable moments. This form of hedonism, of course being undesirable and impractical, led to a more moderate form of hedonism when the Epicureans sought to maximize pleasures, but with some degree of prudence. Stoics, on the other hand, sought to minimize pains.

Jeremy Bentham's term "utility," also with its roots in hedonism, later widened the meaning of pleasure to include "benefits, advantages, profits, good or happiness... [and the absence of] failure, suffering, misfortune or unhappiness" (Tatarkiewicz, 1976, p. 322). Happiness, for utilitarians, was thus equated with both the presence of pleasure and absence of pain. Borrowing from Bentham, modern economists believe that people make choices designed to maximize utility.

Because of the multiplicity of meanings that happiness holds, researchers in this field often avoid the term. However, the term happiness has such currency in public discourse that it is often difficult to dodge. Some researchers prefer to use the term "subjective well-being" (SWB), although happiness is sometimes used synonymously with SWB as well. Echoing the beliefs of Democritus, the term subjective well-being emphasizes an individual's own assessment of his or her own life – not the judgment of "experts" – and includes satisfaction (both in general and satisfaction with specific domains), pleasant affect, and low negative affect.

In the 20th Century psychologists and other scientists became interested in studying happiness, answering the questions – What is happiness? Can it be measured? And what causes happiness? – with empirical methods. In a landmark paper, Jahoda (1958) called for the inclusion of positive states in definitions of well-being, which sparked a paradigmatic shift in conceptions of mental health. No longer was the absence of mental illness sufficient for mental health; happiness became important as well.

Wessman and Ricks (1966) conducted early intensive personality work on happy people. Like many of the early SWB researchers, they were interested in the characteristics of a happy person. Is the happy person well-liked, balanced, et cetera? However, the scientific study of happiness still generated a bit of doubt. When Wilson (1967) wrote about "avowed happiness," his discussion hedged on whether it was real happiness that scientists were measuring, although he did not fully define the state.

A watershed finding in SWB research came when Bradburn discovered that positive affect (PA) and negative affect (NA) are independent (Bradburn, 1969). By demonstrating that positive and negative emotions form separate factors that are influenced by different variables, Bradburn's findings lent empirical support to Jahoda's notion of mental health. In addition, the independence of PA and NA became important to the study of happiness because it suggested that happiness is not unidimensional, but instead is at least two-dimensional. In other words, PA and NA are not simply polar ends of a single continuum, and thus need to be measured separately. Andrews and Withey's (1976) contribution to the science of SWB was to include the third, cognitive component of life satisfaction. At the same time, Campbell et al. (1976) were exploring a fourth form of SWB, domain satisfaction.

In 1984, Diener reviewed the field of SWB, including the various theories and known characteristics of happy individuals at the time. Large national studies of SWB concluded that most Americans were indeed happy, regardless of age, race, sex, income, or education level (Myers and Diener, 1995). Since 1990 there has been an explosion of research in the field, with a large number of SWB studies now occurring in the area of gerontology as well. Neugarten et al. (1961), for example, developed a scale that measures life satisfaction specifically among the elderly.

1.2. Chapter overview

Why is SWB important? First, high SWB leads to benefits (see Lyubomirsky et al., 2002 for a review), not the least of which include better health and perhaps even increased longevity (Danner et al., 2001). Second, people the world over think SWB is very important. In a survey of college students from 17 countries, Diener (2000) found that happiness and life satisfaction were both rated well above neutral on importance (and more important than money) in every country, although there was also variation among cultures. Furthermore, respondents from all samples indicated that they thought about happiness from time to time. Thus, even those from relatively unhappy societies value happiness to some extent. Third, SWB represents a major way to assess quality of life in addition to economic and social indicators such as GNP and levels of health or crime (Diener and Suh, 1997). In fact, SWB captures aspects of national conditions that the other measures cannot. Thus, when used in conjunction with the objective measures, SWB provides additional information necessary to evaluate a society. Fourth, SWB is frequently assessed as a major outcome variable in research on the elderly (George, 1986), and on other target groups. SWB is an important indicator of quality of life and functioning in old age.

The present chapter will review several key areas. However, we will also discuss how the field is moving in new directions. Formerly researchers were searching for the core of SWB, but it is clear that there are multiple components that combine in complex ways, and that no single one of them reflects "true happiness." Instead, SWB must be studied as a multi-faceted phenomenon. People combine the basic building blocks of SWB in different ways.

Some of the topics and questions we will address are as follows:

1. Structure: What are the major components under the umbrella of SWB, and how do they relate to one another?
2. Frequency vs. intensity: Is it the frequency, duration, or intensity of good feelings and cognitions that compose SWB?
3. Temporal sequence and stages: The picture of SWB changes depending on whether one examines moments or longer time frames, such as lifetimes.
4. Stability and consistency: Is there enough temporal stability in people's feelings, and consistency across situations, to consider SWB a personality characteristic? Or is SWB entirely situational?
5. Affect vs. cognition: SWB includes both affective evaluations of one's life (e.g. pleasant feelings, enjoyment, etc.), but also a cognitive evaluation (e.g. satisfaction, meaning, etc.). Which is more important?
6. The functioning mood system: Even happy people experience unpleasant emotions, and the picture of SWB we are advocating does not equate happiness with uninterrupted joy. Adaptive emotions involve being able to react to events, and not being stuck in happy or sad moods.
7. Tradeoffs: Although happiness is desirable, people want to feel happy for the right reasons. Additionally, there are times when people are willing to sacrifice fun and enjoyment for other values.

8. Implications for measurement and research with the elderly: Given the multifaceted nature of SWB, various measures cannot be assumed to be substitutes for one another.

Different measures may provide divergent conclusions about the well-being of the elderly. Thus, the choice of measures should be an informed decision.

2. Hierarchical structure: the components of SWB

In this section, we review the components that make up the domain of subjective well-being. We present these components as a conceptual hierarchy with various levels of specificity (see Fig. 1). At the highest level of this hierarchy is the concept of SWB itself. At this level, SWB reflects a general evaluation of a person's life, and researchers who work at this level should measure various components from lower levels in the hierarchy to get a complete picture of an individual's overall well-being. At the next highest level are four specific components that provide a more precise understanding of a person's SWB. These components – positive affect, negative affect, satisfaction, and domain satisfactions – are moderately correlated with one another, and they are all conceptually related. Yet, each provides unique information about the subjective quality of one's life. Finally, within each of these four components, there are more fine-grained distinctions that can be made. Some researchers, for example, may want to focus on specific negative emotions or satisfaction with specific life domains.

2.1. Positive and negative affect

Pleasant and unpleasant affect reflect basic experiences of the ongoing events in people's lives. Thus, it is no surprise that many argue that these affective evaluations should form the basis for SWB judgments (Frijda, 1999; Kahneman, 1999). Affective evaluations take the form of emotions and moods. Although there are debates about the nature of and relation between these two constructs (Morris, 1999), emotions are generally thought to be short-lived reactions that are tied to specific events or external stimuli (Frijda, 1999), whereas moods are thought to be more diffuse affective feelings that may not be tied to specific events (Morris, 1999). By studying the types of affective reactions that individuals experience, researchers can gain an understanding of the ways that people evaluate the conditions and events in their lives.

Much research on affective evaluations has been focused on the ways that emotions and moods can be categorized, and there are two general approaches to this issue. Some researchers focus on determining whether there are a small number of basic emotions. Researchers who work from this perspective generally try first to identify the basic features of emotions. They can then go on to examine variations in these features in order to determine which emotions are basic. Frijda (1999), for

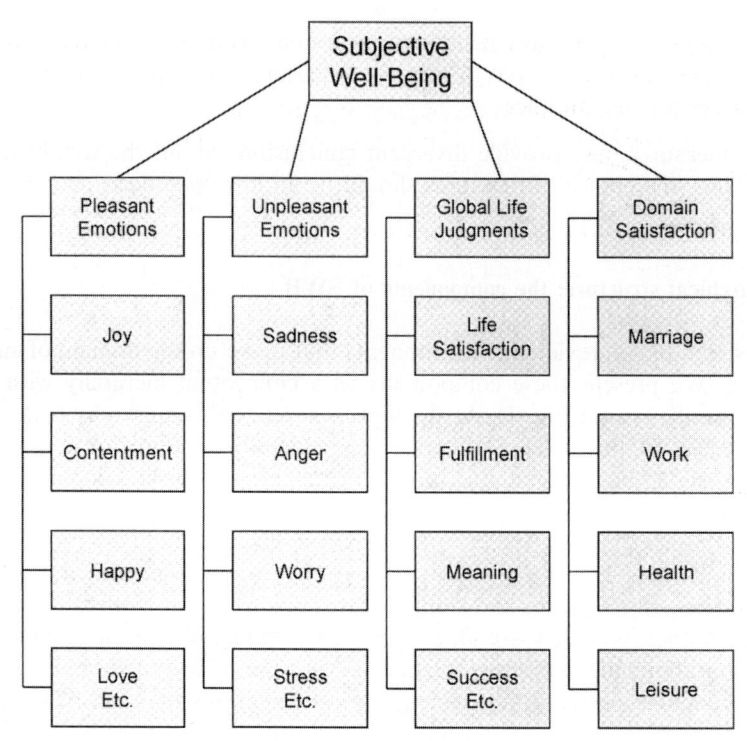

Fig. 1. A hierarchical model of happiness.

example, argued that there are five basic features of emotions. First, emotions involve affect, meaning that they are associated with a feeling of pleasure or pain. Second, emotions include an appraisal of an object or event as good or bad. Third, the elicitation of an emotion is generally associated with changes in behavior toward the environment (or at least with changes in the readiness for specific behaviors). Fourth, emotions often involve autonomic arousal. And finally, emotions often involve changes in cognitive activity.

By examining variation in these features, researchers can classify which emotions are basic. For example, some researchers have argued that a basic emotion will have a distinct action readiness or motivational property (Izard, 1977; Frijda, 1986). Seemingly different emotions with the same action tendency may then be seen as variations of the same basic emotion. Other researchers have avoided analyzing the component parts of emotions, instead relying on criteria such as whether there is a universally recognized facial expression for the emotion (e.g. Ekman et al., 1972). Some of the basic emotions that have been identified are listed under the Positive and Negative Affect headings in Fig. 1 (though see Ortony and Turner, 1990, for a more complete review of the basic emotion literature).

An alternative to the basic emotion approach is the dimensional approach. Researchers working from this perspective have noted that certain emotions and moods tend to be highly correlated both between individuals and within individuals over time. For example, individuals who experience high levels of sadness are also likely to experience high levels of other negative emotions such as fear or anxiety. The fact that these emotions are correlated suggests that they may result from some of the same underlying processes. Thus, according to the dimensional approach, it should be possible to identify certain basic dimensions that underlie the covariation among the various emotions and moods that people experience. Research into the causes and outcomes of emotional experience can then progress by focusing on these underlying dimensions rather than on the individual emotions themselves. Subjective well-being researchers often focus on emotional dimensions rather than specific emotions, because over long periods of time, distinct emotions of the same valence are moderately to strongly correlated (Zelenski and Larsen, 2000).

Most dimensional models of emotions have focused on two underlying dimensions. Russell (1980), for example, argued that the orthogonal dimensions of pleasantness and arousal can be used to describe the variation in emotional experience. According to this model, each emotion can be described by noting the extent to which it is a pleasant emotion and the extent to which it is an aroused emotion. An emotion like excitement, for example, would be a pleasant, highly aroused emotion; whereas an emotion like contentment would be pleasant but much lower in arousal. By plotting emotions on these two dimensions, researchers have developed circumplex models of emotional structure, with most emotions located somewhere on the outer circle formed by orthogonal pleasantness and arousal axes (see Larsen and Diener, 1992, for a discussion of circumplex models; see Fabrigar et al., 1997 and Watson et al., 1999 for recent evidence on the circumplex structure).

Other researchers have argued that although pleasantness and arousal are useful dimensions in a descriptive sense, these axes do not reflect the underlying systems that are responsible for the affect that individuals experience. Watson and Tellegen (1985), for example, argued that the pleasantness and arousal dimensions should be rotated 45 degrees to form separate activated positive and negative affect dimensions. Positive affect is a combination of arousal and pleasantness, and it includes emotions such as active, alert, and excited; negative affect is a combination of arousal and unpleasantness, and it includes emotions such as anxious, angry, and fearful. Like other researchers before him (e.g., Costa and McCrae, 1980), Tellegen (1985) noted that the positive affect dimension is closely aligned with the broad personality trait of extraversion, whereas negative affect is closely aligned with the broad personality trait of neuroticism. Tellegen (1985) argued that together, these extraversion/positive affect and neuroticism/negative affect dimensions reflect two underlying personality systems that are responsible for many of the individual differences in affect and behavior. Thus, he argued, studying these rotated dimensions (rather than arousal and pleasantness) is more likely to prove fruitful when attempting to understand the basic processes underlying personality and emotion.

The disagreements about the structure of affect have led to a sometimes confusing debate about whether positive and negative affect are really separable and independent dimensions (as we have suggested in Fig. 1). Part of the confusion regarding this issue has to do with the fact that the dimensions that are most likely to be independent (the activated positive and negative affect dimensions in Watson and Tellegen's (1985) model) were given names that suggest bipolarity. Watson et al. (1999) recently renamed these constructs as positive activation and negative activation to emphasize the activated nature of these dimensions and to avoid some of this confusion. Yet, the debate is not simply semantic, and there are many unresolved issues regarding the independence of positive and negative affect. Some researchers have suggested that at any given moment, positive and negative affect are bipolar, whereas when aggregated over time they become independent (Diener and Emmons, 1985). According to this view people cannot experience positive and negative emotions simultaneously (Diener and Iran-Nejad, 1986), but over time, people could experience high levels of both. Other researchers have suggested that positive and negative emotions can, in unusual circumstances, be experienced at the same time (Larsen et al., 2001). Whatever the final outcome of this debate, it seems wise to separately assess positive and negative affect, especially in light of the fact that there are often different correlates of the two.

2.1.1. Frequency and intensity of positive and negative affect

A final issue that arises when assessing affective components of well-being is what type of emotional experience we should measure. At any given moment a person may experience either high or low intensity emotions. Is the person who experiences intense positive emotions better off than the person who is only mildly happy most of the time, or is the frequency with which an individual experiences positive emotions the most important factor in determining overall affective well-being? Research shows that the intensity with which one feels emotions is not the same thing as the frequency with which he or she feels these emotions, and these two aspects of emotional experience have distinct implications for well-being.

Schimmack and Diener (1997) used experience sampling methods to demonstrate that emotional intensity can be separated from frequency. Specifically, by assessing moods and emotions repeatedly over time, researchers can assess frequency by summing the number of times a person reports experiencing an emotion. Intensity can be determined by examining the average intensity of that emotion when a person reports feeling it. The importance and validity of these two components can then be determined by comparing these scores with other measures of well-being.

In their investigation of this issue, Diener et al. (1991) suggested that frequency of emotional experience was more important for overall well-being than was intensity. Specifically, they argued that there were both theoretical and empirical reasons for focusing on frequency information. First, at a theoretical level, it seems as though the processes that lead to intense positive emotions are likely often to lead to intense negative emotions, and thus very intense emotions often cancel each other out. Laboratory studies show, for instance, that people who use dampening or amplifying strategies with emotion are likely to use the same strategies with both positive and negative affect (Larsen et al., 1987; Diener et al., 1992). Thus, people who experience positive emotions intensely will likely experience negative emotions intensely, a finding that is supported by research on individual differences in affect intensity (Larsen and Diener, 1987).

A second theoretical reason why intensity should not affect overall levels of well-being is that very intense emotional experiences are very rare. Diener et al. (1991) reviewed evidence showing that extremely intense positive and negative emotions (those that get the highest scores on emotion scales) are very rare when emotions are sampled repeatedly over time. Thus, if these events occur infrequently, they are unlikely to influence overall levels of well-being.

A third reason why researchers might focus on frequency information is that frequency-based measures appear to have better psychometric characteristics. Kahneman (1999), for instance, argued that it is not difficult to determine whether one is feeling positive or negative at any given moment. Reports based on this type of question are likely to be valid and to have a similar meaning across respondents. On the other hand, it is difficult to accurately report how intensely positive or negative one is feeling, and the meaning of an intensity scale may vary across individuals. Intensity reports may mean different things for different people. Research on this issue does suggest that frequency-based measures have more validity than intensity based measures. For example, Thomas and Diener (1990) and Schimmack and Diener (1997) both found that people could recall frequency information better than intensity information. It is not surprising that Diener et al. (1991) and Schimmack and Diener (1997) both found that frequency reports were more strongly related to global well-being measures.

To determine people's general level of affective well-being, frequency measures appear to be theoretically and empirically more desirable than intensity measures. Yet, there are cases where intensity information can be important. Wirtz et al. (in press), for example, found that when people's emotions were sampled multiple times over the course of a spring break vacation, the intensity of their emotions was a better predictor of desire to go on another similar vacation than was the frequency of their emotions. In addition, research suggests that the intensity of emotions may be related to specific personality traits. Eid and Diener (1999) found that intra-personal variability in emotion was related to neuroticism and lower levels of overall happiness. Thus, intensity information can be useful for examining certain questions about emotional well-being.

2.1.2. Recommendations

Although debates about the nature of affective well-being continue, researchers interested in SWB can confidently tap the emotional well-being components by assessing a broad range of positive and negative emotions. Researchers who are interested in recording a general sense of a person's affective well-being will want to examine the separable positive and negative affect dimensions. Researchers who are interested in specific emotions should consider the debates about basic emotions and insure that they include multiple-item measures of these more specific components. We should note, however, that the study of emotions can occur at even more specific levels. Researchers can assess specific emotions, but they can also go on to examine specific situations in which these emotions can be elicited. For example, some individuals may feel anger in some situations but not in others. Researchers must tailor their emotion assessment strategies to the specific research questions in which they are interested. If separate emotions do not produce different results, they can be aggregated. Although the frequency of emotions appears to be more related to long-term happiness, the intensity of emotions will certainly be of interest for many research questions.

Affect reflects a person's ongoing evaluations of the conditions in his or her life. It is easy to see why these dimensions make up an important part of the general subjective well-being construct. It would be hard to imagine a person saying he or she has high well-being if that person experiences high levels of negative affect and low levels of positive affect. Yet, we must caution that affective well-being, alone, does not appear to be sufficient for most people when they provide an overall evaluation of their lives. People do not seem to want purely hedonistic experiences of positive affect. Instead, people want these experiences to be tied to specific outcomes that reflect their goals and values, as we will discuss later in the section on Trade-offs. Thus, domains beyond affective well-being must be assessed to gain a complete understanding of a person's well-being.

2.2. Life satisfaction

The affective components of well-being described above reflect people's ongoing evaluations of the conditions in their lives. We can contrast this type of evaluation with global judgments about the quality of a person's life. Presumably, individuals can examine the conditions in their lives, weigh the importance of these conditions, and then evaluate their lives on a scale ranging from dissatisfied to satisfied. We refer to this global, cognitive judgment as life satisfaction. Because we assume that this judgment requires cognitive processing, much research has focused on the way that these judgments are made.

After years of research, we now know quite a bit about how life satisfaction judgments are made. For example, it appears as though most individuals do not (and perhaps cannot) examine all aspects of their lives and then weight them appropriately. Instead, because this task is difficult, people likely use a variety of shortcuts when coming up with satisfaction judgments (Robinson and Clore, in press; Schwarz and Strack, 1999). Specifically, people are likely to use information that is salient at the time of the judgment. For example, Schwarz and Clore (1983) showed that seemingly irrelevant factors such as the weather at the time of judgment can influence ratings of life satisfaction. This research suggests that current mood can influence ratings of life satisfaction, even if that current mood is not indicative of one's overall levels of affective well-being.

Yet, even with the use of these shortcuts, there is substantial temporal stability in people's life satisfaction judgments (Magnus and Diener, 1991; Ehrhardt et al., 2000). This is because much of the information that is used in making satisfaction judgments appears to be chronically accessible. In other words, people's satisfaction judgments are based on the information that is available at the time of the judgment, but much of that information remains the same over time. If there are domains in people's lives that are extremely important to them, this information is likely to come to mind when people are asked to make judgments about their life satisfaction. In fact, there is evidence that people seem to know what type of information they use when they make life satisfaction judgments. Schimmack et al. (2002), for example, found that those domains that people said were important in making life satisfaction judgments were more strongly correlated with life satisfaction than domains that were rated as being less important. So although the processes by which satisfaction judgments are made can often lead to what may be thought of as mistakes, in many cases people use relevant and stable information, resulting in stable and meaningful satisfaction judgments.

The research on the processes of satisfaction judgments has led to a greater understanding of the relation between affective and cognitive well-being. It appears that people do use their affective well-being as information when judging their life satisfaction, but this is only one piece of information. The weight that this information is given varies across individuals and cultures. Suh et al. (1998), for example, found that participants from individualistic cultures relied on their affective well-being to a greater extent than participants from collectivist cultures when judging life satisfaction. Collectivists, in contrast, relied more on whether or not significant others thought their life was on the right track. Additional information beyond affective well-being is used when constructing life satisfaction judgments. Thus, the association between affective and cognitive well-being will not be perfect, and will vary across samples. Even within a culture, individual differences can moderate what type of information is included in global judgments. For example, the daily experience of pleasure is a greater predictor of life satisfaction for individuals high in sensation seeking than for those low in sensation seeking (Oishi et al., 2001).

Other sources of information that people may use include comparisons with important standards. Campbell et al. (1976) argued that individuals look at various important life domains and compare these life domains to a variety of comparison standards. For example, an individual may compare her income to the income of those around her, to the income she had in the past, or to the income she desires for the future. Interestingly, just as people seem to be very flexible in the type of information that they use when making satisfaction judgments, they also seem flexible in the way they use this information. Diener and Fujita (1997) noted, for example, that social comparison effects are not always consistent across studies or across individuals. Sometimes people may look at individuals who are better off and see these individuals as inspirations (resulting in positive well-being), whereas at other times this type of comparison would lead to a negative comparison and lower levels of well-being.

The advantage of life satisfaction as a measure of well-being is that this type of measure captures a global sense of well-being from the respondent's own perspective. People seem to use their own criteria for making this judgment, and research has begun to identify what these criteria are and how they vary across individuals. Yet, the processes that allow for these individual differences also allow for irrelevant information to be included in satisfaction judgments. People often use whatever information is at hand at the time of judgment, and sometimes this can lead to unreliable or less valid measures. However, on average, the research suggests that although experimental studies can demonstrate the errors that people make, most information that is used in satisfaction judgments is information that is chronically accessible and, presumably, important to the individual.

2.3. Domain satisfactions

The fourth component that is included in our hierarchical model of SWB is domain satisfaction. Domain satisfaction reflects a person's evaluation of the specific domains in his or her life. Presumably, if we were able to assess all the important domains in a person's life, we would be able to reconstruct a global life satisfaction judgment using a bottom-up process. But, as we noted above, the process by which the domain satisfaction judgments are aggregated, and the weight that is given to each domain may vary by individuals. Diener et al. (2002), for example, found that happy individuals were more likely to weight the best domains in their life heavily, whereas unhappy individuals were more likely to weight the worst domains in their life heavily. Thus, domain satisfaction scores do not simply reflect the component parts of a life satisfaction judgment, and they can provide unique information about a person's overall well-being.

More importantly, domain satisfaction will be important for researchers interested in the effects of well-being in particular areas. For example, if a researcher is trying to foster increased well-being at work, job satisfaction may provide a more sensitive measure of these effects than any global well-being scale will. Similarly, researchers who work with certain populations may want to separately assess domain satisfactions that are particularly relevant for that group. Students may be very concerned about grades and learning, whereas the elderly may be more concerned about health and social support. Thus, domain satisfaction scores can provide information about the way individuals construct global well-being judgments; but they can also provide more detailed information about the specific aspects of one's life that are going well or going poorly.

2.4. Convergent and discriminant validity of SWB components

Conceptually, each of the components of well-being represents a distinct way of evaluating one's life. Positive and negative affect reflect the immediate, on-line reactions to the good and bad conditions of one's life. Domain satisfactions reflect the cognitive evaluation of specific aspects of one's life. Life satisfaction reflects a global judgment that is constructed through somewhat idiosyncratic processes across individuals, but which provides useful information about a person's satisfaction with life as a whole. Research on the discriminant validity of these constructs shows that they are not only theoretically distinct, but also empirically separable. Lucas et al. (1996), for instance, used self- and informant-reports of well-being constructs to examine the convergent and discriminant validity of positive affect, negative affect, and life satisfaction. Different methods of measuring the same construct tended to converge, and the correlations across methods of measuring the same construct were usually stronger than the correlations between measures of different constructs. Thus, the empirical evidence suggests that positive affect, negative affect, and life satisfaction are empirically distinct constructs.

2.5. Summary

There are a number of separable components of SWB. To obtain a complete picture of an individual's evaluation of his or her life, more than one component must be measured. For researchers who are interested in attaining a complete evaluation, we recommend that they assess positive affect, negative affect, satisfaction with important domains, and life satisfaction. Depending on the specific research question, additional components may be needed. For example, researchers who are interested in specific emotions like anxiety, anger, joy, or love should make sure to administer reliable and valid measures of these emotions. These researchers may want to focus on the basic emotion literature when choosing measures; whereas researchers who want a general understanding of affective well-being can focus more on the broad affective dimensions. Furthermore, researchers need to consider the time-frame of their measures, an issue to which we now turn.

3. Temporal sequence and stages

In this section we describe the multifaceted nature of SWB with an emphasis on the unfolding of different stages or components over time. These components, ranging from external events to global judgments of one's life, are depicted in Fig. 2. In particular, we highlight the transition between the stages and the divergences among measures of the different stages. Although convergence of measurement is often regarded as the ideal, we will see that discrepancies are also interesting and can inform a theory of SWB.

Our conceptualization begins with two basic premises. First, we have organized our model in terms of sequential stages that unfold over time. Thus, the temporal stages are seen as alternative facets of SWB, and are not identical to one another. Second, no one stage or component can be considered "true" happiness. For instance, both momentary affect and memory for emotions are important to SWB.

At step one, events happen to people, but their effects on long-term well-being are weak (Suh et al., 1996). In fact, all demographics account for less than 20% of variance in SWB (Campbell et al., 1976). Because there are many intervening steps between an event and the construction of a global life satisfaction judgment, events can only have a distal effect on SWB. On the other hand, according to our model, events are expected to have greater influence on online emotional reactions. For example, daily events such as health, family, and social interactions, have an

External Event

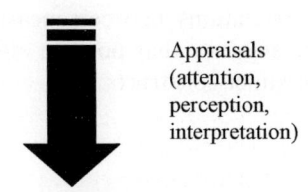

⬇ Appraisals
(attention,
perception,
interpretation)

Online Emotional Reaction

⬇ Encoding,
Repetition,
Rumination,
Reminiscing

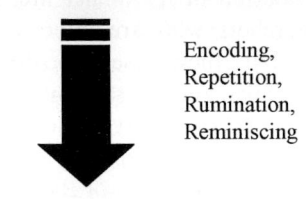

Memory for Emotion

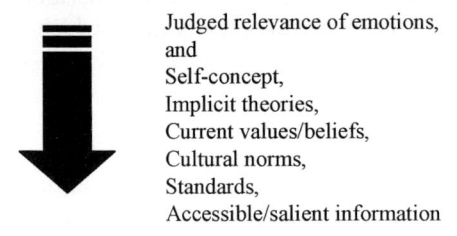

⬇ Judged relevance of emotions,
and
Self-concept,
Implicit theories,
Current values/beliefs,
Cultural norms,
Standards,
Accessible/salient information

Global SWB Judgment

Fig. 2. A temporal stage model of subjective well-being.

impact on the daily mood of nursing home patients (Lawton et al., 1995), but we would not expect daily events to influence global judgments as strongly. In addition, the emotional impact of events will depend largely on people's appraisals, that is, individual differences in attention, perception, and interpretation of the event. Lazarus (1982, 1984) has written extensively on the subject of appraisals, therefore, we will not go into much detail here. For our model, it is sufficient to say that the transition from an event to one's emotional reaction involves evaluating whether the event is good or bad for one's goals and whether one has the resources necessary to cope with the event. Obviously not everyone will react the same way to the same events because events hold different meanings for different people.

The next stage, the on-line emotional reaction, is itself complex and multifaceted. The many aspects of a single emotional experience include physiological responses, nonverbal or behavioral expressions, and the verbal labeling of emotions. Even among these subcomponents of a single temporal stage there are sometimes discrepancies. For instance, a "repressor" might deny feelings of anxiety while showing increased perspiration, heart rate, and so forth (e.g. Weinberger et al., 1979). The verbal on-line measures are postulated to relate to memory for emotions, the next phase, but less so to global evaluations. On-line emotions become encoded in memory by a number of processes, including repetition of emotional information, rumination, and reminiscing, which can influence the degree of relation between on-line experience and the recall of that experience.

Once the on-line emotions are encoded in memory, they do not remain static. Instead, the memory is constantly reconstructed, and this is a critical feature of our model. We treat memory as a separate phenomenon from on-line experience. Some factors involved in the transition from on-line emotion to memory for emotion – that is, factors responsible for the discrepancy between the two stages – include self-concept (Diener et al., 1984; Feldman Barrett, 1997), current beliefs (Levine et al., 2001), implicit theories (Ross, 1989), and cultural norms (Oishi, 2000). To illustrate, when McFarland et al. (1989) asked women to recall their mood during menstruation, they found that women recalled more negative emotion than they previously reported on-line. Furthermore, the amount of negative emotion remembered was moderated by the women's implicit theories about the relation between menstruation and mood. Similarly, Feldman Barrett (1997) found that individuals who scored high on trait measures of neuroticism overestimated in retrospect the amount of negative emotion they experienced online, while individuals high in trait extraversion overestimated the amount of on-line positive emotion. In describing the discrepancy between on-line emotions and memory, Robinson and Clore (2002) noted that two strategies of retrieval can guide recall. Recollections over a wide time frame (e.g. over the past month or year) rely on heuristic information, such as the self-concept. For narrower time frames (e.g. the past hour or day), people use a "retrieve and aggregate" strategy. That is, they recall specific instances of felt emotion and aggregate them to form their retrospective reports. In support of this notion and our model, Scollon et al. (2002) found that recalled reports were predicted by self-concept measures above and beyond on-line emotion.

At the broadest stage are global constructions, including life satisfaction. This stage is influenced by all the previous stages, but again, the degree to which depends on proximity. Thus, on-line experiences can influence global constructions. For example, someone who constantly experiences unpleasant mood would probably evaluate his/her life as unsatisfactory. However the extent to which on-line emotions influence global constructions depends on people's memory for emotions. In support of this, Schimmack et al. (2002) found that not only did hedonic memories correlate with life satisfaction judgments, but changes in memories correlated with life satisfaction as well. In addition to affective information, life satisfaction judgments incorporate several other sources that vary across cultures and individuals. As discussed earlier, these include cultural norms (Suh et al., 1998), and irrelevant but salient information (Schwarz and Clore, 1983). In some sense, global judgments such as life satisfaction, meaning in life, and fulfillment, capture the non-hedonistic meanings of happiness that were advanced by Democritus and Aristotle (even though the global judgments are subjective).

The current picture of SWB is more complex than any one stage can capture. Although each component is influenced by the previous stages, the stages are uniquely influenced by additional factors such as self-concept. Furthermore, there is evidence that the various stages converge moderately, but there are also processes that lead to differences between the stages. Likewise, the different stages of SWB are expected to predict different outcomes. For example, two studies indicate that recalled emotion is a better predictor of behavioral choices than on-line emotion. Wirtz et al. (in press) had students record their on-line emotions during a vacation and found that the degree to which students wanted to take a similar vacation later was strongly predicted by how much fun and enjoyment participants recalled, more so than the amount of fun and enjoyment they reported during the vacation. Similarly, in a study of dating couples, Oishi (2002) found that couples who misremembered interactions with their romantic partner as being more pleasant than in on-line reports were more likely to have intact relationships six months later.

In terms of practical application, the emerging evidence in support of a multi-componential approach to SWB raises new concerns about the measurement of SWB among the elderly. For instance, how should researchers measure the SWB of an elderly person with memory loss? The meaning of global or retrospective measures might be challenged because recollections about past emotions incorporate self-concept information, perhaps to an even greater degree than actual experience. And as memory loss becomes more severe, we predict, the recall of emotions will be more strongly influenced by self-concept. If researchers only rely on retrospective reports, they may be learning more about the self-concept of the elderly than about moment-to-moment experiences.

Philosophically, reconstructive memory also poses an intriguing question: Is happiness the *experience* or the *memory* of pleasant emotions? According to our model, no one measure deserves elevated status. Both the experience and memory (which includes some self-concept information), along with other components, are important. Nor can the different measures be considered substitutes for one another. Often researchers measure a single component or several components to see what correlates most highly with a given outcome measure. Such a practice belies the complexity and inter-relatedness of the different levels of SWB.

What the multi-component approach to SWB suggests is that measures at each stage provide interesting information, but researchers need to understand and specify the components of SWB they are measuring. In some ways, each stage of SWB reflects a different philosophical tradition of happiness. For example, on-line emotion is related to hedonistic views of happiness, whereas global judgments are more closely related to eudaimonia or Democritus's ideas. In the measurement section, we will discuss what researchers need to consider in order to assess SWB. For instance, most researchers would prefer to measure only the recall or global stages of SWB, and we will discuss how valid this practice seems to be.

4. Stability and consistency of SWB

Subjective well-being variables are thought to reflect the actual conditions in a person's life. Thus, when these conditions change, reports of SWB should change accordingly. Yet, because there is some degree of stability in these conditions, we should also expect SWB measures to be relatively stable over time. Furthermore, SWB constructs are influenced by a variety of stable personality factors, a finding that supports the notion that SWB should be relatively stable (Diener and Lucas, 2000), because adult personality is very stable (Costa and McCrae, 1988). In fact, in the literature, there are even debates about whether SWB should be considered a trait or a state (Veenhoven, 1994, 1998; Stones et al., 1995; Lykken and Tellegen, 1996; Ehrhardt et al., 2000). In this section, we review the evidence regarding the stability and consistency of well-being constructs.

There is considerable evidence that SWB variables do exhibit some degree of stability. Magnus and Diener (1991), for example, found that life satisfaction scores exhibited stability coefficients of 0.58 over a 4-year period. Even when different methods of assessment were used to measure life satisfaction (e.g. self- and informant-reports), stability was high ($r = 0.52$). Ehrhardt et al. (2000) examined life satisfaction reports in a large, nationally representative German panel study, and they found stability coefficients of 0.27 across 10 years. For the purposes of this chapter, we reanalyzed this data set (with an additional 5 years of satisfaction reports; see Lucas, Clark, Georgellis, and Diener, in press) and found that stability coefficients did not drop off as the length of the study increased. The correlation between life satisfaction in the first year of the study and life satisfaction in the 15th year was still 0.28. We should also note that this satisfaction measure is a single-item scale, and thus, it probably does not have ideal psychometric characteristics. Across those 15 years, stable between-person variance accounted for 44% of the total amount of variance in these measures. Thus, there is considerable stability in life satisfaction scores over long periods of time; though there are also changes that occur within persons over time.

Additional research shows that positive and negative affect scores are also somewhat stable over time. Watson and Walker (1996), for example, found 6- to 7-year stability coefficients in the range of 0.36 to 0.46 for positive affect and negative affect in a student sample, and Costa and McCrae (1988) found 6-year stability coefficients in the 0.50 range in an adult sample. Costa and McCrae's findings are particularly impressive given that these stability coefficients compared self-reports of affect with spouse ratings of affect. Thus, like Magnus and Diener's (1991) longitudinal study of life satisfaction, stability cannot be explained solely by stability of self-concept or by response artifacts.

The stability of well-being measures does not mean, however, that these measures are insensitive to changing life circumstances. On the contrary, Lucas et al. (in press) and Clark et al. (in press) used the 15-year German panel study described above to show that life satisfaction scores increased following marriage and decreased following widowhood or unemployment. Thus, life circumstances do influence life satisfaction scores, as we would expect. Interestingly, in both the Lucas et al. study and the Clark et al. study, satisfaction scores were very stable from the periods before an event to the periods after the event, suggesting that relative satisfaction scores are stable even in the face of changing life circumstances (also see Costa et al., 1987) that can influence mean levels.

A different way to examine the stability of SWB constructs is to look within persons across situations. If well-being reflects a person's evaluation of his or her life as a whole, we would not expect scores to be completely determined by changing situational factors. Diener and Larsen (1984) examined this question by asking participants to complete mood reports multiple times a day for multiple days. They found that positive affect, negative affect, and life satisfaction were very stable even across diverse situations. For example, positive affect in work situations correlated 0.70 with positive affect in recreation situations, and negative affect in work situations correlated 0.74 with negative affect in recreation situations (similar correlations were found across social vs. alone situations and across novel vs. typical situations). Correlations were even higher for life satisfaction scores, often around 0.95. Thus, well-being is not completely determined by situational factors. A substantial proportion of the variance in well-being reports is stable across situations and even over long periods of time.

We should also note that, to some extent, the consistency of well-being may vary across cultures. Oishi et al. (2002), for example, showed that there is less consistency in affect in samples from Japan than there is in samples from the United States. In other words, people's affect varies to a greater extent across situations in Japan than it does in the United States. Thus, the notion of a happy person may be less meaningful in Japan because there is less person-level variance in SWB scores. Clearly more research is needed, but we recommend that researchers interpret the stability and consistency data cautiously until we can determine the factors that moderate the extent to which people are stable over time and across situations.

5. Affect vs. cognition

SWB includes both an affective (i.e. on-going evaluations of one's life) and a cognitive component (i.e. life satisfaction). Theorists have long debated the degree to which affect and cognition are related (see Zajonc, 1980; Lazarus, 1982, 1984). This controversy bears particular relevance to the study of SWB because it highlights the dependence, and yet separability, of the two systems, suggesting a need to measure affect and cognition separately (even though they are not entirely independent) in order to gain a more complete picture of SWB.

On the one hand, researchers such as LeDoux (2000) argue that some simple emotions such as fear can occur without complex cognitive processing, or as a result of unconscious processing (Zajonc, 1980). Similarly, some people have been shown to deny their subjective feelings, despite showing a physiological reaction to events (Shedler et al., 1993). Both lines of evidence suggest that non-verbal, non-cognitive measures (e.g. eyeblink startle and cortisol) might detect reactions that self-report measures do not.

On the other hand, cognitive appraisals play an important role in shaping our reactions to events. For example, if a student feels responsible for getting a good grade on an exam (appraisal), then she will feel happy about it. As well, cultural norms provide a frame for interpreting events. That is, the emotions a person feels will tend to fit into his or her worldview. Returning to our example, the student who feels responsible for the event of making a good grade on an exam might not label her feeling as pride if her culture regards pride as a sinful emotion. Indeed, cultural norms for emotions are strongly related to reports of subjective experience (see Eid and Diener, 2001), and the rank ordering of societies on measures such as life satisfaction bear considerable resemblance to the rank ordering of societies on emotion norms (see Diener et al., 2000). Thus, self-report measures will detect what individuals label about their subjective feelings, although this is only one aspect of the emotional experience.

An added complication to the affect–cognition debate stems from disagreements about what constitutes cognition (Mathews and MacLeod, 1994). Some theorists argue that cognition includes only higher-order processing; other definitions include lower-order processes such as attention. Although we recognize the importance of attention in affect regulation (see Mathews and MacLeod, 1994; Segerstrom, 2001), of central importance to the present discussion of SWB are the higher-order conscious processes such as cognitive judgments or global evaluations of one's life.

By treating affect and cognition as partially separable constructs, we invite the possibility that one can be satisfied with one's life, and yet experience little pleasant affect, and vice versa. To illustrate, let us consider the SWB of a spouse and caretaker of an Alzheimer's patient. Narrative accounts of individuals who have cared for family members with Alzheimer's disease (e.g. Bayley, 1999) suggest a caretaker's daily life is fraught with frustration and difficulty, with brief and infrequent joys. Despite a preponderance of negative affect, however, the caretaker might still evaluate his overall life positively. This discrepancy between affect and cognitive judgments can occur for several reasons.

First, as discussed in the previous section, people rely on different sources of information when constructing global judgments. Even though enjoyment in a domain tends to correlate with satisfaction in that domain, affective information might be highly important for some people, but irrelevant for others (e.g., Oishi et al., 2001). One possibility is that with certain life tasks such as caregiving or with certain life stages, affect is given less weight in judgments of life satisfaction (cf. Carstensen, 1995), although this remains an empirical question. Second, the individual's culture will provide a framework for interpreting the importance of affect. As noted earlier, cultures differ in the degree to which they rely on affective information in life satisfaction constructions (Suh et al., 1998). But the impact of culture extends further because cultures also clearly differ in what they consider normative tasks. Thus, in a culture in which caring for the elderly is expected, the caretaker might derive a sense of satisfaction from doing the "right thing" and following cultural norms, even though the caretaking is unpleasant.

Third, the works of LeDoux (2000) and Shedler et al. (1993) suggest that the caretaker may be unable or unwilling to articulate his subjective emotional experience. Physiological measures might indicate a different picture, again underscoring the need for multiple measures, including non-cognitive ones.

Finally, people may rely on different standards in judging life satisfaction than in evaluating specific events. For example, daily affect may be determined by whether one is meeting one's lower-level goals, whereas global judgments may be determined by higher-level, more abstract goals. This allows for one's moment-to-moment affect to be quite negative while the bigger picture might reveal a sense of satisfaction for fulfilling some larger goal. Unfortunately, these questions have not yet been empirically tested, and it remains for future research to uncover which standards influence the different types and levels of SWB.

6. The functioning mood system

Although negative emotions are usually unpleasant, theorists have recognized their functionality. For example, fear can motivate us to avoid danger, anger can push us to correct an injustice, and sadness can make us withdraw so that we can renew our resources and make new plans of action after loss. Volumes have been written on the adaptive functions of negative emotions, but much less on the positive side. Recently, Fredrickson (1998, 2001) outlined a "broaden and build model" explaining that the function of positive emotions is to lead to sociability, play, and exploration. Thus, positive emotions help us build our social and material resources, and help us learn new behaviors for the future. Positive emotions occur when things are going well, and when we have the time to engage in actions that will benefit us later.

If emotions are, in many cases, functional and adaptive, and the emotion system has come to us through evolution to guide behavior, it would seem dysfunctional never to experience any negative emotions. In other words, it would also be maladaptive to chronically experience high positive moods all of the time, regardless of the circumstances. After all, the adaptiveness of the emotion system depends on its ability to provide calibrated feedback about one's relation to the environment, and chronic states of any valence would fail to serve that purpose because they are unresponsive to events. Berenbaum et al. (2002) have similarly noted that there is nothing inherently good or bad about emotions of either valence, but rather excesses of either happiness or sadness present problems. A person who can only feel happy would not be able to avoid danger or other bad situations; such a person would be overly expansive and take on new goals even when it is not appropriate. This kind of behavior can best be seen in manics. In extreme form, manics start more projects than they can finish, and they do not exercise caution and good judgment in planning. This is not the picture of happiness that we are advancing. Happiness is not to be equated with mania or uninterrupted ecstasy. Instead, the adaptable happy person should have moods that fluctuate to some degree in reaction to good and bad events.

Indeed the data support both of these notions. First, in studies of thousands of people, we have found that it is very rare for people to be at a 10 on a 10-point scale, or to be at the very top of the Satisfaction With Life Scale (SWLS: Diener et al., 1985). Furthermore, even when people rate themselves as extremely satisfied, we find in follow-up that they are usually not at the top of the scale two years later. That is, people might occasionally move up to a euphoric state, but they do not stay there for long (Diener and Seligman, 2002).

Second, even happy people have pleasant and unpleasant moods. An investigation of 22 individuals who scored in the top 10% on various SWB measures revealed that even these people, although extremely satisfied with life, occasionally had unpleasant affect. Diener and Larsen (1984) found that although people have stable and consistent average moods, their momentary moods fluctuate. Thus, it is possible for happy people to react to events but still maintain an average positive level around which their moods fluctuate. This allows even happy people to react to negative events and not be stuck in a high happy mood.

But clearly chronic unrelieved negative emotion is undesirable and unhealthy. For one thing, people usually do not function well under conditions of severe and prolonged negative affect (Headey and Wearing, 1989; Hays et al., 1995; Hammen, 2002). This state is very unpleasant, and prolonged NA can interfere with quality of life as well as produce a greater likelihood of negative life events. Thus, whereas temporary experiences of negative affect are normal and can be functional, prolonged negative affect is often very dysfunctional.

7. Tradeoffs

Just as the above conception of happiness is not the picture of uninterrupted ecstasy, we believe that people, moreover, do not desire a life of unvariegated joys, at least not without some qualifications. First, people want their happy feelings to be justified. This view marks a clear departure from hedonistic philosophy in which personal enjoyment was considered the ultimate goal (Tatarkiewicz, 1976). Robert Nozick's (1974) philosophical idea of an "experience machine" provides a good example of why good feelings alone are not enough. Nozick (1974) imagines an experience machine that would create the subjective feeling of being engaged in fun, exciting, pleasant activities of one's choosing – for instance, writing a novel, making a new friend, feasting on a fine dinner, or lounging on a tropical beach. The experience machine would provide all the sensations that would ordinarily accompany the activity, but in actuality, the person would be lying in a laboratory hooked up to a computer.

Certainly few people would choose to plug in to the experience machine, even though the feelings it provides are desirable. As Nozick (1974) points out, there is more that matters than people's experiences from the inside. In fact, when we asked college students to rate some hypothetical scenarios and varied aspects of each scenario (such as whether the event occurred in reality or was the product of an experience machine, we found that the reality of events was extremely important, even for intensely pleasant and joyous activities. In particular, when the event involved achievement, momentary pleasure and memory of the event were secondary, but reality was essential. In other words, it would be pointless to plug in to the experience machine to feel as if one has won the Nobel Prize, when, in fact, one has not.

The second limitation on a hedonistic view of happiness is that people are willing, at times, to sacrifice momentary positive affect for other goals that they value. For example, Kim-Prieto (2002) found that Asian and Asian American students were more likely to choose tasks that met their parents' approval or tasks that would lead to achievement over other tasks that were described as fun and personally enjoyable. Thus, some individuals or groups may choose to maximize the non-hedonistic meanings of subjective well-being. Interestingly, Caucasian students preferred tasks that were fun or that maximized personal enjoyment. Other evidence comes from studies of self-improvement. Oishi and Diener (2001) found that when Caucasians were not good at a particular activity, they would switch to a different activity when given the opportunity. On the other hand, Asian Americans often pursued the activity they were not good at, but switched to a different activity if they were good at the first one. Such a strategy might improve one's skills, but would certainly not maximize immediate enjoyment (see also Heine et al., 2001).

8. Implications for measurement

Subjective well-being measures should tap well-being from a respondent's own perspective. For this reason, most studies of SWB have relied on self-report measures of the constructs. However, there are many reasons to be cautious in our interpretation of results based solely on self-report measures. Various response sets and response styles may influence people's ratings. Certain people may appear to be happier than others simply because they use high numbers on a response scale or because they want to look favorable in the eyes of the experimenter. Thus, although self-reports play a central role in SWB research, they must be supplemented with additional measurement techniques to obtain a complete understanding of the construct. In this section, we discuss the theoretical and methodological issues involved in selecting and using SWB measures (for a more detailed discussion, see Larsen and Fredrickson, 1999; Larsen et al., 2002; Lucas, Diener, and Larsen, 2003).

Self-reports of SWB vary considerably in their complexity. A number of studies have shown that even the simplest of these – the single-item measures – can exhibit some degree of reliability and validity. Diener et al. (2002), for instance, showed that a single item measure ("cheerfulness") could predict criterion variables 18 years later. In a separate investigation of this single-item measure, Diener et al. found that it correlated between 0.73 and 0.89 with a multiple-item measure of positive emotions that was assessed multiple times over a 3-month period. Similarly, Lucas et al. (in press) showed that a single-item measure of life satisfaction was relatively stable over time and was sensitive to changes in life events. Thus, if the focus of one's research is to get a relatively reliable and valid measure of well-being and one cannot afford to include a variety of self-report indicators, one can confidently assess these constructs using single-item measures. Of course, multiple item measures will increase reliability and breadth of coverage, and therefore, they are more desirable when one can afford to include them.

There are a number of reliable and valid measures of well-being constructs (see MacKay, 1980; Larsen et al., 1985; Andrews and Robinson, 1991; Stone, 1995; Lucas et al., in press for reviews). Most measure one or more well-being constructs using items with clear face validity. For example, life satisfaction scales may ask respondents the extent to which they agree with statements like: "I am satisfied with my life" or "In most ways my life is close to my ideal" (Diener et al., 1985). Positive and negative affect scales may ask people to indicate the extent to which they experience a series of emotions like "happiness," "sadness," "anger," "affection," or "fear." As indicated in our discussion of the structure of well-being, the different components of well-being can be exhibited in different ways. One could experience a high frequency of positive affect without experiencing affect intensely at any particular moment. Thus, it is often useful to separate frequency from intensity when asking about SWB variables. Similarly, because affect does change from moment to moment, it is important to specify the time frame of well-being reports. If one is interested in relatively short term variation in well-being, one can choose emotion questionnaires that ask only about the past hour, the past day, or the past week. Researchers interested in longer term mood levels, on the other hand, may want to choose scales that ask about mood over the past month, year, or affect in general.

A desirable alternative to asking people to retrospectively judge their happiness is to assess SWB using experience sampling methods (ESM; also known as ecological momentary assessment, Stone et al., 1999). In ESM, participants report their mood multiple times over a relatively long period of time. For example, in some studies, participants may be asked to carry handheld computers that signal an alarm five times a day for seven days. Each time the alarm sounds, the participant completes an emotion report. By using ESM techniques, researchers can study affect as a state and a trait. For example, within-person analyses can elucidate within-person emotional processes. At the same time, an individual's entire set of emotion reports can be averaged to create a reliable trait measure of his or her well-being. Using this type of aggregation process eliminates the need for participants to recall and attempt to derive an overall emotion report. Kahneman (1999) reviewed evidence that individuals have difficulty remembering and aggregating across multiple occasions, and a number of studies have now shown that ESM reports often give different information about a person's overall well-being than do global reports.

The difficulties that people have in accurately recalling their affective experiences suggest that alternative measures should be used when possible. One easily administered alternative to self-report is the informant- or observer-report technique. Although informants may have their own set of biases and response sets, these are likely to be different than the biases and response sets of the target person, and together self- and informant-reports can provide valid information about a person's well-being.

There are two general types of observer reports. In the known-informant approach, friends and family members rate a target person's well-being. Presumably, these known-informants see the target exhibiting well-being relevant behaviors in his or her life, and thus, they should be able to provide information about how happy that target individual is. In general, these informant reports show moderate to substantial convergence with self-report measures (McCrae and Costa, 1989; Diener et al., 1995; Lucas et al., 1996). An alternative to the known-informant approach is the expert-rater approach. Informants who do not know the target can be trained to interpret specific signals of emotional experience (Krokoff et al., 1989; Gottman, 1993). Raters can even be trained to interpret facial expressions of emotions. For example, in the Facial Action Coding System (FACS; Ekman and Friesen, 1978), raters are trained to recognize specific muscle movements that usually co-occur with emotional responses. The expert-rater approach has an important advantage over self-report and the known-informant reports: This technique can be used to attain relatively objective measures of a person's emotional response.

Along the same lines, researchers have looked beyond facial muscle movements to examine other physiological correlates of emotional feelings. Variables such as heart rate, heart rate acceleration, blood pressure, bodily temperature, finger temperature, respiration amplitude, and skin conductance have all been used to measure emotional response (Cacioppo et al., 2000). Other researchers have noted that activity in certain brain regions seems to be associated with both individual differences in emotional levels as well as within-person changes in emotional experience (Davidson, 1992). Thus, electro-encephalograms, PET scans and functional MRIs can be used to measure this differential activity. These measures, like the Facial Action Coding System, can provide relatively objective measures of well-being. However, much more research is needed before these measures can tap the subtle features that can be picked up in self-report measures. For example, many of the objective indicators of emotion seem to be able to distinguish positive emotions from negative emotions (and sometimes certain negative emotions from one another), but distinctions beyond these basic categories are difficult.

A final technique that researchers have used to measure well-being is to examine people's responses to emotion sensitive tasks. Seidlitz and Diener (1993), for example, asked people to recall as many happy experiences from their lives as they could in a short amount of time. Because performance on this task is correlated with well-being measures, it can be used as an alternative measure that is less susceptible to response styles and demand characteristics. Other researchers have exposed participants to word-completion tasks or word recognition tasks (for a review of these cognitive tasks, see Rusting, 1998). Happy people are more likely than unhappy people to complete word stems using positive words and they are quicker to recognize positive words. When social desirability, demand characteristics, or other measurement issues are a concern, these emotion sensitive tasks can provide a useful alternative to self-report measures.

Self-report measures of SWB are likely to remain the most frequently used measures of the constructs. These measures are quick and easy, they are sensitive enough to capture the subtle differences between the various components of well-being, and they have substantial reliability and validity. Yet, they are imperfect.

Researchers should use additional methods of measurement when possible. In addition, researchers who are interested in determining the way that people construct these judgments will need to use multiple self- and non-self-report techniques to understand these processes. Whatever the goal of the research, however, we recommend that people assess the multiple components of well-being separately when possible.

9. Implications for research on aging

Research on SWB over the lifespan offers a unique opportunity for psychologists interested in the processes underlying SWB judgments. SWB judgments are thought to reflect the conditions in one's life, and many of these conditions deteriorate in old age. Thus, studies of aging can provide a useful test of SWB theories. Yet when we examine the empirical evidence regarding age-related changes in SWB, there is somewhat of a paradox (Kunzmann et al., 2000). On the one hand, the objective conditions in one's life do seem to deteriorate. Income levels often decrease and the frequency of negative events including the death of one's spouse and friends and the experience of health problems often increase. Most research finds, however, that SWB levels remain stable over time, and sometimes these levels even increase (see Diener and Suh, 1998; Mroczek and Kolarz, 1998; Kunzmann et al., 2000; Lucas and Gohm, 2000; Lawton, 2001; Pinquart, 2001).

For example, Diener and Suh (1997a) examined age differences in well-being in a sample of approximately 60,000 respondents from 43 nations. They found that life satisfaction increased very slightly, positive affect decreased slightly, and negative affect decreased from age 20 to 60, but then increased slightly among the oldest individuals in their sample. Lucas and Gohm (2000) showed that this effect did not vary substantially when the different nations were studied individually. A number of researchers have replicated these findings, showing little change in life satisfaction, slight declines in positive affect (correlations in the range of -0.05 to -0.12), and initial declines followed by a leveling effect or even subsequent increases in negative affect (Carstensen et al., 2000; Kunzmann et al., 2000). In a recent meta-analysis, Pinquart (2001) found that the average correlations between positive affect and age and between negative affect and age were both negative, but very small: $r = 0.03$ for positive affect and $r = 0.01$ for negative affect. There were also significant quadratic effects: Positive affect decreased more quickly and negative affect began to increase among the very old.

Diener and Suh (1998) suggested that some of the decrease in both positive and negative affect might be due to the measurement of high arousal positive and negative emotions. For example, older adults may feel as much pleasantness, but they may do so with less intensity, or they may be less likely to experience high arousal emotions such as excitement or energy. Pinquart's (2001) meta-analysis supported this hypothesis. Declines in the experience of emotions were greater among high arousal emotion scales than among low arousal emotion scales. Thus, when assessing emotions in older adults, researchers should tap a broad range of high arousal and low arousal positive and negative emotions.

We should also caution that much of the evidence for age changes in subjective well-being comes from cross-sectional studies. Both Kunzmann et al. (2000) and Pinquart (2001) noted that the size of age effects often varies depending on whether cross-sectional or longitudinal methods are used. Because cross-sectional studies conflate age effects with cohort effects, the interpretation of the correlations in these studies is somewhat unclear. Pinquart found that the decline in positive affect was steeper in longitudinal studies than in cross-sectional studies, whereas the decline in negative affect was less steep in longitudinal studies than in cross-sectional studies. Given that these differences across methodologies exist, researchers must be careful in interpreting evidence from cross-sectional studies. However, we should also note that in their examination of a large German panel study, Ehrhardt et al. (2000) found that people responded to the questionnaire differently after repeated measurements. Thus, age-related changes in longitudinal studies may be confounded with practice effects.

A final measurement issue regarding SWB over the life-span is the extent to which changes reflect true differences over time versus changes in the self-concept. Most research that examines age-related changes in SWB relies upon global, retrospective measures. As we noted in the section on measurement, the global measures require participants to be able to accurately remember and aggregate across many moments and many life domains. Older individuals may have a more stable sense of self-concept than younger individuals, and self-reports of emotional experience may reflect this stable self-concept. Similarly, older individuals may not be able to remember and aggregate across multiple experiences as well as younger individuals. Only a few studies have used experience sampling methods to examine the effects of memory on SWB reports of older people. For example, Carstensen et al. (2000) asked participants ranging in age from 18 to 94 years old to complete emotion reports multiple times a day. They found that, consistent with existing literature, reports of negative affect declined until about age 60, and then leveled off after that. Positive affect, in their study, did not show any significant changes across the different age groups.

Although questions about the influence of measurement issues remain, evidence from a variety of methodologies suggests that SWB does not decline very much over time. Thus, we must ask why SWB does not seem to change, even when external life circumstances are declining (Kunzmann et al., 2000). A number of theories have suggested that changes in life circumstances are balanced by changes in emotion regulation. Specifically, research suggests that as individuals mature, they are better able to regulate their emotions (e.g. Gross et al., 1997) or are more motivated to regulate their emotions. Carstensen (1995), for example, argued that as one ages, he or she monitors the amount of time he or she has left before death. This monitoring, in turn, leads to changes in goals. As one becomes more aware of (and closer to) one's mortality, he or she should place a higher premium on experiencing pleasant emotional states. Thus, emotion regulation theories suggest that SWB may, in fact, increase with age, even in the face of declining life circumstances.

Increasingly, researchers are focusing on the functional nature of SWB (Fredrickson, 1998, 2001; Lyubomirsky et al., 2002; Lucas and Diener, 2003).

Researchers should keep this in mind when examining the SWB of older adults. If older adults do experience lower levels of well-being, this may not necessarily signal poor functioning. Instead, it may signal a functional response to real problems. Similarly, although some individuals may place a higher premium on experiencing positive emotions as they age (as Carstensen, 1995, suggested), others may be willing to trade positive well-being for other goals. Thus, researchers must examine changes in well-being within the context of the changing goals that individuals are likely to have as they age.

10. Conclusions: the take-home message(s) and directions for future research

From the early philosophical treatments of happiness to the modern science of subjective well-being, the concept of happiness has evolved considerably. Although subjective well-being can be defined simply as the way that people evaluate their lives, this simple definition belies the complex and multi-faceted nature of the construct. SWB is not a unitary dimension, and there is no single index that can capture what it means to be happy. Instead, SWB reflects a broad collection of distinct components, and to get a complete picture of one's well-being, researchers must understand the various ways that people can evaluate their lives. For example, an older individual may experience more health problems or financial difficulties than a younger individual, and these stressors may cause anxiety and negative emotions on a day-to-day basis. Yet, at the same time, the older individual may have a strong sense of satisfaction with the things he or she has accomplished over the course of an entire lifetime. Researchers who only focus on one component of well-being will not be able to capture the complex nature of these phenomena. A multi-faceted approach to SWB not only suggests the necessity of multiple measures, but the choice of measures should be theoretically meaningful. For example, if researchers are interested in making predictions about people's choices, then they might measure recalled emotions, rather than on-line experiences (Wirtz et al., in press). Similarly, life events may have small effects on global evaluations, but rather larger effects on daily affect (e.g. Lawton et al., 1995).

Naturally, thorough SWB assessments are time-consuming, and this might discourage some researchers, but the payoff can be great in terms of understanding. Just as we do not assess intelligence, mental illness, creativity, or the Big Five with a few quick questions, we cannot expect to measure SWB with a five-minute global assessment. This is not to say that global assessments are useless, because they can provide valid and meaningful information. But they are very incomplete. To be thorough requires more in-depth measurement.

It is not solely for the sake of completeness, however, that we emphasize the multi-faceted nature of well-being. There are also many theoretical reasons for studying the components of well-being separately. We know, for instance, that the different components have different correlates. These findings have led researchers to suggest that distinct processes underlie the various components. Therefore, to develop a theory of these processes, researchers will need to understand the various components separately. Furthermore, although it may seem intuitive that the various components would tap into the same underlying constructs, oftentimes different measures of well-being do not completely converge. Divergent measures need not be cause for despair. Instead, studying the reasons for these divergences can elucidate the processes that lead to the various well-being judgments.

One of the strongest recommendations we can make to SWB researchers and gerontologists is to examine low vs. high intensity emotions separately. If intense emotions are assessed such as PANAS PA (e.g. "active" from Watson et al., 1988) or Bradburn PA items (e.g. "on top of the world"), then the elderly might appear lower in PA. But if low arousal words, such as contentment or happy, are assessed, then we might not see a decline in PA with age (Lawton et al., 1992b; Lawton, 2001). Likewise, there might be no decline in frequency of emotions with age, but a decline in intensity. That is, people might experience anger with the same frequency, but with age, they may experience it less intensely. A similar argument can be applied to the valence of affect, highlighting the need to measure PA and NA separately.

More research on the elderly is needed, and this research should include at least two important aims. First, the structure of SWB needs to be more clearly identified among the elderly (e.g. Lawton et al., 1992a). In fact, more research on many specific populations is needed in order to understand the structure of SWB in various groups (e.g. ethnic/cultural groups). Second, future studies should examine the multi-components of SWB and explore the steps involved in the emotion sequence.

Finally, the evolving conception of SWB suggests that ideal SWB is not to be equated with uninterrupted euphoria. Such a view would place too great an emphasis on hedonism when there are clearly non-hedonistic aspects of SWB as well (e.g., global judgments such as life satisfaction, meaning, and fulfillment). Furthermore, we should consider what is functional, and this includes some negative feelings from time to time. Although pleasant emotions may be desirable, happiness is not the ultimate goal at all times. Rather, individual and cultural differences in the valuing of enjoyment suggest that people are willing to sacrifice feeling happy for other goals. And even when people do seek enjoyment, they want to feel good for the right reasons. Thus, we need to understand people's goals, and consider their feelings within the context of their values.

References

Andrews, F.M., Robinson, J.P., 1991. Measures of subjective well-being. In: Robinson, J.P., Shaver, P.R., Wrightsman, L.S. (Eds.), Measures of Personality and Social Psychological Attitudes. Academic Press, San Diego, pp. 61–114.
Andrews, F.M., Withey, S.B., 1976. Social Indicators of Well-being: America's Perception of Life Quality. Plenum Press, New York.
Bayley, J., 1999. Elegy for Iris. St. Martin's Press, New York.
Berenbaum, H., Raghavan, C., Le, H.-N., Vernon, L.L., Gomez, J.J., 2002. A taxonomy of emotional disturbances. Manuscript submitted for publication. University of Illinois, Urbana-Champaign.

Bradburn, N.M., 1969. The Structure of Psychological Well-being. Aldine, Chicago.
Cacioppo, J.T., Berntson, G.G., Larsen, J.T., Poehlmann, K.M., Ito, T.A., 2000. The psychophysiology of emotion. In: Lewis, M., Haviland-Jones, J.M. (Eds.), Handbook of Emotions, 2nd ed. Guilford, New York, pp. 173–191.
Campbell, A., Converse, P.E., Rodgers, W.L., 1976. The Quality of American Life. Russell Sage Foundation, New York.
Carstensen, L.L., 1995. Evidence for a life-span theory of socioemotional selectivity. Curr. Dir. Psychol. Sci. 4, 151–156.
Carstensen, L.L., Pasupathi, M., Mayr, U., Nesselroade, J.R., 2000. Emotional experience in everyday life across the adult life span. J. Pers. Soc. Psychol. 779, 644–655.
Clark, A.E., Georgellis, Y., Lucas, R.E., Diener, E., in press. Unemployment alters the set-point for life satisfaction. Psychol. Science.
Costa, P.T., McCrae, R.R., 1980. Influence of extraversion and neuroticism on subjective well-being: Happy and unhappy people. J. Pers. Soc. Psychol. 38, 668–678.
Costa, P.T., McCrae, R.R., 1988. Personality in adulthood: A six-year longitudinal study of self-reports and spouse ratings of the NEO Personality Inventory. J. Pers. Soc. Psychol. 54, 853–863.
Costa, P.T., McCrae, R.R., Zonderman, A., 1987. Environmental and dispositional influences on well-being: Longitudinal follow-up of an American national sample. Br. J. Psychol. 78, 299–306.
Danner, D.D., Snowden, D.A., Friesen, W.V., 2001. Positive emotions in early life and longevity: Findings from the Nun Study. J. Pers. Soc. Psychol. 80, 801–813.
Davidson, R.J., 1992. Anterior cerebral asymmetry and the nature of emotion. Brain Cogn. 20, 125–151.
Diener, E., 2000. Subjective well-being: The science of happiness, and a proposal for a national index. Am. Psychol. 55, 34–43.
Diener, E., Colvin, C.R., Pavot, W.G., Allman, A., 1992. The psychic costs of intense positive affect. J. Pers. Soc. Psychol. 52, 492–503.
Diener, E., Emmons, R.A., 1985. The independence of positive and negative affect. J. Pers. Soc. Psychol. 47, 1105–1117.
Diener, E., Emmons, R.A., Larsen, R.J., Griffin, S., 1985. The Satisfaction With Life Scale. J. Pers. Assess. 49, 71–75.
Diener, E., Fujita, F., 1997. Social comparisons and subjective well-being. In: Buunk, B., Gibbons, R. (Eds.), Health, Coping, and Social Comparison. Erlbaum, Mahwah, NJ, pp. 329–357.
Diener, E., Iran-Nejad, A., 1986. The relationship in experience between various types of affect. J. Pers. Soc. Psychol. 50, 1031–1038.
Diener, E., Larsen, R.J., 1984. Temporal stability and cross-situational consistency of affective, behavioral, and cognitive responses. J. Pers. Soc. Psychol. 47, 871–883.
Diener, E., Larsen, R.J., Emmons, R.A., 1984. Person X situation interactions: Choice of situations and congruence response models. J. Pers. Soc. Psychol. 47, 580–592.
Diener, E., Lucas, R.E., 2000. Subjective emotional well-being. In: Lewis, M., Haviland-Jones, J.M. (Eds.), Handbook of Emotions, 2nd ed. Guilford, New York, NY, pp. 325–337.
Diener, E., Lucas, R.E., Oishi, S., Suh, E.M., 2002. Looking up and looking down: Weighting good and bad information in life satisfaction judgments. Pers. Soc. Psychol. Bull. 28, 437–445.
Diener, E., Nickerson, C., Lucas, R.E., Sandvik, E., 2002. Dispositional affect and job outcomes. Social Indicators Research 59, 229–259.
Diener, E., Sandvik, E., Pavot, W., 1991. Happiness is the frequency, not the intensity, of positive versus negative affect. In: Strack, F., Argyle, M., Schwarz, N. (Eds.), Subjective Well-being: An Interdisciplinary Perspective. International Series in Experimental Social Psychology. Pergamon Press, Oxford, England, pp. 119–139.
Diener, E., Scollon, C.K., Oishi, S., Dzokoto, V., Suh, E.M., 2000. Positivity and the construction of life satisfaction judgments: Global happiness is not the sum of its parts. Journal of Happiness Studies 1, 159–176.
Diener, E., Seligman, M.E.P., 2002. Very happy people. Psychol. Sci. 13, 81–84.
Diener, E., Smith, H., Fujita, F., 1995. The personality structure of affect. J. Pers. Soc. Psychol. 50, 130–141.

Diener, E., Suh, E., 1997. Measuring quality of life: Economic, social and subjective indicators. Social Indicators Research 40, 189–216.

Diener, E., Suh, E.M., 1998. Subjective well-being and age: An international analysis. In: Schaie, K.W., Lawton, M.P. (Eds.), Annual Review of Gerontology and Geriatrics, Vol. 8. Springer, New York, pp. 304–324.

Ehrhardt, J.J., Saris, W.E., Veenhoven, R., 2000. Stability of life-satisfaction over time: Analysis of change in ranks in a national population. Journal of Happiness Studies 1, 177–205.

Eid, M., Diener, E., 1999. Intraindividual variability in affect: Reliability, validity, and personality correlates. J. Pers. Soc. Psychol. 76, 662–676.

Eid, M., Diener, E., 2001. Norms for experiencing emotions in different cultures: Inter- and intranational differences. J. Pers. Soc. Psychol. 81, 869–885.

Ekman, P., Friesen, W., 1978. Facial Action Coding System. Consulting Psychologists Press, Palo Alto, CA.

Ekman, P., Friesen, W., Ellsworth, P., 1972. Emotion in the Human Face: Guidelines for Research and an Integration of Findings. Pergamon Press, New York.

Fabrigar, L.R., Visser, P.S., Browne, M.W., 1997. Conceptual and methodological issues in testing the circumplex structure of data in personality and social psychology. Pers. Soc. Psychol. Rev. 1, 184–203.

Feldman Barrett, L., 1997. The relationships among momentary emotion experiences, personality descriptions, and retrospective ratings of emotion. Pers. Soc. Psychol. Bull. 23, 1100–1110.

Fredrickson, B.L., 1998. What good are positive emotions? Rev. Gen. Psychol. 2, 300–319.

Fredrickson, B.L., 2001. The role of positive emotions in positive psychology: The broaden-and-build theory of positive emotions. Am. Psychol. 56, 218–226.

Frijda, N.H., 1986. The Emotions. Cambridge University Press, New York.

Frijda, N.H., 1999. Emotions and hedonic experience. In: Kahneman, D., Diener, E., Schwarz, N. (Eds.), Well-being: The Foundations of Hedonic Psychology. Russell Sage Foundation, New York, pp. 190–210.

George, L.K., 1986. Life satisfaction in later life. Generations 10, 5–8.

Gottman, J.M., 1993. Studying emotion in social interaction. In: Lewis, M., Haviland, J.M. (Eds.), Handbook of Emotions. Guilford, New York. pp. 475–487.

Gross, J.J., Carstensen, L.L., Pasupathi, M., Tsai, J., Skorpen, C.G., Hsu, A.Y.C., 1997. Emotion and aging: Experience, expression, and control. Psychol. Aging 12, 590–599.

Hammen, C., 2002. Context of stress in families of children with depressed parents. In: Goodman, S.H., Gotlib, I.H. (Eds.), Children of Depressed Parents: Mechanics of Risk and Implications for Treatment. American Psychological Association, Washington, D.C., pp. 175–199.

Hays, R.D., Wells, K.B., Sherbourne, C.D., Rogers, W., Spritzer, K., 1995. Functioning and well-being outcomes of patients with depression compared with chronic general medical illnesses. Arch. Gen. Psychiatry 52, 11–19.

Headey, B., Wearing, A., 1989. Personality, life events, and subjective well-being: Toward a dynamic equilibrium model. J. Pers. Soc. Psychol. 57, 731–739.

Heine, S.J., Kitayama, S., Lehman, D.R., Takata, T., Ide, E., Leung, C., Matsumoto, H., 2001. Divergent consequences of success and failure in Japan and North America. An investigation of self-improving motivations and malleable selves. J. Pers. Soc. Psychol. 81, 599–615.

Izard, C.E., 1977. Human Emotions. Plenum, New York.

Jahoda, M., 1958. Current Conceptions of Positive Mental Health. Basic Books, New York.

Kahneman, D., 1999. Objective happiness. In: Kahneman, D., Diener, E., Schwarz, N. (Eds.), Well-being: The Foundations of Hedonic Psychology. Russell Sage Foundation, New York, pp. 3–25.

Kim-Prieto, C.Y., 2002. What's a wonderful life? The pursuit of personal pleasure versus in-group desires. Unpublished master's thesis. University of Illinois, Urbana-Champaign.

Krokoff, L.J., Gottman, J.M., Hass, S.D., 1989. Validation of a global rapid couples interaction scoring system. Behav. Assess. 11, 65–79.

Kunzmann, U., Little, T.D., Smith, J., 2000. Is age-related stability of subjective well-being a paradox? Cross-sectional and longitudinal evidence from the Berlin Aging Study. Psychol. Aging 15, 511–526.

Larsen, R.J., Diener, E., 1987. Emotional response intensity as an individual difference characteristic. J. Res. Pers. 21, 1–39.

Larsen, R.J., Diener, E., 1992. Promises and problems with the circumplex model of emotion. In: Clark, M.S., (Ed.), Review of Personality and Social Psychology: Emotion, Vol. 13. Sage, Newbury Park, CA, pp. 25–59.

Larsen, R.J., Diener, E., Cropanzano, R.S., 1987. Cognitive operations associated with individual differences in affect intensity. J. Pers. Soc. Psychol. 53, 767–774.

Larsen, R.J., Diener, E., Emmons, R.A., 1985. An evaluation of subjective well-being measures. Social Indicators Research 17, 1–17.

Larsen, R.J., Diener, E., Lucas, R.E., 2002. Emotion: Models, measures, and individual differences. In: Lord, R.G., Klimoski, R.J., Kanfer, R. (Eds.), Emotions in the Workplace. Jossey-Bass, San Francisco, pp. 64–106.

Larsen, R.J., Fredrickson, B.L., 1999. Measurement issues in emotion research. In: Kahneman, D., Diener, E., Schwarz, N. (Eds.), Well-being: The Foundations of Hedonic Psychology. Russell Sage Foundation, New York, pp. 40–60.

Larsen, R.J., McGraw, XX, Cacioppo, J.T., 2001.

Lawton, M.P., 2001. Emotion in later life. Curr. Dir. Psychol. Sci. 10, 120–123.

Lawton, M.P., DeVoe, M.R., Parmelee, P., 1995. Relationship of events and affect in the daily life of an elderly population. Psychol. Aging 10, 469–477.

Lawton, M.P., Kleban, M.H., Dean, J., Rajagopal, D., Parmelee, P.A., 1992a. The factorial generality of brief positive and negative affect measures. J. Gerontol. 47, 228–237.

Lawton, M.P., Kleban, M.H., Rajagopal, D., Dean, J., 1992b. Dimension of affective experience in three age groups. Psychol. Aging 7, 171–184.

Lazarus, R.S., 1982. Thoughts on the relations between emotion and cognition. Am. Psychol. 37, 1019–1024.

Lazarus, R.S., 1984. On the primacy of cognition. Am. Psychol. 39, 124–129.

LeDoux, J.E., 2000. Emotion circuits in the brain. Annu. Rev. Neurosci. 23, 155–184.

Levine, L.J., Prohaska, V., Burgess, S.L., Rice, J.A., Laulere, T.M., 2001. Remembering past emotions: The role of current appraisals. Cognit. Emotion 15, 393–417.

Lucas, R.E., Clark, A.E., Georgellis, Y., Diener, E., in press. Re-examining adaptation and the setpoint model of happiness: Reactions to changes in marital status. J. Pers. Soc. Psychol.

Lucas, R.E., Diener, E., 2003. The happy worker: Hypotheses about the role of positive affect in worker productivity. In: Ryan, A.M., Barrick, M. (Eds.), Personality and Work. Jossey-Bass, San Francisco, pp. 30–59.

Lucas, R.E., Diener, E., Larsen, R.J., 2003. Measuring positive emotions. In: Snyder, C.R., Lopez, S.J. (Eds.), The Handbook of Positive Psychological Assessment. American Psychological Association, Washington, D.C., pp. 201–218.

Lucas, R.E., Diener, E., Suh, E.M., 1996. Discriminant validity of subjective well-being measures. J. Pers. Soc. Psychol. 71, 616–628.

Lucas, R.E., Gohm, C.L., 2000. Age and sex differences in subjective well-being across cultures. In: Diener, E., Suh, E.M. (Eds.), Culture and Subjective Well-being. MIT Press, Cambridge, MA, pp. 291–317.

Lykken, D., Tellegen, A., 1996. Happiness is a stochastic phenomenon. Psychol. Sci. 7, 186–189.

Lyubomirsky, S., King, L., Diener, E., 2002. Happiness as a strength: A theory of the benefits of chronic positive affect. Manuscript in preparation. University of California, Riverside.

MacKay, C.J., 1980. The measurement of mood and psychophysiological activity using self-report techniques. In: Martin, I., Venables, P. (Eds.), Techniques in Psychophysiology. Wiley, New York, pp. 501–562.

Magnus, K., Diener, E., 1991. A longitudinal analysis of personality, life events, and subjective well-being. Paper presented at the Sixty-third Annual Meeting of the Midwestern Psychological Association, Chicago (May 2–4).

Mathews, A., MacLeod, C., 1994. Cognitive approaches to emotion and emotional disorders. Annu. Rev. Psychol. 45, 25–50.

McFarland, C., Ross, M., DeCourville, N., 1989. Women's theories of menstruation and biases in recall of menstrual symptoms. J. Pers. Soc. Psychol. 57, 522–531.

McCrae, R.R., Costa Jr., P.T., 1989. Different points of view: Self-reports and ratings in the assessment of personality. In: Forgas, J.P., Innes, M.J. (Eds.), Recent Advances in Social Psychology: An International Perspective. Elsevier Science, Amsterdam, pp. 429–439.

Morris, W.N., 1999. The mood system. In: Kahneman, D., Diener, E., Schwarz, N. (Eds.), Well-being: The Foundations of Hedonic Psychology. Russell Sage Foundation, New York, pp. 169–189.

Mroczek, D.K., Kolarz, C.M., 1998. The effect of age on positive and negative affect: A developmental perspective on happiness. J. Pers. Soc. Psychol. 76, 1333–1349.

Myers, D.G., Diener, E., 1995. Who is happy? Psychol. Sci. 6, 10–19.

Neugarten, B.L., Havighurst, R.J., Tobin, S.S., 1961. The measurement of life satisfaction. J. Gerontol. 16, 134–143.

Nozick, R., 1974. Anarchy, State, and Utopia. Basic Books, New York.

Oishi, S., 2000. Culture and memory for emotional experiences: On-line vs. retrospective judgments of subjective well-being. Unpublished doctoral dissertation, University of Illinois, Urbana-Champaign.

Oishi, S., 2003. The relative importance of daily vs. retrospective judgments of satisfaction in predicting relationship longevity. A poster presented at the fourth annual meeting of the Society of Personality and Social Psychology, Los Angeles, CA.

Oishi, S., Diener, E., in press. Culture and well-being: The cycle of action, evaluation, and decision. Personal and Social Psychology bulletin.

Oishi, S., Diener, E., Scollon, C.N., Biswas-Diener, R., in press. Cross-situational consistency of affective experiences across cultures. J. Pers. Soc. Psychol.

Oishi, S., Schimmack, U., Diener, E., 2001. Pleasures and subjective well-being. Eur. J. Pers. 15, 153–167.

Ortony, A., Turner, T.J., 1990. What's basic about basic emotions? Psychol. Rev. 97, 315–331.

Pinquart, M., 2001. Age differences in perceived positive affect, negative affect, and affect balance in middle and old age. Journal of Happiness Studies 2, 375–405.

Robinson, D., Clore, G.L., 2002. Episodic and semantic knowledge in emotional self-report: Evidence for two judgment processes. J. Pers. Soc. Psychol. 83, 198–215.

Ross, M., 1989. Relation of implicit theories to the construction of personal histories. Psychol. Rev. 96, 341–357.

Russell, J.A., 1980. A circumplex model of affect. J. Pers. Soc. Psychol. 39, 1161–1178.

Rusting, C.L., 1998. Personality, mood, and cognitive processing of emotional information: Three conceptual frameworks. Psychol. Bull. 124, 165–196.

Schimmack, U., in press. Affect measurement in experience sampling research. Journal of Happiness Studies.

Schimmack, U., Diener, E., 1997. Affect intensity: Separating intensity and frequency in repeatedly measured affect. J. Pers. Soc. Psychol. 73, 1313–1329.

Schimmack, U., Diener, E., Oishi, S., 2002. Life satisfaction is a momentary judgment and a stable personality characteristic: The use of chronically accessible and stable sources. J. Pers. 70, 346–384.

Schwarz, N., Clore, G.L., 1983. Mood, misattribution, and judgments of well-being: Informative and directive functions of affective states. Pers. Soc. Psychol. Bull. 18, 574–579.

Schwarz, N., Strack, F., 1999. Reports of subjective well-being: Judgmental processes and their methodological implications. In: Kahneman, D., Diener, E., Schwarz, N. (Eds.), Well-being: The Foundations of Hedonic Psychology. Russell Sage Foundation, New York, pp. 61–84.

Scollon, C.N., Diener, E., Oishi, S., Biswas-Diener, R., 2003. Emotions across cultures and methods. Under review at Journal of Cross-Cultural Psychology. Revise and resubmit.

Segerstrom, S.C., 2001. Optimism and attentional bias for negative and positive stimuli. Pers. Soc. Psychol. Bull. 27, 1334–1343.

Seidlitz, L., Diener, E., 1993. Memory for positive versus negative life events: Theories for the difference between happy and unhappy persons. J. Pers. Soc. Psychol. 64, 654–663.

Shedler, J., Mayman, M., Manis, M., 1993. The illusion of mental health. Am. Psychol. 48, 1117–1131.

Stone, A.A., 1995. Measures of affective response. In: Cohen, S., Kessler, R., Gordon, L. (Eds.), Measuring Stress: A Guide for Health and Social Scientists. Cambridge University Press, New York, pp. 148–171.

Stone, A.A., Shiffman, S.S., DeVries, M.W., 1999. Ecological momentary assessment. In: Kahneman, D., Diener, E., Schwarz, N. (Eds.), Well-being: The Foundations of Hedonic Psychology. Russell Sage Foundation, New York, pp. 26–39.

Stones, M.J., Hadjistavopoulo, T., Tuuko, H., Kozma, A., 1995. Happiness has trait-like and state-like properties: A reply to Veenhoven. Social Indicators Research 36, 129–144.

Suh, E., Diener, E., Fujita, F., 1996. Events and subjective well-being: Only recent events matter. J. Pers. Soc. Psychol. 70, 1091–1102.

Suh, E., Diener, E., Oishi, S., Triandis, H.C., 1998. The shifting basis of life satisfaction judgments across cultures: Emotions versus norms. J. Pers. Soc. Psychol. 74, 482–493.

Tatarkiewicz, W., 1976. Analysis of Happiness. Martinus Nijhoff, The Hague, Netherlands.

Tellegen, A., 1985. Structures of mood and personality and their relevance to assessing anxiety, with an emphasis on self-report. In: Tuma, A.H., Maser, J.D. (Eds.), Anxiety and the Anxiety Disorders. Erlbaum, Hillsdale, NJ, pp. 681–706.

Thomas, D., Diener, E., 1990. Memory accuracy in the recall of emotions. J. Pers. Soc. Psychol. 59, 291–297.

Veenhoven, R., 1994. Is happiness a trait? Tests of the theory that a better society does not make us any happier. Social Indicators Research 32, 101–162.

Veenhoven, R., 1998. Two state-trait discussions on happiness. A Reply to Stones et al. Social Indicators Research 43, 211–225.

Waterman, A.S., 1990. The relevance of Aristotle's conception of eudaimonia for the psychological study of happiness. Theor. Philos. Psychol. 10, 39–44.

Watson, D., Clark, L.A., Tellegen, A., 1988. Development and validation of brief measures of positive and negative affect: The PANAS scales. J. Pers. Soc. Psychol. 54, 1063–1070.

Watson, D., Tellegen, A., 1985. Toward a consensual structure of mood. Psychol. Bull. 98, 219–235.

Watson, D., Walker, L.M., 1996. The long-term stability and predictive validity of trait measures of affect. J. Pers. Soc. Psychol. 70, 567–577.

Watson, D., Wiese, D., Vaidya, J., Tellegen, A., 1999. The two general activation systems of affect: Structural findings, evolutionary considerations, and psychobiological evidence. J. Pers. Soc. Psychol. 76, 820–838.

Weinberger, D.A., Schwartz, G.E., Davidson, R.A., 1979. Low-anxious, high-anxious, and repressive coping styles: Psychometric patterns and behavioral and physiological responses to stress. J. Abnorm. Psychol. 88, 369–380.

Wessman, A.E., Ricks, D.F., 1966. Mood and Personality. Holt, Rinehart, and Winston, New York.

Wilson, W., 1967. Correlates of avowed happiness. Psychol. Bull. 67, 294–306.

Wirtz, D., Kruger, J., Scollon, C.N., Diener, E., in press. What to do on spring break? Predicting future choice based on online versus recalled affect. Psychol. Sci.

Zajonc, R.B., 1980. Feeling and thinking: Preferences need no inferences. Am. Psychol. 35, 151–175.

Zelenski, J.M., Larsen, R.J., 2000. The distribution of basic emotions in everyday life: A state and trait perspective from experience sampling data. J. Res. Pers. 34, 178–197.

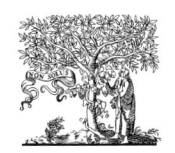

A cultural lens on biopsychosocial models of aging

James S. Jackson*, Toni C. Antonucci and Edna Brown

Institute for Social Research, University of Michigan, P.O. Box 1248, 426 Thompson St., Ann Arbor, MI 48106-1248, USA

Contents

1. Introduction — 221
2. Biopsychosocial model of health — 222
   2.1. A life span model of development — 224
3. The changing nature of aging in America — 225
4. Race, ethnic, and cultural categorizations — 226
5. A revised biopsychosocial model — 228
6. Health and culture: compelling examples — 229
7. Social relations — 230
8. Physical and mental health disparities — 231
9. Ethnic research matrix — 235
10. Conclusions — 236
    References — 237

1. Introduction

Recent advances in biology, behavioral genetics, and the identification of the human genome have been extraordinary. Somewhat paradoxically, this progress has made it even clearer that human beings are not defined by biology alone. As a result, attention among scientists, researchers, and policy makers has increasingly focused on understanding the environmental, social, and psychological complexity of the human organism. We suggest that the biopsychosocial model is especially useful in capturing this complexity. The original biopsychosocial model was proposed by Engel (1977). Recent versions (Clark et al., 1999; Seeman et al., 2001; Lindau et al., 2002) have been updated, however, to take advantage of the additional

---

*Corresponding author. Tel.: 734-763-2491.
E-mail address: jamessj@umich.edu (J.S. Jackson).

biological, psychological, and sociological information that has become available. It is widely recognized that significant understanding of human functioning, health, or well-being will not be achieved without a consideration of the multiple factors known to influence the human organism. In this chapter we focus on the special role of culture and its influence on those biopsychosocial factors that influence development, health and well-being. We begin first with a review of the basic model as it was originally proposed.

2. Biopsychosocial model of health

Although relatively common now, the biopsychosocial model was quite controversial when first introduced to the literature less than 30 years ago by George Engel, Professor of Psychiatry and Medicine at the University of Rochester. In his groundbreaking *Science* article he noted that while the prevalent biomedical model of health represented a considerable step forward from previous "unscientific" notions of health and illness, it did not go far enough. And indeed, the biomedical model did represent a major advancement over historical views, e.g. that illness was a curse from God, caused by evil spirits and demons, or retaliation for past sins. Besides their lack of accuracy, any of these explanations for illness clearly preclude a scientific approach to understanding health and well-being. Similarly, it leaves the health care professional with little role in the treatment of illness, but rather relegates this role to clergy, witch doctors, shaman or medicine men. Although there were intervening views historically, the biomedical model offered a major improvement over previous perspectives in that health and illness were seen to have scientific bases and viable treatment options were developed by health professionals to offer to the public.

The biomedical model represented a combination of disciplinary perspectives with major emphasis on molecular biology as a fundamental basis for understanding human disease with additional insights offered by the biochemical and neurophysiological sciences. While Engel did not dispute the contribution that these disciplines make to our understanding of disease, he strongly disputed the reductionistic view they represented as sufficient to explain disease. He argued that "the language of chemistry and physics" cannot "ultimately suffice to explain biological phenomenon" (p. 130). He suggested that while the biomedical model had been widely and enthusiastically accepted as truly scientific, in fact, like all other models, it is, nevertheless, simply a heuristic, in this case an incomplete one, devised to explain the phenomenon of disease. Engel noted that evidence had been accumulating which made it increasingly evident that the environment, including social, psychological, and physical aspects, influences who becomes sick, the severity of the illness, and who is able to recover. He called for a more inclusive, less ethnomedical scientific model for the study of disease. To this end he proposed the biopsychosocial model, which incorporates all of these influences, i.e. biological, psychological, and social, into an overarching framework designed to take a broader perspective on both the etiology and understanding of disease. It is now widely assumed that this model is appropriate, not only for understanding disease, but also as a broader context for possibly understanding human behavior, health, and well-being.

As Engel noted, despite the biomedical model's emphasis on physical elements to study illness, it has been common for the clinician, both historically and currently, to consider behavioral, psychological, and social criteria in the identification and treatment of disease. Engel argued for a multidimensional model that incorporates all these factors. The model is designed to include both somatic diseases, such as diabetes, and mental diseases, such as schizophrenia. He identified several characteristics of the biopsychosocial model that offer important advantages over the prior widely accepted biomedical model. He noted that the biopsychosocial approach incorporates into the diagnostic process the biochemical aspects of a disease but also the complex array of psychological, social, and behavioral factors often critical to the identification and treatment of illness. Similarly, the biopsychosocial model establishes a link between identified biochemical processes and the behavioral manifestations of the disease as experienced by the patient and those around him or her. For most people, the biochemical process is not how they experience or identify a disease. Rather most people experience a disease in terms of what they can or cannot do, what obligations they are unable to meet, or the prevalent emotions they experience.

The biopsychosocial model links these previously separated aspects of health and illness. Thus, a biochemical indication of illness which is not represented behaviorally, socially, or psychologically in the individual's life in any identifiable form must and should be treated differently than an illness with only behavioral, social, or psychological manifestations but no, as yet identified, biochemical aberration. At the same time both manifestations need to be recognized and receive the attention they require, rather than one being recognized as a "real" illness and the other considered somehow less real. The biopsychosocial model also acknowledges that non-physiological characteristics of the person, including life circumstances, may change the individual's physiological response and susceptibility to an illness, as well as the development and course of the illness they experience. As we face an increasingly diverse population both in terms of demographic and social characteristics, the potency of this argument becomes ever more compelling.

In accordance with, or perhaps in spite of, the identification of the human genome, and in recognition of the changing demographics and life span experiences of many groups, our focus on older people and the aging experience suggests that it is time once again to revisit Engel's biopsychosocial model. While identification of the human genome has helped to clarify some genetic determinants of disease, more often it has made clear that no single gene accounts for most illnesses or behaviors. We propose that it is now time to explicitly infuse the biopsychosocial model with both a life span developmental framework and recognition of the role of culture in the aging process. We need time to revise the biospsychosocial model in order to incorporate the significantly improved empirical evidence that can serve to uniquely inform the original model. We begin with the incorporation of a life span approach to human development.

2.1. A life span model of development

As changing demographics require increased focus on older ages, lessons learned from the life span model of development are particularly germane. Unfortunately, the basic tenets of the life span framework have not been explicitly applied to the biopsychosocial model. At about the same time Engel was proposing the biopsychosocial model, Baltes et al. (1980) articulated a life span approach to human development that in many ways complements the biopsychosocial model presented above. Baltes, Reese, and Lipsitt described the basic determinants of development as separate biological and environmental factors but recognized that they could also interact to affect development. In addition, they outlined three major influences on development. The first is normative, age-graded systems. These are the usual, average developmental systems that occur over time. They described this as normal, ontogenetic development, basically the experiences of each individual as they move through infancy, childhood, adolescence, and adulthood. The second influence is normative, history-graded systems. These involve the particular historical or evolutionary period in which the individual develops. They describe evolutionary changes or historical events that occur in one particular historical period such as economic depressions, wars, epidemics. In our life time, people of different ages have experienced the first and second World Wars, the Great Depression, the AIDS epidemic and now SARS. The third and final system Baltes, Reese, and Lipsitt described refer to non-normative systems. These are individual life events that are not usual or customary but have a significant affect on a particular individual in his or her lifetime. Examples of these include medical trauma, divorce, institutionalization, and death of a close relative. Although these are idiosyncratic, they are noteworthy because they significantly affect the course of an individual's life, sometimes physically, sometimes emotionally, often simultaneously. Baltes et al. (1979, 1980) explicitly suggested that age graded influences are very important early in life and decrease in importance later in life, while history-graded influences become increasingly important in later childhood, adolescence and early adulthood, but are less important in old age, and non-normative influences become increasingly important with age.

In many ways, Baltes (1997) more recent work on the incomplete ontogeny of human development and his proposal to recognize the influence of culture in human development represents an important extension of the original work. In this latest consideration of life span developmental theory, Baltes uses the concepts of selection, optimization, and compensation as illustrative of the adaptive strategies people use in order to maximize their competency. He notes that with the challenges of age one has increased need to select, optimize, and compensate in order to achieve designated goals. At the same time it is noteworthy that culture is infused in every element of this process. What one selects, how one chooses to optimize, and what one considers appropriate forms of compensation are all culturally influenced, if not determined. As one ages this influence accumulates and appears to have an ever-increasing influence on the experience of aging. In the earlier work (Baltes et al., 1980) culture could be understood under the generic heading of environmental influences, but in more recent work (Baltes, 1997) it occupies a much more dominant role. In fact, Baltes argues that while culture becomes increasingly important with age, its actual influence on development decreases with age. The degree to which one agrees with this proposition appears to depend upon the specific characteristic of interest. Thus, biological and physical development are said to dominate in childhood where culture has minimum impact. Within most Western cultures this appears to be true. But of course, one might imagine a culture where one group is disfavored, e.g. girls, and thus provided only very limited access, e.g. to nutritional resources, thus limiting the biological or physical development that might otherwise dominate. Similarly, among older people what one values may be determined by culture and how one copes with biological or physical loses might also be influenced by culture – some of which would optimize and others of which might minimize normal or successful adaptation to the challenges one often faces with age.

We believe that it is necessary to incorporate both the life span framework and the role of culture into the biopsychosocial model, especially as it applies to aging. Recent adaptations and criticisms of the model may help pave the way for this fusion.

3. The changing nature of aging in America

America has always been a nation of immigrants. Several factors will change the face of America in the future. Our population will age dramatically. The ethnic and racial composition of the country will change significantly. Earlier waves of migration came from Europe, China, and Africa, new waves are coming from Central and Latin America, the Middle East, and Southeastern Asia. While the country is aging rapidly, the rate of aging is faster among the ethnic and racial minority "new" immigrant groups (Angel and Hogan, 1991; Siegel, 1993; Stanford and DuBois, 1993).

As we focus on the aging process through a cultural lens, this changing racial and ethnic minority population will represent unique groups of aging individuals. As culture has affected their lifetime experiences, it will also affect their aging experiences. The biopsychosocial model will be fundamentally affected by the cultural lens through which they view aging, both cumulatively and contemporaneously. These immigrant groups have unique histories. For example, Cuban immigrants fled Castro and arrived in the United States feeling forcibly expelled from their homeland. They arrived in a country that was similarly anti-Castro and sympathetic to their plight. Middle-Easterners escaped dictators, war, and oppression but, at least currently, are aging in a considerably less sympathetic, if not hostile, United States. Asians, for example, Koreans, also fled a homeland torn by war and remain embedded in communities with specific cultural values that guide their expectations about aging. The life span experiences of these individuals may include immigrating as children and spending 60 years in the United States, learning another language, living in urban vs. rural communities, being among a minority vs. majority culture. Some immigrants have left a higher standard of living; others came to the United States to seek a higher standard of living. But particularly relevant to the aging experience is the fact that all immigrants have been influenced by their physical characteristics, their family and friendship relationships, and the communities within which they live, i.e. their biopsychosocial development. And, while we focus on minority racial and ethnic groups, these biopsychosocial influences are no less important for the majority group. In this case, recognizing the significant influence on minority groups only serves to highlight the role of these factors for aging among all people.

4. Race, ethnic, and cultural categorizations

How the concepts of culture, race, and ethnic group are defined and categorized in a biopsychosocial model of aging and human development is of critical importance (Wilkinson and King, 1987; Jackson, 1993; Jackson et al., 1995). We also need to know about the conditions under which race, ethnicity, socio-cultural, and socio-economic factors may serve as important resources in the coping and adaptation of ethnic elders to their relatively disadvantaged circumstances (Dressler, 1985; Wilkinson and King, 1987; Dressler, 1991). Culture has been defined in many different ways (Jackson et al., 1990, 1995). We employ Swidler's (1986, 2001) definition of culture as a symbolic vehicle of meaning, including beliefs, ritual practices, art forms and ceremonies, as well as informal practices such as language, gossip, stories, and rituals of daily life. This definition emphasizes the role of culture in providing strategies of action, continuity in the ordering of these actions through time, and a template for constructing action. We believe that this perspective on culture is a useful framework for understanding its role in aging and aging-related social and biological processes (Jackson et al., 1990). Ethnicity is defined within a larger societal context and several distinctly different definitions of ethnicity exist. Yinger's (1985) definition stresses the common and shared origins of the group and participation in shared activities in which common origins, language, ancestral homeland, and culture are critical ingredients. Current theories of ethnicity postulate that the development and persistence of ethnicity – the crystallization of solidarity and identification – are dependent upon structural conditions in society (Nielsen, 1985). In contrast, older pluralist notions of ethnicity held that shared cultural heritage was the major basis for ascriptive group identity.

Several researchers have taken a self-identifying approach to the definition of ethnicity (Jackson et al., 1995). This view emphasizes the dynamic interactions among cultural traits, socialized patterns of social behavior and environmental influences. For example, Barth (1969) defines ethnicity as "... a population that has membership that identifies itself, and is identified by others as constituting a category distinguished from other categories of the same order" (p. 11). This definition is presumed to be on the basis of racial or cultural markers, like language, religion or customs (Nielsen, 1985). The definition is minimal in that the many attributes usually associated with ethnicity, e.g. biological self-perpetuation, shared values and bounded interactions are not necessarily definitional requirements (Nielsen, 1985).

Race also should be defined within the larger cultural context. There is growing agreement that whatever the biological reality of race categorizations, racial differences derive social significance from cultural diversity (Yinger, 1985). Many researchers (e.g., Cooper (1984, 1991)) propose that the concept of race has no scientific meaning and that social definitions of race and ethnicity are only important for determining environmental causes of observed differences between groups. Research in behavioral medicine, for example, has revealed that cultural and lifestyle differences among racial groups play an independent role in accounting for behavioral and health outcomes (Williams et al., 2003).

The term "minority group" proposed by Wirth (1945) is closely linked to definitions of ethnicity but has the added dimensions of inequality and discrimination in their treatment by majority group members. Taylor (1979) proposed that for black Americans in the United States, more attention is needed on the role of migration, urbanization, and ethnic identity more broadly. The recent arrival of Haitian immigrants as well as immigrants from other Caribbean and African countries highlights the historical fact of the diversity among African-Americans. This diversity may be best captured in ethnic rather than racial terms.

Exemplifying the issue of intra-group heterogeneity, the term Hispanic masks large differences among several major groups. For example, Cuban elderly constitute a smaller proportion of the Hispanic population than Puerto Ricans, but have nearly twice the proportion of individuals over the age of 65. On the other hand, Mexican descent Hispanics constitute nearly two-thirds of the total population of Hispanics but only about half of the total Hispanic elderly population. Significant differences exist in the material advantages of these different groups and in their social-historical backgrounds, political affiliations and orientations.

Similarly, the term Asian/Pacific Islanders also masks vast differences in backgrounds and national origins. They are also experiencing large increases among their respective older populations. Similar to Hispanics, the proportions of those over age 65 in the various subpopulations vary greatly, from about 7% among Japanese Americans to 2% among Vietnamese. These large differences in the proportions of elderly Asian/Pacific Islander subpopulations are fueled by past immigration policies, and the nature and make-up of current and projected rates of immigration and fertility.

The proportion of American Indians, Eskimos, and Aleuts 65 years of age or older has also shown a large jump. Between 1970 and 1980 the proportion of the total American Indian population over the age of 65 increased by more than one half. Similar to Americans of African, Hispanic and Asian descent, the term American Indian encompasses vast differences in language, life-style, world-views, and socio-economic resources among many different nations. And these factors have differential effects on the aging experience.

The tendency of most researchers to address race and ethnicity as demographic characteristics rather than as distinct predisposing cultural and social environment orientations (Jackson et al., 1990, 1995) has precluded the types of research and analyzes that examine the contributory role of socio-cultural factors to health behaviors within racial and ethnic groups (James, 1984; Myers, 1984). Many researchers have even questioned the appropriateness and validity of socio-economic status and other socio-cultural measures (e.g. occupation, coping resources, and lifestyle factors) when making comparisons across race and ethnic groups (Markides, 1990; Markides et al., 1990).

As we suggest in this chapter, a life-course, biopsychosocial framework is needed to explore how environmental stressors influence and interact with group and personal resources to both impede and facilitate the quality of life of successive cohorts of ethnic elders (Baltes, 1987). Notable improvements in the life situations of ethnic elders, particularly health, have occurred over the last 40–50 years, however, many ethnic groups of color in the United States continue to suffer greater disadvantaged circumstances than whites (Jackson and Sellers, 2001).

Finally, we emphasize in this chapter the need to separate the constructs of minority group, race, ethnicity and culture (e.g. Holzberg, 1982; Rosenthal, 1986) as we move toward viable biopsychosocial life-course development models of aging. We suggest that ethnicity and culture be viewed as mutable and changeable over the lifecourse for different cohorts, with continuity over time and generations (Jackson et al., 1990, 1995). Race is an externally imposed social construction; ethnicity is a self and other imposed group construction; and, cultural distinctiveness, the particular patterning of artifacts, beliefs, and values across generations, have to be conceptualized as more than just "variables." Instead they should be conceptualized as potential individual and group resources, providing psychological, social, and personal identity, and group cohesion for ethnic elders as they age.

5. A revised biopsychosocial model

Accumulating evidence over the last several years has made the biopsychosocial model increasingly compelling as an important approach to the investigation of aging phenomenon. The most recent consideration of the model was proposed by Seeman and Crimmins (2001). The goal of this revision was to more explicitly incorporate both macro and micro level physical and socio-cultural environmental influences. We incorporate concepts that recent empirical evidence argues are critically influential. Thus, personal demographics, such as age, gender, and ethnicity, as well as socioeconomic status, influence numerous aspects of the biopsychosocial model. Critical among these are social relationships, psychological characteristics such as efficacy, mastery and self-esteem, and behavioral factors, such as exercise, smoking, and diet. These different influences can affect numerous biological pathways such as the cardiovascular system, the metabolic system and the immune system, all of which in turn affect health outcomes. We highlight this complex model because it provides a clear theoretical representation of how culture, especially including ethnic and racial behaviors, traditions or customs, influence health and well-being. Sociodemographic factors and how these might be significantly altered by culture, as well as social relations and psychological characteristics, such as feelings of empowerment or efficacy are all known to influence biological pathways and, therefore, health outcomes. Recent empirical evidence indicating how the cultural environment affects the health of specific majority or minority groups is especially compelling. We turn to that evidence next.

6. Health and culture: compelling examples

Contrary to popular stereotypes, new Hispanic and Asian American immigrants actually have relatively better health than United States born individuals of Hispanic or Asian-American ancestry. However, as these immigrant groups have increased exposure to and participation in American traditions and behaviors, they also increasingly face health problems. One example is dietary. Adopting common American dietary customs is likely to lead to an increase in nutritionally deficient foods that are often associated with health problems. As foreign-born minorities adapt to American life-styles and habits there is some evidence that their health begins to decline (Yee and Gelfand, 1992; Elo and Preston, 1997). This dietary pathway is one possible cause for the finding, which some would consider counterintuitive.

In addition to unhealthy diets, some immigrant minorities are also exposed to a level of racial discrimination not necessarily found in their countries of origin. Repeated encounters of discrimination can be devastating to physiological and psychological health (Adler and Ostrove, 1999). Reactions and responses to discrimination range from anger and hostility to passivity and helplessness and can also lead to significant health problems. However, the effects are not universal. In some cases achieving higher levels of socioeconomic status can serve as a buffer or protection against stress, and is thus associated with better health outcomes. Individuals with higher socioeconomic status have access to more resources, such as high quality health care, than lower socioeconomic status individuals. However, the buffering effects of socioeconomic status or protection associated with better health outcomes appears not to have the same positive effect for African-Americans and women as it does for white men (Adler and Ostrove, 1999). The biopsychosocial model provides an effective means with which to examine the complexity of how various environmental and personal factors interact to affect health outcomes over the life-course.

Clark et al. (1999) also used a modified biopsychosocial model to explain the health impact of living within a culture of racial discrimination. Empirical evidence had been contradictory but they propose that for African-Americans the affect of racism on health outcomes varies by sociodemographic factors, e.g. level of socioeconomic and type of racism (overt or covert). Clark et al. argue that psychological factors can serve as resources (i.e. perceived control and self-esteem) or as detriments (i.e. hostility) that affect health outcomes. These psychological factors have been associated with cardiovascular health. For example, research suggests that African-Americans who repress anger may be at risk for negative health outcomes, including stroke and heart disease (Johnson and Crowley, 1999). In addition to general coping responses to the perception of racism as a stressor, African-Americans may use coping responses that are particularly germane for dealing with racism. However, these coping responses do not necessarily lead to better outcomes. Clark et al. suggest that psychological responses to stress include helplessness and anger that may, in turn, lead to additional negative responses such as substance abuse. Negative psychological responses have deleterious effects on the body's physiological functioning. Thus, Clark et al. (1999) argue that many African-Americans live in a culture of racism and discrimination which both influences the psychological resources available to them as well as their physical and mental health.

The various components of a biopsychosocial model help to explain the link between cultural, environmental, psychological, social, and biological forces over the life span. These effects both accumulate and potentially change over time. For example, during early and mid life African-Americans have higher mortality rates and poorer health status than White Americans. However, those differences in morbidity begin to converge and, although this interpretation is still controversial, mortality rates are thought by many to actually "crossover" during old age. One explanation for this change is that older African-Americans have learned effective coping strategies for dealing with negative life consequences. Another explanation is a survival of the fittest view, which posits that these older survivors are the healthiest African-Americans and are, therefore, the fittest. An examination of the biopsychosocial model across the life span, especially the examination of this model within different cultural contexts, provides a useful tool for examining factors that contribute to the "mortality crossover" phenomenon. In the next two sections we review briefly work on social relations and health disparities, suggesting ways in which the biopsychosocial model might apply.

7. Social relations

The biopsychosocial model assumes a critical role occupied by social relationships but this too varies by culture. A great deal of research has focused attention on social relations and health, in general, and among older people, in particular (Cohen and Syme, 1985; House et al., 1989; Antonucci, 1985, 2001; Levy and Pescosolido, 2002). We apply that work specifically to this reconsideration of the biopsychosocial model within a cultural context. As Antonucci and Jackson (1987) hypothesized, one role of social relations is to convey to an individual feelings of self-worth and efficacy required to maintain health and well-being. Interestingly, a body of research has been accumulating which addresses this point and documents the ways in which the cultural milieu influences social exchanges, health and well-being. For example, social support has been shown to be especially important to minority elderly and low socioeconomic status individuals. Phenninx et al. (1998) found that emotional support was associated with less depressive symptoms in elderly individuals. The effect was stronger for elderly with chronic illnesses than for those without disease. In other areas, having a dependable support network may make the difference in affording child care, receiving health care, or maintaining employment. The ability to borrow money or to have access to transportation for emergencies from family and friends may be the critical link between environmental stressors and health. For example, middle-aged men of lower socioeconomic status who report feeling supported by their children are as healthy as men of higher socioeconomic status (Antonucci et al., 2003). One might argue that the culture that encourages the exchange of goods, services, and favors among individuals can have a positive influence on psychological and physical health, as well as the aging experience more generally.

8. Physical and mental health disparities

In a recent chapter we suggested the need to develop better national health policies directed to the growing United States ethnic and racial minority populations (Jackson and Sellers, 2001). These policies must be responsive to life-course considerations and realities of family life, if we are to improve the health of underrepresented minority populations, especially blacks and Latinos. Recent research on discriminated-against minorities has focused on three major themes – heterogeneity, vulnerabilities due to societal mal-treatment, and family strengths (e.g. Beckman and Mullen, 1997; Miles, 1999). A life-course framework is needed to explore how socio-historical context influences and interacts with individual and group resources to both impede and facilitate the quality of life and health of successive cohorts of African-Americans over the group life-course, and in the nature of their individual human development experiences (Baltes, 1987; Burton et al., 1991; Smith and Kington, 1997a). For example, relationships between socio-ecologic factors, such as high crime rates, family dysfunction, high noise levels and social isolation, and negative health factors (e.g. hypertension) can affect all members of families and communities, thus possibly initiating poorer health among younger, as well as older African-Americans (Berkman and Mullen, 1997; Smith and Kington, 1997a). A life-course perspective illuminates the fact that current and aging cohorts of underrepresented race/ethnic minorities have been exposed to the conditions that will profoundly influence their social, psychological, and health statuses from childhood to adulthood and older ages in the years and decades to come (Baltes, 1987; Barresi, 1987; Jackson and Sellers, 1996).

For the most part, African-Americans and other race/ethnic groups have been portrayed in the scientific literature in a simplistic and undifferentiated manner. Recent studies show these groups as diverse and heterogeneous populations, possessing a wide array of group and personal resources (Stanford, 1990; Jackson, 1993; Farley, 2000). A continuing gender imbalance, segregated geographic distribution, and disproportionate numbers in poverty, among other factors, will have profound effects on family structure, health status, and the well-being of many of these groups in the 21st century (Miles, 1999; Siegel, 1999).

As we noted earlier, ethnic and racial categories derive their interpretations from: (1) the socio-historical and current circumstances that different groups with well-defined physical characteristics face, and (2) the "own-" and "other-group" attitudes and behaviors toward members who belong to these categories (Jackson and Sellers, 1996; Dressler and Bindon, 2000; Jackson, 2000; Jackson and Sellers, 2001). While some genetic and biological factors may vary with the categorization of peoples of African descent (e.g. sickle cell anemia, hypertension, and lupus), for example, we believe that the fundamental nature of being an underrepresented race/ethnic minority derives from both self- and other-definitions, and continuing discrimination and maltreatment (Jackson and Sellers, 1996; Neel, 1997; Dressler and Bindon, 2000; Jackson and Sellers, 2001). It is not yet clear how race and ethnic group categorizations fit in biopsychosocial models of health, human development, and life-course development (e.g. Wilkinson and King, 1987; Williams and Jackson, 2000). However, it is particularly important to integrate into models of health, health promotion and disease prevention, the conditions under which race, ethnicity, sociocultural, and socioeconomic factors may serve as important resources in coping processes and adaptation to environmentally disadvantaged circumstances (Dressler, 1985; Wilkinson and King, 1987; Dressler, 1991).

Compared to Americans of European descent, at every point of their life span, African-Americans (and many Latino and Native American groups) have greater morbidity and mortality (Jackson, 1991; Braithwaite and Taylor, 1992; Jackson and Sellers, 1996; Smith and Kington, 1997b; LaVeist, 2000; Jackson and Sellers, 2001). Among African-Americans, as with most racial-ethnic groups in the United States, cancer and cardiovascular disease are the two leading causes of death (LaVeist, 2000). Hypertension is particularly deadly. Hypertension afflicts one out of every three African-Americans and blacks have a 60% greater risk of death and disability from stroke and coronary disease than whites. In particular, black women have three times the rate of high blood pressure compared to white women (National Center for Health Statistics, 1999) and are twice as likely as white women to die of hypertensive cardiovascular disease (National Center for Health Statistics, 1999). Similarly, cancer incidence rates for blacks are 6–10% higher than whites.

Mortality statistics are equally troubling. The infant mortality rate for blacks is 20 deaths per 1000, twice the rate that occurs among whites (LaVeist, 2000). The average life expectancy for whites is approximately 76.8 years, compared to 70.3 years for blacks (LaVeist, 2000), with an almost 10-year difference between white (73.8) and black men (66.1). African-American overall cancer mortality rates are 20–40% higher than the general population (National Cancer Institute, 1989). Another important area is the assessment and treatment of serious mental disorders among African-American and Latino populations. The impediments to research in this area include the lack of knowledge about culturally appropriate cognitive and mental health assessment (Lichtenberg, 1998; Manly et al., 1998, 1999; Wall et al., 1998; Mast et al., 2001), and the lack of effective recruitment of African-American and Latino participants into the ongoing studies (Welsh et al., 1994; Fillenbaum et al., 1998).

In sum, many race/ethnic groups, especially blacks, are at disproportionate risk for negative health outcomes when compared to European Americans (Smith and

Kington, 1997b) and face significant challenges as they age. A number of factors may contribute to these disparities, ranging from biological dispositions (Baquet and Ringen, 1987) to dietary habits (Hargreaves et al., 1989), to a failure to receive adequate health care (Jones and Rice, 1987; Williams and Rucker, 2000). The specific mechanisms, however, that produce these differential outcomes are less clear (Williams, 1999; LaVeist, 2000). Given complex socio-historical contexts, it may be less useful in determining exact mechanisms to compare *between* racial and ethnic group outcomes than *within* groups. For example, black/white comparisons may be less illuminating than the examination of various intra-group social and cultural factors as possible sources of risk and resilience for African-American men, women and children (Jackson, 1991; Jackson and Sellers, 1996; Dressler and Bindon, 2000).

It is important to continue to develop frameworks within which the nature of the economic, social, and health circumstances of racial/ethnic groups can be explained and understood in the context of historical and current structural disadvantage and blocked mobility opportunities (Jackson et al., 1990a,b; Jackson, 1991). This framework contextualizes individual and group experiences by birth cohort, period events, and individual aging processes (Riley and Loscocco, 1994; Riley, 1994a,b; Riley and Riley, 1994a,b). It is clear, however, that blacks and other underrepresented race/ethnic minorities have, and do, arrive in adulthood and older ages with extensive histories of disease, ill health, and varied individual adaptive reactions to their poor health (Smith and Kington, 1997b). The available cohort data for cause-specific mortality and morbidity across the life-course over the last few decades indicates that there are accumulated deficits that perhaps place black, Latino and Native American middle-aged and older people at greater risk than comparable chronologically aged whites (Jackson, 1991). Similarly, the fact that blacks may actually outlive their white counterparts in the very older ages suggests possible selection factors at work that may result in hardier older blacks (Gibson and Jackson, 1987, 1991; Manton and Stollard, 1997). These selection factors may act on successive cohorts of blacks in a "sandwich-like" manner leaving alternate cohorts of middle-aged and older blacks of relative wellness and good functional ability. The cohort experiences of blacks undoubtedly play a major role in the nature of their health experiences over the life-course in terms of the quality of health care from birth, exposure to risk factors, and the presence of exogenous environmental factors. Another contributing factor is the stressor role of prejudice and discrimination across the life-course, even though it may differ in form and intensity as a function of birth cohort, period and age (Cooper et al., 1981; Baker, 1987; Dressler, 1991; Williams and Williams-Morris, 2000).

The role of socioeconomic status (SES) has been touted as a major risk factor and implicated in the effects of other risk factors in mortality and morbidity (Haan and Kaplan, 1985; Smith and Kington, 1997a,b; Williams, 1999). Impressive evidence exists that SES plays a major role in a wide variety of diseases such that increasing SES is associated with better health and lowered morbidity (Adler and Ostrove, 1999). This effect has been shown at both the individual and ecological levels on blood pressure, general mortality, cancer, cardiovascular heart diseases (CHD), and cerebrovascular disease, diabetes, and obesity (James, 1985). What has not been shown is how SES status from conception, birth or early in the life-course, affects these health outcomes in adulthood and older ages (Smith and Kington, 1997b; Williams, 1999). Perhaps, over the full life-course, advantaged blacks would be considerably more similar to their white counterparts than less advantaged blacks (Jackson, 1993); but current middle to high SES blacks would be at an intermediate position, and the full life-course disadvantaged blacks would continue to show worse health status conditions than their comparable low SES white counterparts (Smith and Kington, 1997a).

The effects of socioeconomic status on the health of black Americans require additional research (Adler and Ostrove, 1999). Contemporary cohorts of blacks and other race/ethnic groups being born today are at considerable risk. For example, studies reveal that black Americans are most likely to spend the majority of their childhood in low income, single female-headed households. Poverty in turn places black Americans at risk for inadequate diets, fewer educational opportunities, greater exposure to crime, and limited opportunities for occupational advancement (Massey and Denton 1993; Wilson, 1996). Job prospects will be poor in young adulthood and a large proportion will die or suffer chronic disease prior to reaching middle adulthood. Only a comparative few will have the advantage of inter-generational economic transfers from parental sources (Oliver and Shapiro, 1995). Even for those born into contemporary middle-class homes (since this is an often fragile situation for most blacks), providing a tangible legacy for children, even college funding, is problematic (Oliver and Shapiro, 1995). Recent data suggests that blacks at every family income level (Williams and Collins, 1995) have lower wealth than comparable whites. At the lowest income quintile, whites have ten thousand dollars in wealth while comparable black families have one dollar. In every new generation of African-Americans, wealth is thus recreated and consumed. This results in structural disadvantage that increases risk for poor health over the life-course.

In the face of severe structural, social, and psychological constraints, one wonders how black Americans and other underrepresented groups do as well as they do. Studies that address the coping skills, capacity, and adaptability of racial and ethnic minority groups at different points in the life-course are particularly important (Jackson, 1991). It is possible that the most important race and ethnicity effects, if they do occur, are probably in the form of interactions with other structural or cultural factors (e.g. religion, socio-economic status, and world views) (Jackson et al., 1990a; Markides et al., 1990; Jackson, 2000). Blacks and other underrepresented groups may utilize, over the individual life-course, different mechanisms than whites to maintain levels of productivity, physical and mental health, and effective functioning (Williams and Williams-Morris, 2000).

In sum, the African-American and other race/ethnic life-course experiences, perhaps more so than in the majority population, highlight the continuities and discontinuities of a life-course perspective on health. From birth to death, for example, African-Americans are at greater risk for debilitating social, psychological, and physical conditions that negatively influence the quality of individual and family life and, in many instances, results in "premature" death: greater fetal death rates; greater homicide statistics in adolescence and mid-life; and, greater risk of death from chronic health conditions early in old age (Smith and Kington, 1997b; Miles, 1999). However, not all blacks and underrepresented ethnic/racial minorities are born into such circumstances. For example, though its relative proportions are debated (Vanneman and Cannon 1987), there exists a sizeable black middle-class and some blacks in the United States can look forward to relatively comfortable styles of living over their life-courses (Farley, 2000). This heterogeneity is intertwined with categorical group membership and consequent experiences of ethnic/racial discrimination.

A biopsychosocial life-course perspective suggests the need to consider human development, historical context, and structural position as factors that influence the health of present and future cohorts of blacks and other race/ethnic individuals. Different birth cohorts, historical and current environmental events, and individual differences in development and aging processes interact with one another to affect physical and mental health. Racial group membership plays an important part in physical and mental health, and cultural resources provide important coping and adaptive mechanisms in alleviating the distinct socioeconomic and psychological disadvantages of categorical racial membership (Stanford, 1990; Jackson, 1993; Williams and Williams-Morris, 2000). The unique social history and the nature of their group and individual developmental experiences all serve to place new cohorts of racial/ethnic Americans from birth to death at disproportionate risk for poor physical and mental health (LaVeist, 2000). This can be seen in population statistics, e.g. continuing disproportionate rates of mortality, disintegrating neighborhoods, number of women and children in poverty, joblessness, and unemployment (Jackson, 2000). Individual efforts are not enough to improve the health of underrepresented race/ethnic populations. Without significant interventions, the future health of individuals from these populations is clear and it is dismal (Richardson, 1996).

9. Ethnic research matrix

In a prior chapter (Jackson et al., 1995), we proposed an "Ethnic Research Matrix" as a useful approach to life-course model that seriously considered cultural, ethnic, racial and ethnic differentiation in aging experiences. We think that this matrix also makes sense within the proposed biopsychosocial model of aging. The lack of comparable data among and across groups makes it almost impossible to contrast biological, social and physical and mental health status and functioning among and within ethnic elderly groups. It is clear that age and ethnicity make a difference in the epidemiology and pathophysiology of mental and physical health; an understanding of their exact role, however, awaits further study (e.g. Kessler et al., 1992). We suggest that an Ethnic Research Matrix (Vasques, 1986; Jackson et al., 1995) is needed that takes as its defining elements: ethnicity, national origin, racial group membership, gender, social and economic statuses, age, and acculturation; possible mediators (e.g. coping reactions); and, physical and mental health outcomes. Methodological concerns of sampling and measurement must be standardized within the constraints imposed by issues of cultural sensitivity and meaningfulness (Markides et al., 1990). The Ethnic Research Matrix would be adjusted for important cohort and socio-historical occurrences and must be guided by a biopsychosocial life-course framework. A longitudinal cohort-sequential design (Baltes, 1987) that included an intergenerational family component (Jackson and Antonucci, 1993) would be ideal. This matrix would provide a powerful framework for analyzing physical and mental health disorders, coping and adjustment responses, utilization patterns and a variety of individual and group outcomes. Its implementation may ultimately lead to an understanding of what, how, and when, aspects of race, ethnicity, culture, aging and the life-course influence (and are influenced by) biological, physiological and physical, mental and cognitive functioning.

10. Conclusions

The last half century has witnessed new knowledge about aging of biological, sensory, behavioral, physiological, and cognitive systems related to aging (Lonergan, 1991). For example, we now know that all people do not age the same way; individuals differ greatly in age related declines (and increments) in physical, behavioral and cognitive functioning. Research clearly suggests that some aging processes are modifiable (Rowe and Kahn, 1987). In addition, observed functional differences across individuals are greatly influenced by societal, environmental, and health related statuses, and most importantly the background and makeup of the individual.

Cognitive declines are not universal with age; some intellectual abilities are actually maintained or improve with age; positive social and psychological change is possible in older adults; intergenerational models of aging and human development are of critical importance in understanding individual aging trajectories; period events and cohort membership play a determining role in aging processes; and, it is necessary to conceptualize age-related change and processes within an individual, family, and societal life-course framework. In this chapter we have speculated on the possibility of extending the life-course framework to encompass an integrated framework of development and aging that includes historical, cohort, and cultural influences on successful social and psychological aging among racial and ethnic elders as part of a biopsychosocial model.

In most cases, older minority adults show relatively poorer status. On the other hand, based upon current estimates of mortality and life expectancies, older minority populations have grown and will continue to do so (Jackson and Sellers, 2001). Some data indicate that some minority populations of advanced ages, for example blacks (e.g. Gibson and Jackson, 1992), may be more robust in comparison to whites, perhaps reflecting different aging processes and selection over time for hardier individuals (Manton, et al., 1987). However, at every point earlier in the individual life span most members of racial and ethnic groups are at greater mortality and morbidity risk than whites (Jackson and Sellers, 2001).

There is a good scientific rationale for increased attention to racial, ethnic group, and cross-cultural perspectives in research on aging (Holzberg, 1982; Gelfand and Barresi, 1987; Lonergan, 1991). Theories of social and psychological aging, physical and mental health research paradigms, service delivery models and public policies have to be increasingly responsive to the growing racially and ethnically diverse proportions of our older population (Bestman, 1986; Angel and Hogan, 1991; Gatz and Smyer, 1992; Siegel, 1993). Culture and life style differences are of fundamental importance in the behavioral science constructs, theories, and interventions that are employed (Holzberg, 1982; Jackson, 1985; Lonergan, 1991; Jackson et al., 1995). Some studies have shown how recognition and inclusion of cultural and racial considerations in service delivery programs can increase the effectiveness and reduce the cost of delivering services to racial and ethnic populations (Jackson et al., 1992; Jackson and Sellers, 2001). It is also our belief that the infusion of racial minority and ethnic content has positive effects on our understanding of the health status and health needs of the nation's elderly more generally, regardless of whether the direct focus of that work is on racial and ethnic groups (Cooper et al., 1981; Jackson et al., 1990; Jackson and Sellers, 2001)

Although there is some convergence toward a risk and resources, life-course model of ethnicity that utilizes modern biopsychosocial theories of culture and acculturation (Jackson, et al., 1990), the empirical literature has not kept pace with this perspective. The work that we have briefly reviewed suggests directions that new health and behavioral and social science research might take in this area. Theoretical frameworks of ethnicity and culture are beginning to emerge (Jackson et al., 1995) that will lead to more and better empirical studies. Race, ethnicity, and cultural effects on biological and social functioning over the life-course are not readily accounted for by current theories of aging (e.g. social class, stratification, modernization, age leveling, minority status, disengagement, or activity) (Jackson et al., 1990; Markides et al., 1990; Jackson and Sellers, 2001). A biopsychosocial, life-course approach has significant promise for research. Future studies, perhaps utilizing the proposed conceptual and methodological biopsychosocial, ethnic research matrix, may yield increased refinements and more extensive emphasis on the important contextual variables of race, culture, ethnicity, gender, and social and economic statuses, within a life-course framework (Lonergan, 1991; Jackson et al., 1993; Stanford and DuBois, 1993), that we believe are needed for scientific and public policy advancements.

References

Adler, N.E., Ostrove, J.M., 1999. Socioeconomic status and health: What we know and what we don't know. In: Adler, N., Marmot, M., McEwen, B., Stewart, J. (Eds.), Socioeconomic Status and Health in Industrial Nations. Annals of the New York Academy of Sciences, New York, pp. 3–15.

Angel, J.L., Hogan, D.P., 1991. The demography of minority older populations. In Task Force on Minority Aging (Eds.), Minority Elders: Longevity, Economics, and Health. The Gerontological Society of America, Washington, D.C., pp. 1–13.

Antonucci, T.C., 2001. Social relations: An examination of social networks, social support, and sense of control. In: Birren, J.E., Schaie, K.W. (Eds.), Handbook of the Psychology of Aging. Academic Press, San Diego, CA, pp. 427–453.

Antonucci, T.C., 1985. Personal characteristics, social networks, and social behavior. In: Binstock, B.H., Shanas, E. (Eds.), Handbook of Aging and the Social Sciences. Van Nostrand Reinhold, New York, pp. 94–128.

Antonucci, T.C., Ajrouch, K.J., Janevic, M.R., 2003. The effect of social relations on the SES-health link in men and women aged 40 and over. Soc. Sci. Med. 56, March, 949–960.

Antonucci, T.C., Jackson, J.S., 1987. Social support, interpersonal efficacy and health. In: Carstensen, L.L., Edelstein, B.A. (Eds.), Handbook of Clinical Gerontology. Pergamon, New York, pp. 291–311.

Baker, F.M., 1987. The Afro-American life cycle: Success, failure and mental health. J. Natl. Med. Assoc. 7, 625–633.

Baltes, P.B., 1997. On the incomplete architecture of human otntogeny: Selection, optimization and compensation as foundation of developmental theory. Am. Psychol. 52, 366–380.

Baltes, P.B., 1987. Theoretical propositions of life-span developmental psychology: On the dynamics between growth and decline. Dev. Psychol. 23, 611–626.

Baltes, P.B., Cornelius, S.W., Nesselroade, J.R., 1979. Cohort effects in developmental psychology. In: Nesselroade, J.R., Baltes, P.B. (Eds.), Longitudinal Research in the Study of Behavior and Development. Academic, New York, pp. 61–88.

Baltes, P.B., Reese, H.W., Lipsitt, L.P., 1980. Life-span developmental psychology. Annu. Rev. Psychol. 31, 65–110.

Baquet, C., Ringen, K., 1987. Health policy: Gaps in access, delivery and utilization of the Papsmear in the United States. Milbank Q. 65(2), 322–347.

Barth, F., 1969. Ethnic Groups and Boundaries: The social Organization of Culture Difference. Little, Brown & Co, Boston, MA.

Barresi, C.M., 1987. Ethnic aging and the life course. In: Gelfand, D.E., Barresi, C.M. (Eds.), Ethnic Dimensions of Aging. Springer, New York, pp. 18–34.

Braithwaite, R.L., Taylor, S.E. (Eds.), 1992. Health Issues in the Black Community. Jossey-Bass, San Francisco.

Burton, L.M., Dilworth-Anderson, P., Bengtson, V.L., 1991. Creating culturally relevant ways of thinking about diversity. Generations 15, 67–72.

Clark, R., Anderson, N.B., Clark, V.R., Williams, D.R., 1999. Racism as a stressor for African-Americans: A biopsychosocial model. Am. Psychol. 54, 805–816.

Cohen, S., Syme, L., 1985. Issues in the study and application of social support. In: Cohen, S. (Ed.), Social Support and Health. Academic Press, San Diego, CA, pp. 3–22.

Cooper, R., 1984. A note on the biological concept of race and its application in epidemiological research. Am. Heart J. 108, 715–722.

Cooper, R., 1991. Celebrate diversity – or should we? Ethn. Dis. 1, 3–7.

Dressler, W., 1985. Extended family relationships, social support, and mental health in a Southern black community. J. Health Soc. Behav. 26, 39–48.

Dressler, W.W., 1991. Social class, skin color, and arterial blood pressure in two societies. Ethn. Dis. 1, 60–77.

Dressler, W.W., Bindon, J.R., 2000. The health consequences of cultural consonance: Cultural dimensions of lifestyle, social support and arterial blood pressure in an African-Americana community. American Anthropologist 102(2), 244–260.

Elo, I.T., Preston, S.H., 1997. Racial and ethnic differences in mortality at older ages. In: Martin, L.G., Soldo, B.J. (Eds.), Racial and Ethnic Differences in the Health of Older Americans. National Academy Press, Washington, DC, pp. 10–42.

Engel, G., 1977. The need for a new medical model: A challenge for biomedicine. Science 196, 129–136.

Farley, R., 2000. Demographic, economic, and social trends in a multicultural America. In: Jackson, J.S. (Ed.), New Directions: African Americans in a Diversifying Nation. National Policy Association, Washington, D.C., pp. 11–44.

Fillenbaum, G.G., Peterson, B., Welsh-Bohmer, K., Kukull, W.A., Heyman, A., 1998. Progression of Alzheimer's Disease in black and white patients. Neurology 51, 154–158.

Gelfand, D.E., Barresi, C., 1987. Current perspectives in ethnicity and aging. In: Gelfand, D., Barresi, C. (Eds.), Ethnic Dimensions of Aging. Springer Publishing Co, New York, pp. 5–17.

Gibson, R.C., Jackson, J.S., 1992. The Black oldest old: health, functioning, and informal support. In: Suzman, R., Willis, D., Manton, K. (Eds.), The Oldest Old. Oxford University Press, New York, pp. 321–340.

Hargreaves, M.K., Baquet, C., Gamshadzahi, A., 1989. Diet, nutritional status and cancer risk in American blacks. Nutr. Cancer 12(1), 1–28.

Holzberg, C.S., 1982. Ethnicity and aging: Anthropological perspectives on more than just the minority elderly. Gerontologist 22, 249–257.

House, J.S., Landis, K.R., Umberson, D., 1989. Social relationships and health. Science 241, 540–545.

Jackson, J.S., 1993. Racial influences on adult development and aging. In: Kastenbaum, R. (Ed.), The Encyclopedia of Adult Development. Oryx Press, Phoenix, AZ, pp. 18–26.

Jackson, J.S. (Ed.), 2000. New Directions: African-Americans in a Diversifying Nation. National Policy Association, Washington, D.C.

Jackson, J.S., Antonucci, T.C., 1993. Survey research methodology and life-span human development. In: Cohen, S., Reese, H. (Eds.), Life-span Developmental Psychology: Methodological Innovations. Erlbaum Associates, New York, pp. 65–94.

Jackson, J.S., Sellers, S., 1996. African-American health over the life-course: A multi-dimensional framework. In: Kato, P.M., Mann, T. (Eds.), Handbook of Diversity Issues in Health Psychology. Plenum Press, New York, pp. 301–317.

Jackson, J.S., Sellers, S.L., 2001. Health and the elderly. In: Braithwaite, R., Taylor, S.E. (Eds.), Health and the Elderly, 2nd ed. Jossey Bass Inc, San Francisco, pp. 81–96.

Jackson, J.S., Antonucci, T.C., Gibson, R.C., 1990. Cultural, racial, and ethnic minority influences on aging. In: Birren, J.E., Schaie, W. (Eds.), Handbook of the Psychology of Aging, 3rd ed. Academic Press, New York, pp. 103–123.

Jackson, J.S., Antonucci, T.C., Gibson, R.C., 1995. Ethnic and cultural factors in research on aging and mental health: A life-course perspective. In: Padgett, D.K. (Ed.), Handbook on Ethnicity, Aging and Mental Health. Greenwood/Praeger Press, New York, pp. 22–46.

Jackson, J.S., Burns, C., Gibson, R.C., 1992. An overview of geriatric care in ethnic and racial minority groups. In: Calkins, E., Ford, A.B., Katz, P.R. (Eds.), Practice of Geriatrics, 2nd ed. W.B. Saunders Company, Philadelphia, PA, pp. 57–64.

Jackson, J.S., Chatters, L.M., Taylor, R.J. (Eds.), 1993. Aging in Black America. Sage Publications, Newbury Park, CA, pp. 21–35.

Johnson, R.E., Crowley, J.E., 1999. An analysis of stress denial. In: Neighbors, H.W., Jackson, J.S. (Eds.), Mental Health in Black America. Sage, Thousand Oaks, CA, pp. 62–76.

Jones, W., Rice, M.F., 1987. Health care issues in Black America: policies, problems and prospects. New York: Greenwood Press. J. Int. Neuropsychol. Soc. 5, 191–202.

Levy, J.A., Pescosolido, B.A., 2002. Social Networks and Health. JAI Press, New York.

Lindau, S.T., Laumann, E.O., Levinson, W., Waite, L., 2002. Synthesis of scientific disciplines in pursuit of health: The interactive biopsychosocial model. Unpublished Paper. University of Chicago, Chicago IL.

Lichtenberg, P.A., 1998. Mental Health Practice in Geriatric Healthcare Settings. Haworth Press, New York.

Lonergan, E.T. (Ed.), 1991. Extending Life, Enhancing Life. National Academy Press, Washington, DC.

Manly, J.J., Jacobs, D.M., Sano, M., Bell, K., Merchant, C.A., Small, S.A., Stern, Y., 1998. Cognitive test performance among nondemented elderly African-Americans and whites. Neurology 50, 1238–1245.

Manton, K.G., Patrick, C.H., Johnson, K.W., 1987. Health differentials between blacks and whites: Recent trends in mortality and morbidity. Milbank Q. 65, 129–199.

Manton, K.G., Stollard, E., 1997. Health and disability differences among racial and ethnic groups. In: Martin, L.G., Soldo, B.J. (Eds.), Racial and Ethnic Differences in the Health of Older Americans. National Academy Press, Washington, DC, pp. 43–104.

Markides, K.S., Liang, J., Jackson, J.S., 1990. Race, ethnicity, and aging: Conceptual and methodological issues. In: George, L.K., Binstock, R.H. (Eds.), Handbook of Aging and the Social Sciences, 3rd ed. Academic Press, New York, pp. 112–129.

Massey, D., Denton N., 1993. American Apartheid: Segregation and the Making of the underclass. Harvard University Press, Cambridge.

Mast, B.T., Fitzgerald, J., Steinberg, J., MacNeill, S.E., Lichtenberg, P.A., 2001. Effective screening for Alzheimer's Disease among older African-Americans. Clin. Neuropsychol. 15, 196–202.

Miles, T.P. (Ed.) 1999. Full-color Aging: Facts, Goals, and Recommendations for America's Diverse Elders. Gerontological Society of America, Washington, D.C.

Myers, H.F., 1984. Summary of workshop III: Working group on socioeconomic and sociocultural influences. Am. Heart J. 108, 706–710.

National Cancer Institute, 1989. Cancer among Blacks and other minorities: statistical profiles. Public Health Service, Hyattsville, MD.

National Center for Health Statistics, 1999. Health, United States. Hyattsville, MD: Public Health Service.

Neel, J.V., 1997. Are genetic factors involved in racial, and ethnic differences in late-life health? In: Martin, L.G., Soldo, B.J. (Eds.), Racial and Ethnic Differences in the Health of Older Americans. National Academy Press, Washington, DC, pp. 210–232.

Nielsen, F., 1985. Toward a theory of ethnic solidarity in modern societies. Am. Sociol. Rev. 50, 133–149.

Oliver, M., Shapiro, T., 1995. Black Wealth/White Wealth: A New Perspective on Racial Inequality. Routledge, NY, pp. 335–349.

Phenninx, B., vanTilburg, T., Boeke, J., Deeg, D., Kriegsman, D., van Eijk, J., 1998. Effects of social support and personal coping resources on depressive symptoms: Different for various chronic diseases? Health Psychol. 17, 551–558.

Richardson, J., 1996. Aging and health: African-American elders, 2nd ed. (Stanford Geriatric Education Center Working Paper Series, Number 4: Ethnogeriatric Reviews). Stanford, CA: Stanford Geriatric Education Center, Division of Family & Community Medicine, Stanford University.

Riley, J.W., Riley, M.W., 1994b. Beyond productive aging: Changing lives and social structure. Aging Int., 15–19.

Riley, M.W., 1994a. Changing lives and changing social structures: Common concerns of social science and public health. Am. J. Public Health 84, 1214–1217.

Riley, M.W., 1994b. Aging and society: Past, present and future. Gerontologist 34, 436–446.

Riley, M.W., Loscocco, K.A., 1994. The changing structure of work opportunities: Toward an age integrated society. In: Abeles, R.P., Gift, H.C., Orey, M.C. (Eds.), Aging and the Quality of Life. Springer, New York, pp. 235–252.

Riley, M.W., Riley Jr., J.W., 1994a. Age integration and the lives of older people. Gerontologist 34, 110–115.

Rosenthal, C.J., 1986. Family supports in later life: Does ethnicity make a difference. Gerontologist 26, 19–24.

Rowe, J.W., Kahn, R.L., 1987. Human aging: Usual and successful. Science 237, 143–149.

Seeman, T.E., Crimmins, E., 2001. Social environment effects on health and aging: Integrating epidemiologic and semographic approaches and perspectives. In: Weinstein, M., Hermalin, A. (Eds.), Population Health and Aging: Strengthening the Dialogue Between Epidemiology and Demography. Annals of New York Academy of Sciences, New York, pp. 88–117.

Seeman, T.E., Lusignolo, T.M., Albert, M., Berkman, L., 2001. Social relationships, social support, and patterns of cognitive aging in healthy, high-functioning older adults: Macarthur studies of successful aging. Health Psychol. 20(4), 243–255.

Siegel, J.S., 1993. A Generation of Change: A Profile of America's Older Population. Russell Sage, New York.

Siegel, J.S., 1999. Demographic introduction to racial/Hispanic elderly populations. In: Miles, T.P. (Ed.), Full-Color Aging: Facts, Goals, and Recommendations for America's Diverse Elders. Gerontological Society of America, Washington, D.C., pp. 1–20.

Smith, J.P., Kington, R., 1997a. Demographic and economic correlates of health in old age. Demography 34(1), 159–170.

Smith, J.P., Kington, R.S., 1997b. Race, socioeconomic status, and health in late life. In: Martin, L.G., Soldo, B.J. (Eds.), Racial and Ethnic Differences in the Health of Older Americans. National Academy Press, Washington, DC, pp. 105–162.
Stanford, E.P., DuBois, B.C., 1993. Gender and ethnicity patterns. In: Birren, J.E., Sloane, R.B., Cohen, G. (Eds.), Handbook of Mental Health and Aging, 2nd ed. Academic Press, San Diego, CA, pp. 99–117.
Swidler, A., 1986. Culture in action: Symbols and strategies. Am. Sociol. Rev. 51, 273–286.
Swidler, A., 2001. Talk of Love: How Culture Matters. University of Chicago Press, Chicago, IL.
Taylor, R.L., 1979. Black ethnicity and the persistence of ethnogenesis. Am. J. Sociol. 84, 1401–1423.
Vanneman, R., Cannon, L., 1987. The American Perception of Class. Temple University Press, Philadelphia.
Vasques, J., 1986. The ethnic matrix: Implications for human service providers. Explorations in Ethnic Studies 9, 1–22.
Wall, J.R., Deshpande, S.A., MacNeill, S.E., Lichtenberg, P.A., 1998. The fuld object memory evaluation, a useful tool in the assessment of urban geriatric patients. Clin. Gerontol. 19, 39–50.
Welsh, K.A., Ballard, E., Nash, F., Raiford, K., Harrell, L., 1994. Issues affecting minority participation in research studies of Alzheimer's Disease. Alzheimer's Disease and Associated Disorders 8, 38–48.
Wilkinson, D.T, King, G., 1987. Conceptual and methodological issues in the use of race as a variable: Policy implications. The Millbank Quarterly 65(Supplement 1), 56–71.
Williams, D., 1999. Race, socioeconomic status, and health: The added effects of racism and discrimination. In: Adler, N., Marmot, M., McEwen, B., Stewart, J. (Eds.), Socioeconomic Status and Health in Industrial Nation. Annals of the New York Academy of Sciences, New York, pp. 173–188.
Williams, D.R., Collins, C., 1995. U.S. socioeconomic and racial differences in health. Annu. Rev. Sociol. 21, 349–386.
Williams, D.R., Jackson, J.S., 2000. Race/ethnicity and the 2000 Census: Recommendations for African-American and other black populations in the United States. Am. J. Public Health 90(11), 1728–1730.
Williams, D.R., Rucker, T.D., 2000. Understanding and addressing racial disparities in health care. Health Care Finan. Rev. 21(4), 75–90.
Williams, D.R., Williams-Morris, R., 2000. Racism and mental health: The African-American experience. Ethn. Health 5(3/4), 243–268.
Williams, D.R., Neighbors, H., Jackson, J.S., 2003. Racial/ethnic discrimination and health: Findings from community studies. Am. J. Public Health 93(2), 7–15.
Wilson, W., 1996. When work disappears: The world of the new urban poor. Random House, New York.
Wirth, L., 1945. The problems of minority groups. In: Linton, R. (Ed.), The Science of Man in the World Crisis. Columbia University Press, New York.
Yee, B.W., Gelfand D., 1992. Trends and forces: Influence of immigration, migration, and acculturation on the fabric of aging in America. In: Percil, E., Stanford, Fernando, Torres-Gil, M. (Eds.), Diversity: New Approaches to Ethnic Minority Aging. Baywood, Amityville, N.Y., pp. 5–14.
Yinger, J.M., 1985. Ethnicity. Annu. Rev. Sociol. 11, 151–180.

List of Contributors

Paul T. Costa, Jr., Ph.D   National Institute on Aging
Laboratory of Personality and Cognition
5600 Nathan Shock Drive
Baltimore, MD 21224
Phone: 410-558-8220
Fax: 410-558-8108
Email: paulc@lpc.grc.nia.nih.gov

Ilene C. Siegler, Ph.D, M.P.H   Professor of Medical Psychology
Department of Psychiatry and Behavioral
Sciences, Box 2969
Duke University Medical Center
Durham, NC 27710
Phone: 919-684-6352
Fax: 919-681-8960
Email: ics@duke.edu

Daniel L. Schacter, Ph.D.   Department of Psychology
Harvard University
William James Hall, 33 Kirkland St.
Cambridge, MA 02138
Phone: 617-495-3855
Fax: 617-496-3122
Email: dls@wjh.harvard.edu

Benton H. Pierce   Department of Psychology
Harvard University
33 Kirkland Street
Cambridge, MA 02138
Phone: 617-495-3856
Fax: 617-496-3122
Email: pierce@wjh.harvard.edu

Jon S. Simons, Ph.D.   Institute of Cognitive Neuroscience
University College London
Alexandra House, 17 Queen Square
London WC1N 3AR
United Kingdom
Phone: +44 20 7679 1144
Fax: +44 20 7813 2835
Email: jon.simons@ucl.ac.uk

David J. Madden, Ph.D.   Psychiatry Department
Duke University School of Medicine
Box 2980
Durham, NC 27710
Phone: 919-660-7537
Fax: 919-684-8569
Email: djm@geri.duke.edu

Wythe L. Whiting, Ph.D.   Asst. Professor of Psychology
Le Moyne College
Syracuse, NY 13214
Phone: 315-445-4341
Fax: 720-221-6578
Email: wlw@geri.duke.edu

Merrill F. Elias, PhD MPH   Professor of Epidemiology in
Mathematics and Statistics
Statistics and Consulting Unit
Department of Mathematics and Statistics
Boston University
Boston, MA 02215
Phone: 617-353-8092
Fax: 617-353-4767
Email: maineeffects@aol.com

Michael Robbins, PhD   Research Associate Professor of Psychology
Department of Psychology
University of Maine
Orono, Maine 04469-5742
Phone: 207-581-2051
Fax: 207-581-6128
Email: michael.robbins@umit.maine.edu

Marc M. Budge, BScMed, MBBS, FRACP   Associate Professor of Geriatric Medicine
Australian National University Medical School
Canberra, Australia ACT 0200
Phone: 61-2-6244 4027
Fax: 61-2-6244 4036
Email: marc.budge@act.gov.au

Penelope K. Elias, PhD   Research Assistant Professor
Statistics and Consulting Unit
Department of Mathematics and Statistics
Boston University
Boston, MA 02215

List of Contributors

	Phone: 617-353-8092 Fax: 617-353-4767 Email: pelias100@aol.com
Barbara A. Hermann, MS	Graduate Research Assistant in Psychology Department of Psychology University of Maine Orono, Maine 04469-5742 Phone: 207-581-2002 Fax: 207-581-6128 Email: barbara.hermann@umit.maine.edu
Gregory A. Dore	Research Assistant in Psychology Department of Psychology University of Maine Orono, Maine 04469-5742 Phone: 207-581-2097 Fax: 207-581-6128 Email: gregory.dore@umit.maine.edu
Susan Turk Charles, Ph.D.	Assistant Professor Department of Psychology and Social Behavior University of California, Irvine 3340 Social Ecology II Irvine, CA 92697-7085 Phone: 949-824-1450 Fax: 949-824-3002 Email: scharles@uci.edu
Laura L. Carstensen, Ph.D.	Department of Psychology Stanford, University Jordon Hall Stanford, CA 94305 Phone: 650-723-3102 Fax: 650-725-5699 Email: llc@psych.stanford.edu
Kali H. Trzesniewski, Ph.D.	Psychology Department One Shields Ave. University of California Davis, CA 95616-8686 Phone: 530-754-8287 Fax: 530-752-2087 Email: mailto:kftrzesniewski@ucdavis.edu Webpage: http://psyweb2.ucdavis.edu/grads/kali

List of Contributors

Richard W. Robins

Associate Professor
Associate Editor, JPSP: PPID
Department of Psychology
University of California
Davis, CA 95616-8686
Phone: 530-754-8299
Fax: 530-752-2087
Website: http://psyweb2.ucdavis.edu/labs/robins/

Brent W. Roberts

Associate Professor
Associate Editor, Journal of Research in Personality
Department of Psychology
University of Illinois
603 East Daniel Street
Champaign, IL 61820
Phone: 217-333-2644
Fax: 217-244-5876
Email: broberts@s.psych.uiuc.edu

Avshalom Caspi, Ph.D

Box Number P080
SGDP Centre
Institute of Psychiatry
De Crespigny Park
London SE5 8AF
UK
Phone: 44-(0)207-848-0936
Fax: 44-(0)207-848-5262
Email: spjwavc@iop.kcl.ac.uk

Ed Diener, Ph.D.

Alumni Professor of Psychology
603 E. Daniel Street, University of Illinois
Champaign, IL 61820
Phone: Secretarial Assistant,
Kris Eaton: 217 244-5985
Fax: 217 244-5876
Email: Ediener@s.psych.uiuc.edu
Journal Web Page: http://www.psych.uiuc.edu/~jpsped

Christie Napa Scollon

Department of Psychology
University of Illinois at Urbana-Champaign
603 East Daniel Street
Champaign, IL 61820
Fax: 217-244-5876
Email: scollon@s.psych.uiuc.edu

Richard E. Lucas	Department of Psychology
	Michigan State University
	East Lansing, MI 48824
	Phone: 517-432-4360
	Fax: 517-432-2476
	Email: lucasri@msu.edu
James S. Jackson, Ph.D.	Institute for Social Research
	University of Michigan
	Room 5010 ISR
	426 Thompson Street
	PO Box 1248
	Ann Arbor, MI 48106-1248
	Phone: 734-763-2491
	Fax: 734-615-3212
	Email: jamessj@umich.edu
Toni C. Antonucci, Ph.D.	Survey Research Center
	5100 ISR
	426 Thompson Street
	Ann Arbor, MI 48106-1248
	Phone: 734-763-5846
	Fax: 734-647-0861
	Email: tca@umich.edu
Edna Brown, Ph.D.	Survey Research Center
	5080 ISR
	426 Thompson Street
	Ann Arbor, MI 48106-1248
	Phone: 734.936.3075
	Fax: 734.647.0861
	Email: eebrown@umich.edu

Advances in
Cell Aging and Gerontology

Series Editor: Mark P. Mattson
URL: http://www.elsevier.com/locate/series/acag

Aims and Scope:

Advances in Cell Aging and Gerontology (ACAG) is dedicated to providing timely review articles on prominent and emerging research in the area of molecular, cellular and organismal aspects of aging and age-related disease. The average human life expectancy continues to increase and, accordingly, the impact of the dysfunction and diseases associated with aging are becoming a major problem in our society. The field of aging research is rapidly becoming the niche of thousands of laboratories worldwide that encompass expertise ranging from genetics and evolution to molecular and cellular biology, biochemistry and behavior. ACAG consists of edited volumes that each critically review a major subject area within the realms of fundamental mechanisms of the aging process and age-related diseases such as cancer, cardiovascular disease, diabetes and neurodegenerative disorders. Particular emphasis is placed upon: the identification of new genes linked to the aging process and specific age-related diseases; the elucidation of cellular signal transduction pathways that promote or retard cellular aging; understanding the impact of diet and behavior on aging at the molecular and cellular levels; and the application of basic research to the development of life span extension and disease prevention strategies. ACAG will provide a valuable resource for scientists at all levels from graduate students to senior scientists and physicians.

Books Published:

1. P.S. Timiras, E.E. Bittar, *Some Aspects of the Aging Process*, 1996, 1-55938-631-2
2. M.P. Mattson, J.W. Geddes, *The Aging Brain*, 1997, 0-7623-0265-8
3. M.P. Mattson, *Genetic Aberrancies and Neurodegenerative Disorders*, 1999, 0-7623-0405-7
4. B.A. Gilchrest, V.A. Bohr, *The Role of DNA Damage and Repair in Cell Aging*, 2001, 0-444-50494-X
5. M.P. Mattson, S. Estus, V. Rangnekar, *Programmed Cell Death, Volume I*, 2001, 0-444-50493-1
6. M.P. Mattson, S. Estus, V. Rangnekar, *Programmed Cell Death, Volume II*, 2001, 0-444-50730-2
7. M.P. Mattson, *Interorganellar Signaling in Age-Related Disease*, 2001, 0-444-50495-8
8. M.P. Mattson, *Telomerase, Aging and Disease*, 2001, 0-444-50690-X
9. M.P. Mattson, *Stem Cells: A Cellular Fountain of Youth*, 2002, 0-444-50731-0
10. M.P. Mattson, *Calcium Homeostasis and Signaling in Aging*, 2002, 0-444-51135-0
11. T. Hagen, *Mechanisms of Cardiovascular Aging*, 2002, 0-444-51159-8
12. M.P. Mattson, *Membrane Lipid Signaling in Aging and Age-Related Disease*, 2003, 0-444-51297-7
13. G. Pawelec, *Basic Biology and Clinical Impact of Immunosenescence*, 2003, 0-444-51316-7
14. M.P. Mattson, *Energy Metabolism and Lifespan Determination*, 2003, 0-444-51492-9
15. P. Costa, I.C. Siegler, *Recent Advances in Psychology and Aging*, 2004, 0-444-51495-3